SHOULDER ARTHROSCOPY

SHOULDER ARTHROSCOPY

Stephen J. Snyder, M.D.

Southern California
Orthopedic Institute
Van Nuys, California

McGraw-Hill, Inc.

HEALTH PROFESSIONS DIVISION

New York   St. Louis   San Francisco   Auckland   Bogotá   Caracas   Lisbon   London   Madrid
Mexico City   Milan   Montreal   New Delhi   Paris   San Juan   Singapore   Sydney   Tokyo   Toronto

SHOULDER ARTHROSCOPY

Copyright © 1994 by McGraw-Hill, Inc. All rights reserved.
Printed in the United States of America. Except as permitted
under the United States Copyright Act of 1976, no part of
this publication may be reproduced or distributed in any
form or by any means, or stored in a data base or retrieval
system, without the prior written permission of the
publisher.

1234567890 KGP KGP 9876543

ISBN 0-07-059526-7

This book was set in Caslon by
Arcata Graphics/Kingsport.
The editors were Jane Pennington and Peter McCurdy;
the production supervisor was Rick Ruzycka;
the cover designer was Marsha Cohen/Parallelogram. Phil James prepared the index.
Arcata Graphics/Kingsport was printer and binder.

Library of Congress Cataloging-in-Publication Data

Snyder, Stephen J.
    Shoulder arthroscopy / Stephen J. Snyder.
       p.   cm.
    Includes bibliographical references and index.
    ISBN 0-07-059526-7
    1. Shoulder joint—Endoscopic surgery.   2. Shoulder joint—
Abnormalities—Diagnosis. I. Title.
    [DNLM: 1. Shoulder Joint—surgery. 2. Arthroscopy—methods. WE
810 S675h 1993]
RD557.5.S63   1993
617.5'72059—dc20
DNLM/DLC
for Library of Congress   93-31088
                              CIP

This book is dedicated to my wife, Ann, with loving thanks for all her encouragement, support, patience, and counsel.

Contents

Preface

The purpose of this book is to offer the reader, in a monograph, the current arthroscopic surgical techniques used by the shoulder team at the Southern California Orthopedic Institute in Van Nuys, California.

The initial chapters of the book review the most basic, but important, concepts of operating room preparation and patient care and positioning prior to shoulder arthroscopy. This section is valuable for in-service training of the operating room staff to develop a shoulder arthroscopy protocol that will facilitate application of surgical techniques while protecting the patient from inadvertent injury while under anesthesia.

The next few chapters present a rigid step-by-step method for entering the shoulder for diagnostic arthroscopy and bursoscopy, highlighting the salient anatomic features that must be understood and differentiated from the more unusual anatomic variations. The importance of developing a technique for safe and correct portal placement that will ensure a detailed anatomical review is presented.

The more advanced areas of shoulder arthroscopic surgery are then discussed in detail. Treatment of arthritis and biceps tendon problems, acro-mioclavicular joint disease, instability, rotator cuff problems, and calcific tendinitis are all discussed.

In each chapter, a brief review of the important features of the common history and physical examination are presented along with the appropriate x-ray and MRI studies. The individual chapters illustrate, using step-by-step artwork sequences coupled with arthroscopic photographs, the techniques for surgical treatment of those conditions amenable to arthroscopic repair. In addition, related surgical techniques, such as mini-open rotator cuff repair or biceps tenodesis, are presented. In each case, the instruments recommended for the operation are identified by name and manufacturer. A "Surgeon's Preference Card" is included for each procedure and can be copied for the operating room staff.

Chapter 14 presents a collection of unusual applications of shoulder arthroscopy that is hoped to stimulate the reader's imagination, exploring the endless possibilities available to a skillful arthroscopic shoulder surgeon. The final chapter reviews the potential risks that can accompany shoulder arthroscopy and discusses the appropriate steps to minimize them.

It is my hope that this book will serve to stimulate additional interest in shoulder arthroscopy and aid arthroscopists, from the novice to the expert, in their quest for better diagnosis and treatment of shoulder pathology. It is my belief that the arthroscope has opened an entirely new realm for shoulder evaluation and treatment, and that, in the future, it will continue to be an important tool in the armamentarium of the complete shoulder surgeon.

Introduction

The task of composing a monograph devoted to my preferred technique for shoulder arthroscopy and related surgery was not an overwhelming one. The work involved in writing and revising the chapters of this book, although time-consuming, actually proved valuable and satisfying. From the time of my first shoulder arthroscopic experience, in 1981, I believed that this new and radical technique of evaluating the anatomy of the shoulder was destined to be more than a curiosity for the shoulder surgeon. I spent many restless nights after arthroscoping my first patient with an anterior dislocation, reviewing in my mind the seemingly endless possibilities for arthroscopic repair of shoulder pathology. The same was true after finding loose bodies, rotator cuff damage, and many other types of joint injury. In addition, the beauty of the glenohumeral and bursal anatomy, complete with its previously undescribed (and therefore misunderstood) variation, always caused considerable excitement. Since nature usually has a mechanical or functional reason for its anatomical architecture, my curiosity was, and continues to be, piqued at every encounter with a new variation.

Early in the development of my shoulder arthroscopy practice, I had the good fortune to meet Dr. James Esch, of Oceanside, California, when we both attended an international arthroscopy meeting in London in 1982. Dr. Esch was feeling the same frustrations as I, being unable to find a proper forum in which to discuss his interests in shoulder arthroscopy. We vowed then to develop a two-pronged educational system that would not only help us, but would also promote understanding and technical expertise throughout the orthopaedic community. Dr. Esch had previously hosted an informal meeting of arthroscopic surgeons in the San Diego area; the participants reviewed videotapes and discussed shoulder arthroscopy. Since that time, the San Diego Shoulder Arthroscopy Course has grown into an annual event, drawing hundreds of enthusiastic attendees each year.

For my part, I agreed to become the founder and editor of a videotape magazine that would permit interested physicians around the world to participate in a high-level exchange of new techniques and curious cases of shoulder arthroscopy. This "Shoulder Arthroscopy Study Group" (SASG) has had the honor of circulating original tapes by some of the pioneers in shoulder arthroscopy, including Drs. Harvard Ellman, Lanny Johnson, Burt Elrod, Michael Gross, Frank Wilson, Eugene Wolf, and Richard Caspari, and, of course, a few from our group at the Southern California Orthopedic Institute (SCOI). The study group now includes members from six countries outside the United States and continues to offer a video forum in which shoulder arthroscopy devotees can share their original thoughts and ideas with their peers.

The Arthroscopy Association of North America has also taken up the task of improving the level of shoulder arthroscopy education. The Education and Program committees, with the blessing of the Board of Directors, have elevated the shoulder to an equal level with the all-important knee in their educational programs. The numbers of participants registering for shoulder courses have increased exponentially as new techniques have become feasible and equipment available. The proliferation of technical devices geared specifically to the shoulder has also been remarkable.

With all this excitement during the past decade and all the dedicated minds working to improve and perfect shoulder arthroscopy techniques, there is still a long way to go. I do not consider the ideas expressed in the chapters of this book to be the final answers to any aspect of shoulder arthroscopy. I have chosen to put these ideas together in one volume as a 10-year milestone, but I expect the 15- and 20-year markers may be completely different. My hope is that surgeons, especially in the field of instability surgery, will not accept the current state of the art. There must be a better way to evaluate capsular tension and adjust for congenital and traumatic laxity.

The teachings of Neer, Matsen, Rockwood, Nobuhara, and Rowe, as well as the other pioneers of open shoulder surgery, must never be forgotten. The problem of the rotator interval—with its propensity for scarring and limited motion, or stretching and posterior/inferior laxity—should be considered along with the other, more traditional, aspects of instability.

Adhesive capsulitis is another pathologic enigma that I have made no attempt to discuss in this book. At the time of this writing, new concepts have been advanced by Dr. Daryl Ogilvie-Harris and Dr. Thomas Neviaser that may open up new avenues of arthroscopic treatment for this difficult problem.

Progress in treatment of the rotator cuff, with the many new developments listed in Chap. 11, has been very promising. Since that chapter was written, additional new devices have been created which should make the stitching and anchoring of the torn cuff very reliable and much easier to accomplish. The work of Dr. Stephen Burkhart, from Texas, on the arthroscopic treatment of severe, and sometimes irreparable, cuff lesions has greatly enhanced our understanding of these difficult problems.

Several additional, and seemingly insurmountable, problems still exist. Treatments for arthritis and severe chondromalacia re-main beyond our abilities. Behind the scenes, there are preliminary discussions about cartilage grafting and fascial arthroplasty techniques that may benefit the unfortunate patients who suffer from these conditions. The absorbable suture anchors, although not yet generally available, should make these techniques much more viable in the near future.

Early in my quest for better instrumentation to allow application of new arthroscopic techniques in the shoulder, I came to see that unless a surgeon became personally involved with the technical engineers and marketing people at the arthroscopic equipment companies, there was very little likelihood that any significant new instruments would be developed. I was fortunate to meet, and continue to work with, many outstanding members of the development teams for most of the leading arthroscopic equipment makers. A significant number of the products mentioned in this book have been developed at my suggestion, or at the suggestion of other orthopaedic surgeons; many hours of meetings, with subsequent laboratory and clinical tests, have been necessary to refine the tools that are currently available. I have endeavored to present only the safest and most effective techniques, regardless of whether I was involved in their development.

Acknowledgments

I wish to thank a few of the people who have made this monograph possible. Dr. James M. Fox, my senior partner at SCOI, took me aside during my second year in practice and said, without smiling, that if I didn't get going on shoulder arthroscopy he would have to do it. Dr. Marc J. Friedman was always there to listen patiently while I expounded on a "crazy" new idea and to offer a thoughtful and sensible critique as a professional and a friend. Dr. Ronald Glousman has been my friend and "little brother" in shoulder surgery for 10 years; he has helped me with the understanding of biomechanics of throwing trauma to the shoulder and has helped to support many clinical investigations. Drs. Wilson Del Pizzo, Richard Ferkel, and Ronald Karzel have helped me to pursue the many unanswered questions in shoulder arthroscopy with zeal and enthusiasm, as well as helping evaluate new equipment and ideas.

My three "nudges"—my secretary, Catherine Fick; my manuscript typist, Eleanor O'Brien; and my surgical nurse, Kelly Kapp—have always been there to remind me of important deadlines, and to encourage me when the enormity of the job threatened to get me down. Mr. Robert Williams is the medical illustrator, video technician, and photographer at Valley Presbyterian Hospital; Bob's talent can skillfully illustrate on paper even the most complex surgical and anatomical details of the shoulder, and he was always available for a last minute drawing emergency. The "three Chrises" and Lois, in SCORE (the research arm of SCOI), always found time to capture one more video slide or x-ray for me and never complain. I thank all of the visitors and former fellows who have spent time at SCOI offering the stimulus of their keen interest in the field, without which I certainly could not have developed many of these new ideas. And last, but not least, I must thank my sons Eric and Nathan, who set up my research computer and helped input the shoulder data that became the backbone for the manuscript; without their help I would still be working with my scraps of yellow paper, frustrated beyond belief.

1

Learning Shoulder Arthroscopy

Introduction

When a young surgeon finishes a residency program, he or she is usually fairly well educated in basic arthroscopic techniques for the knee. It has become obvious to us at SCOI, from interviews with fellowship applicants, that most residency programs are severely deficient in regard to the teaching of shoulder arthroscopy. Since many practicing orthopaedic surgeons also wish to add shoulder arthroscopy to their surgical armamentarium, a real need exists for an ongoing educational process at all levels. The purpose of this introductory chapter is to present the various options available for learning shoulder arthroscopic techniques. Let us hope that the options will increase as these techniques become more common, and that soon the orthopaedic residency training programs will prepare their graduates as well for the shoulder as they do now for the knee.

Who Should Learn Shoulder Arthroscopy?

Without question, any surgeon who has a sincere desire to practice the highest-quality shoulder surgery should learn at least basic diagnostic shoulder arthroscopy. Over the past 12 years, both the normal and the pathological anatomy of the shoulder have been completely redefined because of the visualization afforded by the arthroscope. Many difficult clinical situations that previously could not be understood are now routinely diagnosed and, often, definitively treated using arthroscopic techniques. It is *not* my belief that all shoulder surgeons need to become *expert* shoulder arthroscopists, but those who are unable to offer their patients the additional diagnostic benefits of arthroscopy are missing an important opportunity, both for themselves and for their patients. The general orthopaedic surgeon in private practice, on the other hand, must decide what level of sophistication he or she wishes to achieve. I believe that any surgeon can learn and perform excellent diagnostic arthroscopy and bursoscopy; but without appropriate training and experience the more advanced procedures, such as rotator cuff repair, acromioclavicular joint stabilization, and shoulder instability surgery, probably should not be attempted. This recommendation, in my opinion, is no different than for any other form of surgery, be it arthroscopic or open. It seems obvious that a general orthopaedic practitioner should be able to pin a fractured hip or perform a routine total hip replacement but probably should not perform a complicated arthroplasty revision surgery without advanced training and experience.

Starting the Learning Process

The foundation for shoulder arthroscopy should begin with a thorough review of the anatomy and biomechanics of the shoulder. Since there are definite risks to the neurovascular anatomy in shoulder arthroscopy, the locations of important structures must be clearly understood. Any good anatomy textbook with a comprehensive shoulder section is adequate for review of the important anatomy at risk. Additionally, any basic textbook of arthroscopic surgery, such as *Operative Arthroscopy,* by John B. McGinty et al. (Raven, New York, 1991), will have a useful review section on pertinent shoulder anatomy.

Journals and Periodicals

Over the past 5 years the numbers of journal articles published concerning shoulder arthroscopy have increased dramatically. Although no journal is yet dedicated solely to shoulder arthroscopy, many journals routinely include such articles (see Table 1-1). *Arthroscopy: The Journal of Arthroscopic and Related Surgery* is the primary source of the most current printed materials. Recent papers presented at meetings of the Arthroscopy Association of North America (AANA) are published; others are presented in abstract form.

The new *Journal of Shoulder and Elbow Surgery* does not offer a great number of arthroscopic articles; I believe, however, that the interested surgeon will benefit from those that are included. Additionally, the excellent papers on open surgical technique enhance the reader's understanding of the more conventional open techniques that complement the shoulder arthroscopy. In the future, as more medium- and long-term results become available, I expect that this journal will be a valuable source for more reports on arthroscopic techniques. The abstracts of the papers presented at the Annual Closed Meeting of the Association of Shoulder and Elbow Surgeons are published in this journal.

An excellent two-volume review on shoulder arthroscopy was published in *Operative Techniques in Orthopaedics* and edited by Dr. Freddie H. Fu. In these two volumes, Dr. Fu has assembled a comprehensive collection and review of the current state of shoulder arthroscopy with multiple invited authors.

TABLE 1-1   Available Journals and Periodicals

Arthroscopy: The Journal of Arthroscopic and Related Surgery
   Raven Press, Ltd., 1185 Avenue of the Americas, New York, NY 10036
Journal of Shoulder and Elbow Surgery
   Mosby Yearbook, Inc., 11830 Westline Industrial Dr., St. Louis, MO 63146–3318
Operative Techniques in Orthopaedics, vol 1, no. 2 and vol 1, no. 3
   W. B. Saunders Co., the Curtis Center, Independence Square West, Philadelphia, PA 19106–3399
Orthopedic Clinics of North America, vol 24:1, January 1993
   W. B. Saunders Co., The Curtis Center, Independence Square West, Philadelphia, PA 19106–3399

Although the review is now a little outdated, many of the techniques described are still valuable and worth reviewing.

The January 1993 volume of *Orthopedic Clinics of North America* is dedicated to an updated multi-author review of state-of-the-art shoulder arthroscopy in 1992. Ronald P. Karzel and I, as guest editors, invited an outstanding group of authors to contribute to the work. The multi-author format allows presentation of diverse ideas, and the reader has the opportunity to explore and contrast the various authors' arthroscopic approaches to a variety of shoulder problems.

Videotape Instruction in Shoulder Arthroscopy

The learning of shoulder arthroscopy via a videotape format can be very beneficial for both the novice and the experienced orthopaedist. An excellent starting point is the Video Learning Center at the Annual Meeting of the American Academy of Orthopaedic Surgeons (AAOS). The selection of tapes available for viewing and purchase is excellent and ranges from basic shoulder arthroscopy to some of the most complicated arthroscope-assisted surgical procedures. Additionally, several private sources offer videotapes for sale (see Table 1-2).

Many of the arthroscopic instrument companies also supply videotapes, either free or at a nominal cost, demonstrating various advanced surgical procedures. These tapes are frequently on display at the technical exhibits at the various orthopaedic and arthroscopy meetings and are usually listed in the technical brochures and catalogues that accompany the products.

Shoulder Arthroscopy Conferences

Many excellent courses are offered yearly where shoulder arthroscopy is a featured topic (see Table 1-3). The AANA has two such courses. In March the annual course is held, featuring both original manuscripts and special topic symposia. Although the other aspects of arthroscopy are also included, the shoulder topics usually are well represented. Specialized instructional courses are also available, and 90-minute shoulder topics are presented on both mornings. The fall AANA course is a hands-on practicum. The cadaver laboratory experience is excellent. The didactic portion of the course is geared toward the practical applications of arthroscopic techniques; live surgical demonstrations by invited faculty members round out the presentation.

At the Specialty Day course of the AANA, during the annual AAOS meeting, at least 30 percent of the program is dedicated to shoulder arthroscopy. This meeting offers an ideal

---

TABLE 1-2   Available Videotapes on Shoulder Arthroscopy

American Academy of Orthopaedic Surgeons (AAOS)
   6300 North River Road, Rosemont, IL 60018
Instrument Makar
   P.O. Box 885, Okemos, MI 48805
Research Center of Virginia
   7660 Parham Rd., #100, Richmond, VA 23229
San Diego Shoulder Arthroscopy Update, 1993 Videotape Sale
   Contact Rebecca Rimmer, San Diego Shoulder Arthroscopy, Inc., 3905 Waring Rd., Oceanside, CA 92056
SCOI Techniques of Shoulder Arthroscopy, 1993 (updated annually)
   Contact SCORE, 6815 Noble Ave., Van Nuys, CA 91405
The Video Journal of Orthopaedics
   Contact Medical Video Productions, 450 N. New Ballas Rd., Suite 266, St. Louis, MO 63141

TABLE 1-3   Available Shoulder Arthroscopy Courses

American Adademy of Orthopaedic Surgeons (AAOS)
   6300 North River Rd., Rosemont, IL 60018
Arthroscopy Association of North America (AANA)
   2250 East Devon Ave., Suite 101, Des Plaines, IL 60018
American Orthopaedic Society for Sports Medicine (AOSSM)
   2250 East Devon Ave., Suite 115, Des Plaines, IL 60018
James C. Esch, M.D.—10th Annual San Diego Shoulder Arthroscopy Course
   3905 Waring Road, Oceanside, CA 92054
James Guhl, M.D.
   3267 S. 16th St., Suite 101, Milwaukee, WI 53215
Wesley Nottage, M.D.—Shoulder Arthroscopy Cadaver Workshop
   23961 Calle de Magdalena, Suite 349, Laguna Hills, CA 92653
Lonnie Paulos, M.D.
   5848 S. 300 East, Salt Lake City, UT 84107
Southern California Orthopedic Institute (SCOI)
   Contact SCORE, 6815 Noble Ave., Van Nuys, CA 91405
Tuckahoe Orthopedics
   7660 Parham Rd., #100, Richmond, VA 23229

---

opportunity for an update on current shoulder arthroscopic topics. The best original papers from the annual AANA meeting are presented, along with symposia on timely topics, often related to the chosen papers.

The American Orthopaedic Society for Sports Medicine (AOSSM) also holds an annual open meeting. Many current shoulder arthroscopic topics are presented, along with related topics, by leading sports medicine shoulder surgeons. In addition, AOSSM holds a Specialty Day course at the annual AAOS meeting. The topics presented are usually slanted toward the use of shoulder arthroscopy in the treatment of sports injuries; many new and innovative concepts are presented not just for surgery, but also for rehabilitation pre- and postoperatively.

Also at the AAOS, the Instructional Course lectures are excellent. The lectures on shoulder arthroscopy, usually organized in a series, most often include segments on basic arthroscopic principles, instability, the rotator cuff, acromioclavicular (AC) joint problems, and other timely topics. Usually, two or three instructors are chosen to present these courses, which offer an opportunity for questions and answers as well as a didactic learning experience.

Several private courses have been very helpful for surgeons wishing to learn shoulder arthroscopy. The "San Diego Shoulder Update" is probably the most well known. This course, headed by Dr. James C. Esch, has been held in the La Jolla area since 1982. The course has been instrumental in the introduction of many surgeons to shoulder arthroscopy. The curriculum is updated yearly. The popular shoulder cadaver lab offers the opportunity for each participant not only to practice shoulder arthroscopy techniques, but also to perform an anatomical dissection on the specimen to evaluate the surgical treatment.

Each year the AAOS cosponsors several shoulder courses. One such course is cosponsored by the American Shoulder and Elbow Surgeons. Although this course does not feature shoulder arthroscopy alone, it always includes a segment on shoulder arthroscopy along with an excellent program on open shoulder surgery. Additional courses that include cadaver workshops are sponsored by Dr. Richard Caspari and the Research Institute of Virginia; Dr. Wesley Nottage, in Laguna Hills, California; Dr. James Guhl, in Chicago (although Dr. Guhl is located in Milwaukee, the course is held in Chicago); and Dr. Lonnie Paulos, in Salt Lake City, Utah.

We at SCOI traditionally sponsor a spring arthroscopy course. The course, usually held in the Palm Springs area, offers a choice of various arthroscopic surgical experiences including shoulder, knee, ankle, wrist, hand, and elbow. A cadaver lab is also available, along with workshops and lecture sessions.

Visitations and Tutorials

Another way to observe shoulder arthroscopy is through planned visitations to shoulder arthroscopy centers throughout the country. Although it may be time-consuming, the experience of direct observation of a surgical technique, with concomitant discussion with the presenting surgeon, is often a very valuable experience. The sports medicine tutorial system established by the American Orthopaedic Society for Sports Medicine offers an organized visitation to various centers on a yearly basis. Information can be obtained through the office of the AOSSM.

Fellowships

The ultimate learning experience for shoulder arthroscopy is to take a postgraduate fellowship. Although no such fellowships exist purely for shoulder arthroscopy, many of the sports medicine fellowships include the shoulder as well as the knee, ankle, and elbow. These positions range from 6 months to 1 year in duration and are variable in content, depending on the institution or individual sponsoring the program. Information concerning fellowships is available through the Advisory Council for Orthopaedic Resident Education (ACORE), 222 South Prospect Avenue, Park Ridge, IL 60068. Additionally, listings of fellowships in arthroscopy can be found in the classified sections of *The Journal of Bone and Joint Surgery, The Journal of Arthroscopy and Related Surgery,* and *The American Journal of Sports Medicine.*

Arthroscopic Learning Center

The Arthroscopy Association of North America is in the process of developing a permanent learning center dedicated to the teaching of arthroscopic skills. The center, to be located in the home office building of the American Academy of Orthopaedic Surgeons, is currently under construction and is expected to be available for use by the fall of 1993. The purpose of the center is to offer an all-inclusive learning experience for the interested physician. A videotape library, didactic lectures, and a practical laboratory with cadaver and dry model surgery will be offered (Fig. 1-1). Information on the Learning Center

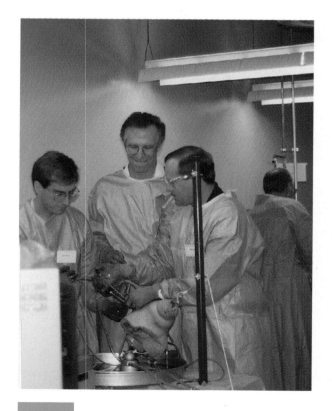

Figure 1-1

A training session sponsored by the Mitek Company was held at the DonJoy, Inc., research facility, in Carlsbad, California, to develop and improve shoulder arthroscopy skills. Drs. Marc Friedman (center) and Ronald Karzel (left) were involved with the author in training future instructors for the AANA cadaver labs.

may be obtained by writing the office of AANA, at 2250 East Devon Avenue, Suite 101, Des Plaines, IL 60018.

Practicing Shoulder Arthroscopy

It is always a good idea, when starting a new technique like shoulder arthroscopy, to work as an assistant with a surgeon who is already skilled in the technique. If this is not possible, then it is certainly worthwhile, once the techniques have been practiced in the cadaver lab, to begin simple diagnostic arthroscopy before performing open shoulder surgery. The diagnostic arthroscopy will soon enhance the pathological diagnosis; as experience grows, the arthroscopic surgical techniques can be added.

In my opinion, the first 30 or more shoulder arthroscopies should include both diagnostic glenohumeral and bursal anatomy review, and only simple surgical procedures, such as debridement. I believe that it requires at least 30 cases to become comfortable with the arthroscope before more difficult surgical manipulations are attempted. It is valuable to practice passing instruments into the bursa and locating and correlating glenohumeral and bursal anatomy using suture marker techniques. This will enhance the diagnostic quality of the exam and, in addition, will allow excellent practical experience for the surgeon. When the surgeon is comfortable with the diagnostic and simple operative procedures, the appropriate videotape selections for the desired surgical procedure should be reviewed. Any necessary equipment and instruments should be procured in advance of the case and tested, preferably on cadaver materials. Additionally, techniques such as arthroscopic suturing, knot tying, and implantation of bone anchors can be practiced in a simulated situation in the office prior to their use on the patient in surgery.

2

Operating Room Set-Up for Shoulder Arthroscopy

Introduction

When a surgeon plans to perform shoulder arthroscopy it is important to have the entire surgical team prepare for the case in advance. This chapter will describe a model operating room set-up designed specifically for the implementation of shoulder arthroscopy. It is intended for use not only by the surgeon and assistant but by the entire operating room staff, including the nurses and scrub and video technicians. It is suggested that an "inservice" be performed with the entire team before the first procedure is begun, so that each person is aware of his or her assignments and responsibilities. This should ensure that the procedure will go smoothly.

Operating Room Environment

Any standard operating room is suitable for shoulder arthroscopy. Laminar flow systems are not necessary; in fact, the noise that they make is distracting. High-quality operating room lights are necessary, especially when a mini-open surgery will follow the arthroscopic procedure.

Pre-Prep Table

A pre-prep table is prepared in advance. It includes the following items, which the surgical team will use to isolate the surgical field and perform the surgical skin preparations.

1. Plastic U-drape with adhesive backing, no. 10–15 (3M Co., St. Paul, Minn.)

2. Small rectangular plastic drape with adhesive edge, no. 10–10 (3M Co., St. Paul, Minn.)

3. Betadine prep set

4. Prep razor

5. 2-in adhesive tape (for hair removal)

6. Electrosurgical grounding pad

Operating Room Layout (Figs. 2-1 and 2-2)

The operating room table should be situated in the center of the room, but should be angled so that the anesthesiologist is positioned well away from the head of the table—approximately 45 degrees toward the anterior side of the lateral-positioned patient. The video equipment, including a television monitor, a light source, and a recording machine, is best situated on a portable cart located on the anterior side of the table, facing the surgeon. If a video printer is used, it should be located near the video cart but well away from all surgical fluids. The instrument table is located on the back side of the operating table, behind the surgeon. On this table are stored all the auxiliary arthroscopic equipment, such as basket punches, arthroscopic knife handles, extra arthroscopic cannulae, and specialty instruments.

The first Mayo stand is placed within the surgeon's reach on the posterior side of the table. This tray holds all of the instruments that the surgeon will need to prepare the shoulder and then introduce the arthroscopic cannula and scope. (See Table 2-1 and Fig. 2-3.)

A second Mayo stand is prepared for use on the anterior side of the table. This tray holds the mechanical and electrical equipment, including the arthroscope and pump tubing that will be used during the arthroscopic procedure. (See Table 2-2 and Fig. 2-4.)

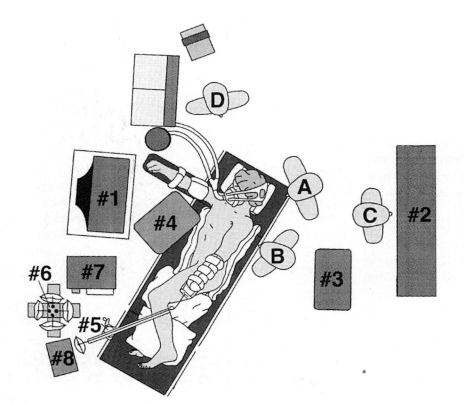

Figure 2-1

An overview of the operating room layout for all shoulder arthroscopic surgeries with the patient in the lateral decubitus position (see text). A, surgical assistant; B, surgeon; C, scrub nurse; D, anesthesiologist. 1, video cart with television monitor, video recorder, camera and light source, and shaver power system; 2, auxiliary instrument table; 3, Mayo stand no. 1; 4, Mayo stand no. 2; 5, traction apparatus for arm support; 6, adjustable irrigation tower; 7, electrosurgical power unit; 8, arthroscopic pump.

Figure 2-2
Any standard operating room can be used for shoulder arthroscopy, but the proper placement of the equipment and operating room table is important.

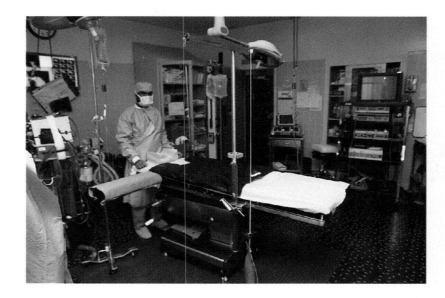

TABLE 2-1   Mayo Stand No. 1

1. 10-mL syringe with surgical irrigant
2. 50-mL syringe with extension tubing connected
3. Beaker filled with surgical irrigant
4. Knife handle with no. 11 blade
5. Skin-marking pencil
6. 18-gauge 2 1/2-in. spinal needle
7. Arthroscopic cannula system with blunt trochars
8. Guide rod and switching stick
9. No. 1 PDS suture with needle removed (marker suture)

Figure 2-3
Mayo stand no. 1 contains all the equipment that the surgeon needs to outline the anatomy and enter the shoulder (see text).

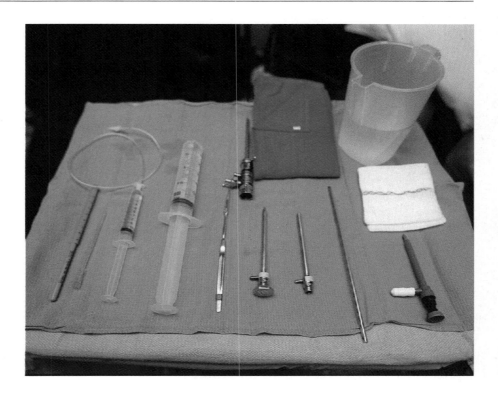

TABLE 2-2   Mayo Stand No. 2

1. Motor unit for shaver system
2. Electrosurgical hand piece with subacromial electrode tip (if decompression is planned)
3. Appropriate blades for the surgery planned (shavers or abraders)
4. Arthroscope and bridge assembly with attached light source and tubing for pump
5. Remote controls for pump and video recorder

Shoulder Traction Apparatus

Proper support of the shoulder during arthroscopy requires the use of a safe and effective traction apparatus to apply appropriate suspension and allow easy positioning of the arm. In addition, the device used to grip the forearm and hand should be anatomically safe, with appropriate padding or molding to avoid pressure areas on bony prominences and neurovascular structures. A convenient method used at SCOI consists of an arm and forearm sleeve, made of presterilized foam with five circumferential Velcro straps, called the STaR Sleeve (shoulder *traction and rotation*) from Arthrex, Inc. (Naples, Florida) (see Fig. 3-13). The traction apparatus should be firmly attached to the operating table, so that if the table is moved, the device will move in concert with it. The ideal device should allow easy adjustment for both abduction and forward flexion and should have a low-friction pulley system and free-hanging weights to avoid inadvertent traction injury to the arm. The application of two-point traction, when it is needed for shoulder stabilization surgery, is possible with the Two Way Traction Shoulder Holder, from Arthrex, Inc. (Naples, Florida) (Fig. 2-5).

Arthroscopic Fluid Irrigation Stand and Arthroscopic Pump System

The arthroscopic fluid irrigation stand and arthroscopic pump system are placed next to the video cart. There should be adequate space between them to reduce to a minimum

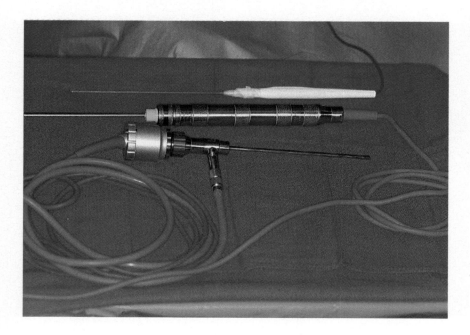

Figure 2-4
Mayo stand no. 2, situated on the front side of the table, contains the mechanical and electrical equipment as well as the remote controls for the pump and video equipment.

Figure 2-5
The traction apparatus should be fixed to the operating table. It should allow easy positioning of the arm between 10 and 70 degrees of abduction and between 0 and 30 degrees of forward flexion.

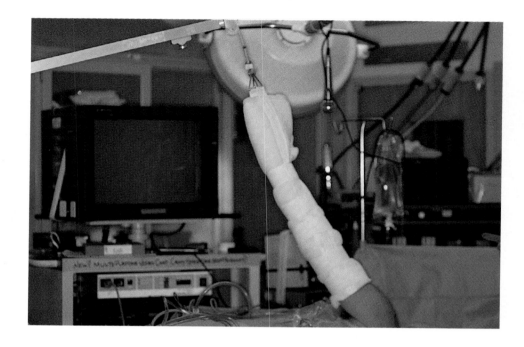

the possibility of fluids leaking onto the electrical equipment. The pump mechanism is supported on a stand within easy view of the surgeon, usually at the foot of the table. We have used an arthroscopic pump system for shoulder arthroscopy for five years and believe it to be a valuable asset. The pump we prefer is supplied by 3M, Inc. (St. Paul, Minnesota) (Fig. 2-6). This pump incorporates the fluid inflow line and the pressure sensor system into the bridge of the arthroscope (Fig. 2-7). This arrangement ensures accurate pressure readings at all times. (A false measurement might occur if the inflow and the pressure sensor were connected to separate cannulae.) Also, a gravity outflow tube is included; it is useful during all abrasion and decompression surgery.

The 3-L irrigation bags are hung near the arthroscopic pump. We use a specialized arthroscopic irrigation pole that allows the positioning of each bag at a variable height above the floor. This unit facilitates the circulating nurse's job by allowing him or her to elevate and lower each bag of irrigant independently of the others. If gravity flow is being

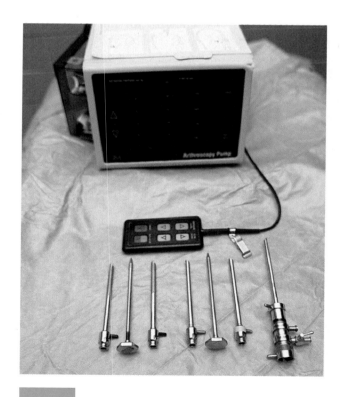

Figure 2-6
The pump used for shoulder arthroscopy should have a remote control that can be sterilized and placed on Mayo stand no. 2, within easy reach of the surgeon.

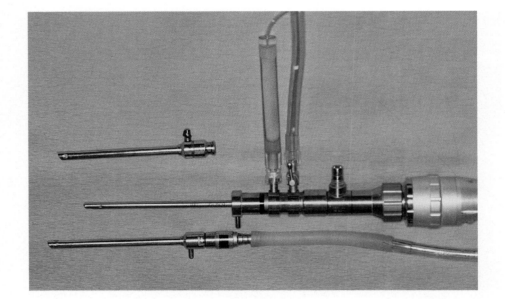

Figure 2-7
The 3M pump offers convenience and safety. One notable feature is that the inflow and pressure sensor tubing are both attached to the bridge assembly of the arthroscope.

used, it is easy to lower one arm of the pole to replace an empty bag while leaving the other bags at the desired higher level. Also, by staggering the heights of the individual bags a continuous fluid flow is guaranteed. Two or more bags can be opened at the same time with this system; when the upper bag is depleted the next lower bag begins to flow with no interruption. The system we prefer is supplied by Allen Medical Systems (Cleveland, Ohio) (Fig. 2-8).

Levelert Fluid Monitoring System

Often the circulating nurse is extremely busy during an arthroscopic case and therefore is unable to watch the irrigation fluid level continuously. If the irrigation bags become depleted, the procedure is interrupted until the fluid can be started again. A helpful device for assisting with the monitoring of the irrigation bags is the Levelert fluid depletion monitor, from Dyonics, Inc. (Andover, Massachusetts) (Fig. 2-9). This system consists of four sensor units connected to an alarm box mounted on

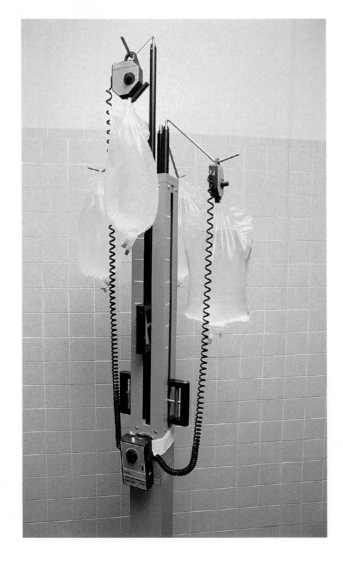

Figure 2-8
The Allen IV and irrigation tower permits each irrigation bag to be adjusted or lowered individually to maintain high-pressure flow, even during replenishment of an empty bag.

Figure 2-9
The Levelert fluid depletion alarm (Dyonics, Inc.) hangs on the IV pole to suspend the irrigation bags and warns the staff before a "fluid depletion emergency" can occur.

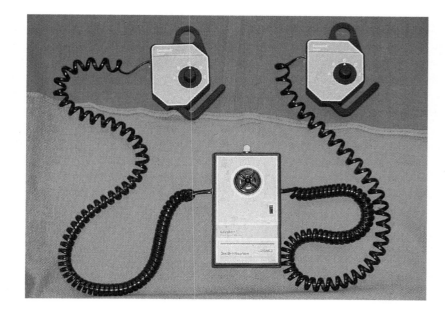

the irrigation stand. An individual bag is suspended from the arm of a sensor so that when fluid in that bag reaches a prescribed level near depletion, a warning chime is sounded to alert the operating room staff. This chime gives the surgical team adequate time to hang an additional bag of fluid if it is needed for the uninterrupted progress of the procedure.

The suction system is also placed on the anterior side of the table, for easy access for emptying and servicing by the circulating nurse. The suction should include a two-canister collection system, so that when one canister is being emptied the other is still in service. A single suction tube from the canister to the table is adequate, but it is helpful to have a Y connector with two extension tubes to the operative field. This arrangement saves time in the transition from one suction instrument to the other.

Positioning Aids

Since the patient will often be placed in a lateral decubitus position for arthroscopy, several unique positioning aids should be available (Table 2-3 and Fig. 2-10). A Vacupak beanbag with one U-shaped end is placed on the table with the base of the U at the level of the patient's scapula. A useful "axillary roll" can be made by wrapping a 1-L bag of intravenous solution in a cotton towel. A foam head-and-neck support with a cutout for the ear should be available for use by the anesthesiologist after the patient is turned. Two kidney rests are also used, one on each side of the table, to support the pelvis in the lateral position. Additionally, two soft pillows are used between the patient's legs to prevent strain on the hips and knees and excess pressure on the bony prominences. Flat foam

TABLE 2-3   Table Positioning Aids

1. U-shaped Vacupak beanbag, 3 ft long
2. Axillary roll (a 1-L IV bag covered with a towel)
3. Kidney rest supports for OR table (2)
4. Contoured foam head-and-neck support
5. Arm board
6. Pillows (2)
7. Foam pads for ankles, knees, and arms

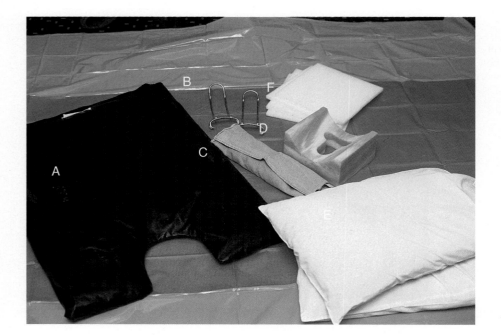

Figure 2-10
Positioning aids for shoulder arthroscopy should include: *A,* 3-ft Vacupak beanbag to hold the patient in the lateral position on the operating table; *B,* two curved 8-in kidney rest supports; *C,* axillary roll; *D,* contoured foam head-and-neck support; *E,* two soft pillows; and *F,* six flat, soft foam pads.

padding is also needed for protection of the dependent peroneal nerve and ankle areas, as well as for the elbow and wrist of the contralateral arm.

Once the room set-up is complete and the instruments and arthroscopic equipment are ready, the patient may be brought into the operating room.

3

Patient Preparation and Positioning for Shoulder Arthroscopy

Operating Room Admission

The patient is brought into the operating room when the surgical team has completed the room set-up and the instruments are ready. The patient is positioned on the operating table in a comfortable position with the U of the beanbag at the level of the axilla. The head is supported with a pillow, and warm blankets are used for comfort. To put the patient at ease, it may be helpful to have a member of the surgical team—especially someone who is known to the patient—point out the various components of the arthroscopic equipment, such as the video camera, the recorder, and the arthroscope. It is important that the surgical team maintain a quiet sense of decorum and professionalism so that the patient feels relaxed and confident.

Anesthesia

The anesthesiologist chosen for shoulder arthroscopy should be well versed in the special needs of this procedure. These include:

1. Use of interscalene nerve block for regional anesthesia

2. Hypotensive control of blood pressure to minimize bleeding and aid visualization

3. Necessity of managing and monitoring the patient from a remote position away from the head of the table

4. Placement of leads and monitors to avoid the surgical field

5. Protection of the head, neck, and airway with the patient in the lateral decubitus position

The choice of anesthesia should be determined before the patient enters the operating room. The anesthesiologist should review the options with the patient after taking a thorough history and reviewing the medical records. The ability to offer the patient an interscalene block for either surgical anesthesia or postsurgical pain control is a valuable asset. At SCOI, the usual anesthetic includes the combination of a preoperative interscalene block and a general balanced anesthesia. The block is best performed in the preoperative area, where there are adequate nursing personnel and monitoring equipment to observe the patient. If this is not available then the block can be performed in the operating room, just prior to the administration of the general anesthetic. The ECG electrodes are positioned well away from the involved shoulder. Once the anesthetic is completed and the vital signs are stable, the patient is ready for positioning.

Patient Positioning for Arthroscopic Surgery

Correct positioning of the patient on the operating table is important to ensure his or her safety while allowing the best possible access to the shoulder joint and bursa for the surgical procedure. The circulating nurse should review the surgeon's preference card and speak with the surgeon to ascertain the preferred position for the planned surgical procedure. All members of the surgical team have the responsibility to protect the patient from potential harmful effects of the surgical position. The operating room circulating nurse is responsible for coordinating the details for restraints, extremity supports, and safe patient transfer. Besides providing optimum exposure and access to the operative site, the surgical position must sustain circulatory and respiratory function, protect neurovascular structures, and afford as much comfort as possible before and after the anesthetic induction.

Shoulder arthroscopy may be performed in either the "beach chair" position or the lateral decubitus position. At SCOI the beach chair position is seldom used, except for a diagnostic arthroscopic procedure prior to an open anterior capsular reconstruction procedure. In the beach chair position, also known as the modified Fowler's (sitting) position, most of the patient's weight is on the dorsum of the body (Fig. 3-1). The body must be carefully aligned with the hinge breaks in the OR table to prevent abnormal pressure. The table back is elevated while the hips and knees are flexed. A donut headrest is used to support

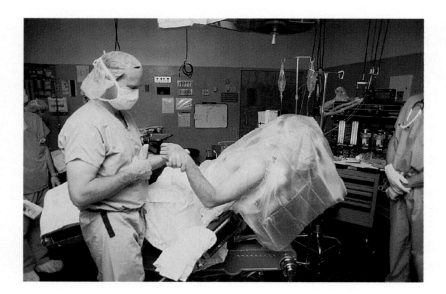

Figure 3-1
The beach chair position is sometimes used for diagnostic arthroscopy prior to a planned open anterior reconstruction.

Figure 3-2
The standard arthroscopy position is the lateral decubitus position, with the torso tilted posteriorly approximately 30 degrees.

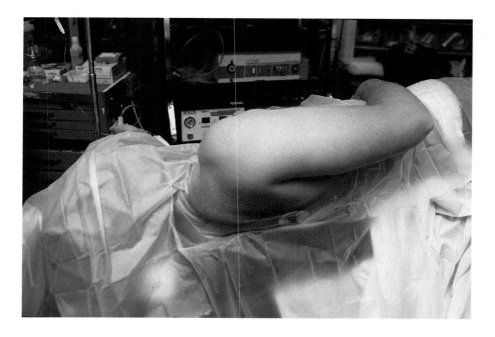

the head and neck with the head turned a few degrees away from the involved shoulder. The head should be secured to the table with adhesive tape crossing the forehead over a protective pad. The nonoperative arm rests on a pillow in the patient's lap or is tucked carefully at the patient's side with protective foam padding. A pillow is placed beneath the knees and legs to prevent pressure on the heels. After placing a blanket over the patient's thighs the safety strap is applied. A plastic U-drape is used proximally, and a barrier drape is used distally to isolate the surgical field. These should be placed to allow wide exposure of the shoulder from the base of the neck to the midthorax on the surgical side while protecting the patient's head from contamination by the surgical fluids.

The lateral decubitus position is most often used for shoulder arthroscopy, particularly when performing surgery in the glenoid humeral joint, subacromial bursa, or AC joint (Fig. 3-2). This position is also ideal for performing the "mini-open" rotator cuff repair or

Figure 3-3
The head and neck are supported in line with the spine by a contoured foam pillow.

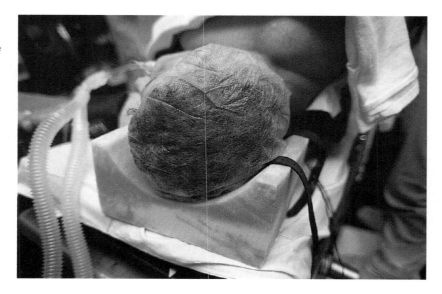

biceps tenodesis. The patient is turned to lie on the nonoperative side with the help of four members of the surgical staff as well as the anesthesiologist. The anesthesiologist controls the turn; the surgeon and the assistant are positioned on either side of the torso. A third person stands at the foot to control the legs. On a signal from the anesthesiologist, the patient is lifted and turned with the appropriate side uppermost. The patient's head is placed on a contoured foam pillow and the table adjusted to avoid any stress on the neck (Fig. 3-3). An axillary roll is placed beneath the dependent thorax when the body is elevated (Fig. 3-4). Foam-rubber padding is placed beneath the dependent elbow, knee, and ankle, and pillows are placed between the knees and legs (Fig. 3-5). The kidney rests are moved into position, and the Vacupak beanbag is molded around the patient's torso in such a way that the body tilts posteriorly approximately 15 degrees. This position is held while the air is evacuated with suction from the beanbag (Fig. 3-6). The surgeon should make a final check of the positioning aids and protective pads to be certain that the bony prominences are protected.

An electrosurgical ground pad is placed

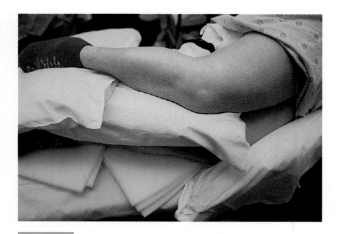

Figure 3-5
The lower leg and ankle are protected by foam pads; two pillows are placed beneath the slightly bent knees.

over the muscular area of the lateral thigh. The table is then turned and the lights adjusted so that the surgeon has access to the entire superior and posterior aspect of the patient. This usually involves turning the head of the table in a posterior direction approximately 45 degrees. A towel is placed on the side of the patient's head for protection. The surgical field is isolated with a plastic U-drape extending from the base of the neck down the anterior and posterior hemithorax. A second plastic barrier drape is used at about midthorax level to connect the legs of the U-drape. This technique outlines a wide surgical field

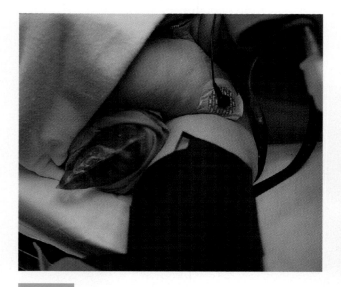

Figure 3-4
An axillary roll consisting of an IV bag covered with a towel should be placed beneath the dependent hemithorax to protect the axillary contents.

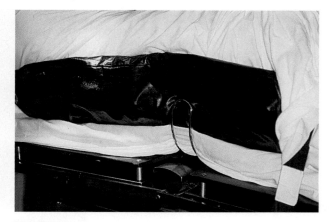

Figure 3-6
The beanbag is contoured around the patient's laterally tilted torso and supported with kidney rests.

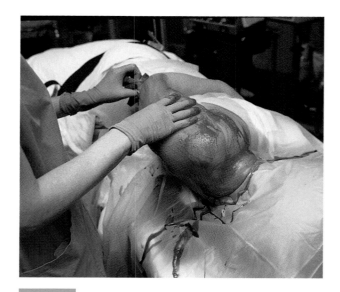

Figure 3-7
The surgical field is isolated with a plastic U-drape. The skin preparation includes the entire hand, arm, and shoulder.

and protects the patient from fluid contamination (Fig. 3-7).

Shoulder Stability Examination

The lateral decubitus position is ideal for examining the patient's shoulder stability (Fig. 3-8). The surgeon stands behind the patient and supports the involved arm with one hand above the elbow, holding the shoulder in a 90 degrees abducted position. The surgeon's other hand grasps the humeral head, using the middle finger and thumb. The weight of the arm is allowed to compress the glenohumeral joint. The humeral head is gently moved in an anterior and posterior direction, the surgeon sensing any catching or subluxing as it crosses the lip of the glenoid. The arm can then be rotated both internally and externally to determine the effect of tightening or relaxing of the ligamentous tissues on shoulder stability. Inferior traction also can be applied, and the subacromial gap visualized. If necessary for documentation or confirmation of instability, an axillary x-ray exposure can be made with anterior or posterior stress applied to the shoulder in this position. Inferior traction can also demonstrate a subacromial gap, if one is present, on x-ray.

Draping

Once the surgical team has scrubbed and gowned, the draping procedure can commence. The arm and exposed shoulder and hemithorax area are prepped by a surgical technician. Alcohol is used to clean an area around the periphery of the field to allow for better drape adherence. First, a 3/4-length

Figure 3-8
All shoulders should be examined for range of motion and stability prior to arthroscopy. The lateral position is ideal for performing stability testing.

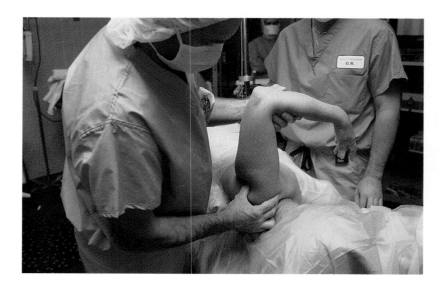

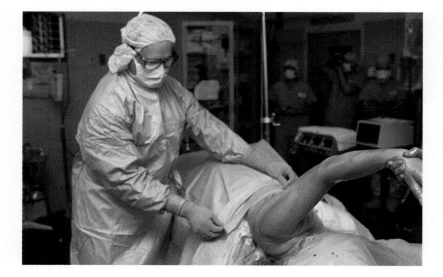

Figure 3-9
The first drape applied is a 3/4-length sheet which covers from the midthorax to the bottom of the table.

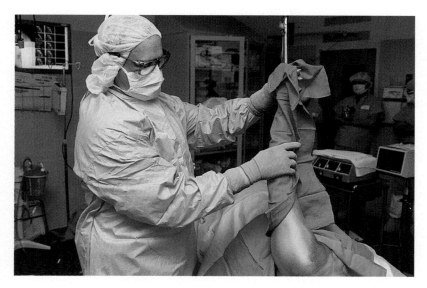

Figure 3-10
Three sterile towels are used to blot dry the surgical field and the arm and hand.

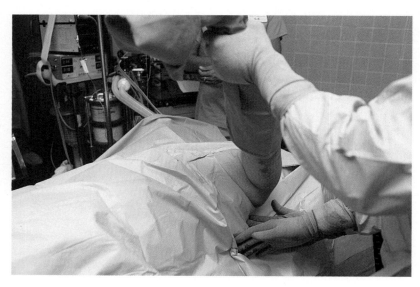

Figure 3-11
The lower drape has a plastic U-shaped upper edge with adhesive backing.

drape is applied from the foot of the table to the midthorax, covering the inferior aspect of the operating field (Fig. 3-9). The arm is held by the surgical assistant with a dry sterile towel. The surgeon next lays a second drying towel in the axilla and a third towel over the upper aspect of the shoulder and the base of the neck (Fig. 3-10). After the skin is blotted and the drying towels discarded, the second drape is applied.

At SCOI, we use a shoulder drape pack supplied by the Baxter Convertor Custom Sterile Division (McGraw Park, Illinois). This pack includes a body drape that covers the lower two-thirds of the table and has an upper U-shaped plastic end with adhesive backing (Fig. 3-11). The upper drape has a built-in fluid collection pouch on the anterior, posterior, and superior aspects connected to a dependent drainage system (Fig. 3-12). This draping set is easy to apply and protects the patient from fluid contamination while collecting excess liquids in the pouch. Two drainage tubes are attached to the connectors on the lower end of the pouch and inserted into a gravity reservoir.

The arm is then placed in a sterilized foam traction sleeve (STaR Sleeve) (Arthrex, Inc., Naples, Florida) (Fig. 3-13). It is supported in a position of approximately 70 degrees of abduction and 10 degrees of flexion. For an average-sized patient, 10 lb of weight is adequate for arm support; but a few pounds more

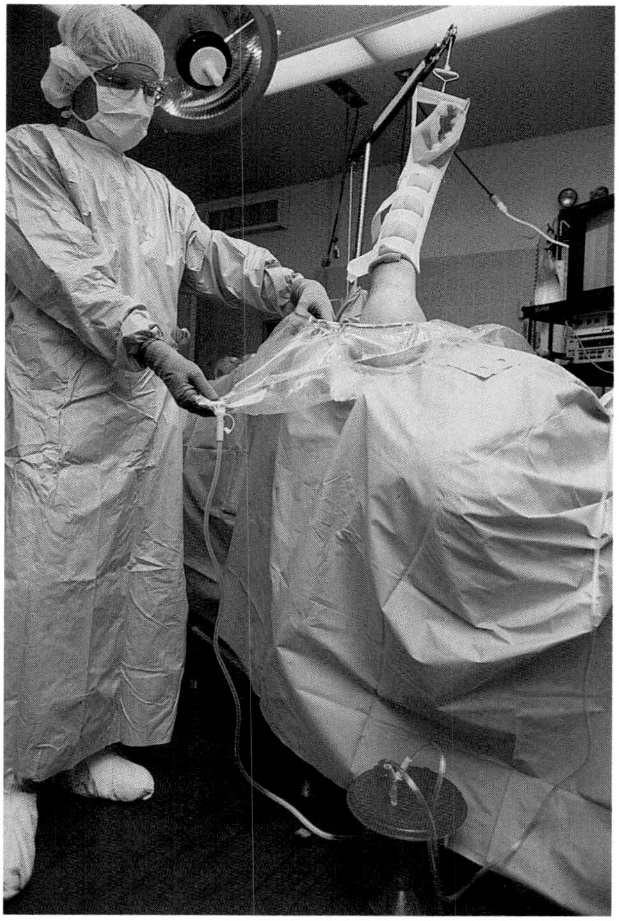

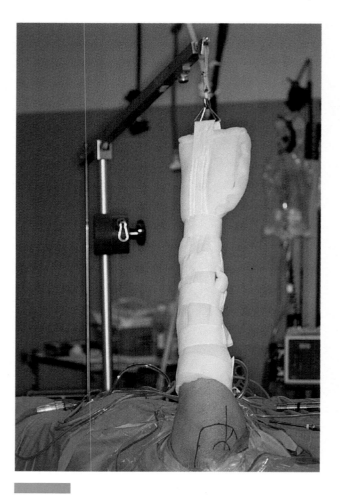

Figure 3-12
The upper drape has built-in fluid collection pouches on the anterior and posterior sides, each with a connector for a drainage tube.

Figure 3-13
The arm is wrapped in a sterilized foam traction sleeve, which is attached to an overhead traction device.

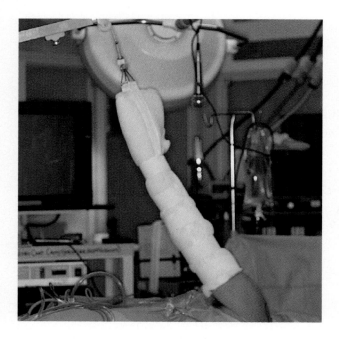

Figure 3-14
In the final position for shoulder arthroscopy, the arm is supported in 70 degrees of abduction and 10 degrees of flexion.

or less can be added as necessary, depending on patient size and arm weight (Fig. 3-14).

When the patient's positioning is completed, the pump tubing is connected to the irrigation bags and the arthroscope, and the no. 1 and no. 2 Mayo stands, with appropriate instruments, are moved into position. Once the video equipment is connected and the power instruments checked, the arthroscopic procedure can begin.

4

Diagnostic Arthroscopy of the Shoulder: Normal Anatomy and Variations

Introduction

Diagnostic arthroscopic evaluation of the shoulder is performed with the patient in the lateral decubitus position on the operating table and with the arm supported in 70 degrees of abduction and 20 degrees of forward flexion. The basic diagnostic procedure consists of visualizing and video-recording all of the anatomical features in the glenohumeral joint and subacromial space, from both the anterior and posterior portals. At SCOI we have developed a checklist of anatomical areas, including 15 points in the glenohumeral joint and 8 points in the subacromial space, which we use on every case to ensure a complete evaluation. By using this rigid stepwise evaluation procedure we can ensure that the anatomy review is complete in each case and that no pathological situation goes unnoticed. This chapter will describe the techniques we use to visualize the glenohumeral anatomy.

Also, anatomical variants in the glenohumeral joint will be identified and discussed.

Surface Anatomy Outline

With the arm suspended in traction, a marking pencil is used to outline the surface anatomy. The supraclavicular fossa is first palpated, and the surgeon's thumb is inserted into this area just posterior to the AC joint and medial to the acromial edge. This area is outlined with a sterile skin-marking pen.

Next, the acromial and clavicular outlines are traced. *When these reference lines are drawn they should be "around the corner" of the bone—not on the most superficial subcutaneous bony prominence.* In other words, the important anatomical point is the inferior margin of these bones, because that is the area from which the entry points and surgical incisions for the joint and bursa are measured

(Fig. 4-1). To locate the correct position a "pincher" grasp is used, with the thumb in the supraclavicular notch and the index finger feeling for the inferior aspect of the acromion, beginning at the posterior lateral angle. Once this area is located, an ink dot is drawn on the skin. The index finger then proceeds across the lateral aspect of the acromion to the anterior lateral corner, and this point is marked with ink. Next, the S-shaped clavicle is outlined to the midclavicular area. Finally, the thick spine of the scapula, posteriorly, is outlined. The AC joint is then marked. Its posterior edge is located at the anterior margin of the suprascapular notch, and its direction can usually be identified by palpation. Once these points are correctly identified on the skin, the marking pencil is used to connect them, giving an accurate superficial rendering of the underlining bony anatomy.

An important bursal orientation line is drawn next. Beginning at the posterior edge of the AC joint (the anterior edge of the supraclavicular fossa), a line is drawn perpendicular to the lateral border of the acromion, extending distally from that point approximately 4 cm down the arm. This line should divide the acromion into an anterior two-fifths and posterior three-fifths. Beneath the anterior

acromion lies the subacromial bursal cavity. The biceps tendon is located near the anterior lateral edge of this bursal space; the posterior bursal curtain is usually located just posterior to this line. The line is also used as a reference for inserting a bursal palpating probe, as well as for creating the lateral subacromial operating portal for decompression and Mumford procedures. Additionally, if a mini-open rotator cuff repair is performed, the incision made uses this important orientation line as a guide.

Glenohumeral Arthroscopy

The first step in arthroscopic evaluation of the glenohumeral joint is to gently insert a spinal needle into the glenohumeral joint in the position of the posterior portal. This point is chosen after palpation of the posterior shoulder anatomy and balloting of the humeral head. The exact position cannot be simply measured from the surface anatomy, but must be determined after consideration of the thickness of the soft tissues around the shoulder and the size of the bony anatomy. In the average-sized individual, the entry point is approximately 2 cm inferior and 1 cm medial to the posterolateral acromial angle. For patients with thicker muscle and adipose tissue or larger bony structures, the point will be farther inferior and medial. A $2\frac{1}{2}$-in 18-gauge spinal needle with a stylet is carefully inserted through the skin and into the capsule at this point. Care must be taken not to move the needle around too much, since the tip can injure the articular surface of the humeral head. Usually a distinct "pop" is felt as the capsule is penetrated. The stylet is removed and the joint injected with surgical irrigant using a 10-mL syringe (Fig. 4-2). This small syringe allows the surgeon to sense resistance to the injection flow. If resistance is felt, the needle is repositioned until a free flow of fluid is achieved. The syringe is removed. Backflow of fluid from the needle ensures that it is correctly positioned in the joint. Once this is established, a 50-mL syringe with an extension

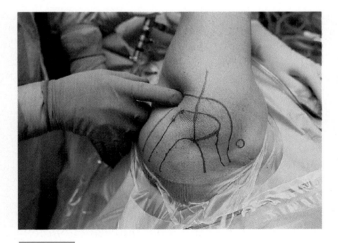

Figure 4-1
The bony anatomy is outlined with a sterile skin-marking pencil. The difference between the superficial bony landmarks and the correct "around-the-corner" position can be seen in this photograph.

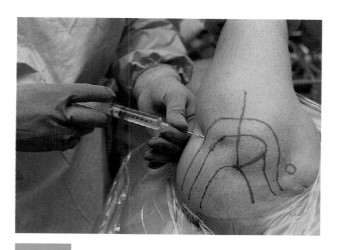

Figure 4-2

The posterior portal is created by first inserting a spinal needle and distending the joint with a 10 mL syringe full of irrigant.

tubing is connected to the needle and the joint distended to its maximum. This usually takes an additional 20 to 30 mL of fluid. After removal of the needle, a 5-mm stab wound is made through the skin with a no. 11 knife blade, following the direction of the skin lines. *No attempt is made to pierce the muscular tissues or capsule at any time with the knife.*

The arthroscopic cannula, with a blunt-tipped obturator, is inserted through the posterior stab wound and worked through the muscle until the posterior humeral head is palpated; sharp-tipped obturators are never used in the shoulder (Fig. 4-3). With the non-

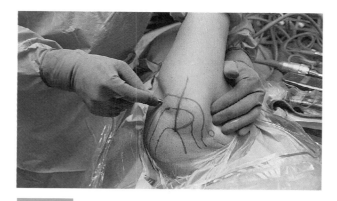

Figure 4-3

A small stab wound is created through the skin, and an arthroscopic cannula is inserted with a blunt-tipped obturator.

dominant hand palpating the anterior surface of the shoulder joint, the humeral head is balloted back and forth until a sense of the joint line's location is appreciated. By directing the cannula to slide medially and slightly superior off the humeral head, a step-off is felt at the edge of the head. The cannula is advanced through the capsule, and usually a definite "pop" is felt. When the obturator is removed, a gush of fluid flows from the cannula. Sometimes, especially with large capsular or rotator cuff lesions, vigorous fluid backflow will not be seen, despite proper cannula placement in the joint. It is important to insert the arthroscope into the cannula to assess its location visually before a second puncture is performed, since the cannula may be in the joint despite the absence of fluid backflow.

A common error made by the beginning arthroscopist is attempting to insert the cannula at a point too lateral or too proximal. It should be remembered that the joint line is inferior and medial to the posterolateral corner. If difficulties are encountered, the reference anatomy should be rechecked and the spinal needle reinserted a little more medial and inferior. Care should be taken not to move below the joint into the axillary area, where serious neurovascular damage might occur.

Anterior Portal Creation

With the arthroscope inserted into the posterior cannula, the joint is distended with fluid by means of the arthroscopic pump or gravity inflow, and the biceps tendon is visualized. The anterior portal is created by passing the tip of the arthroscope to a point just inferior to the biceps tendon. Once past the biceps tendon, the tip of the arthroscope is angled a few degrees superior and lateral and is held against the anterior capsule. The scope is removed, and a taper-tipped guide rod is inserted into the cannula to puncture the anterior capsule and tent the skin. A small stab wound is made adjacent to the tip of the guide rod, which ideally is located approximately 2 cm inferior and 1 cm medial to the anterior edge of the acromion, near the AC joint. The guide rod is passed through this puncture, and

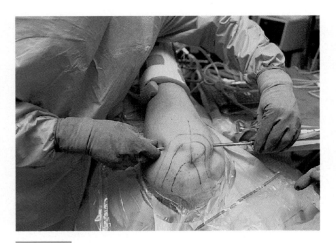

Figure 4-4
The anterior portal is created using a transarticular rod, passing through the posterior cannula and exiting anteriorly, just below the biceps tendon.

a second cannula is inserted over the tip of the rod and worked into the joint (Fig. 4-4). Connected to this anterior cannula is a gravity drainage tube. The arthroscope is reinserted posteriorly, and the location of the anterior cannula is verified. Following this, the video recorder is activated and the 15-point glenohumeral review is begun.

Glenohumeral Joint Evaluation/15-Point Anatomy Review (see Tables 4-1 and 4-2)

The arthroscopic evaluation is always performed with the video image rotated so that the glenoid is on the lower half of the television monitor. Keeping this rotation throughout the anatomy examination makes it easier for the entire surgical team to understand the anatomy review. Ten points in the 15-point anatomy review are visualized in a sequential manner from the posterior portal (Fig. 4-5); the remaining five points are visualized from the anterior portal. Let us now consider each of the 15 points in detail.

Position 1 includes the biceps tendon and its superior labral anchor (Fig. 4-6). The biceps tendon is visualized and carefully evaluated throughout its intra-articular passage. Using the anterior cannula, the biceps tendon can be palpated and pulled a few millimeters into the joint to aid in evaluation of the segment of the tendon that resides in the intertubercular groove. In addition, the superior labral attachment of the biceps tendon is inspected and palpated. If this area appears loose, traction on the biceps tendon may cause the superior labrum to arch away from the usual glenoid attachment and may indi-

TABLE 4-1   First Part of 15-Point Anatomy Review—Visualizing from Posterior Portal

1. Biceps tendon
2. Posterior labrum and capsule attachment
3. Inferior axillary recess and inferior capsular insertion to humeral head
4. Inferior labrum and glenoid articular surface
5. Supraspinatus tendon of rotator cuff
6. Posterior rotator cuff insertion and bare area of humeral head
7. Articular surface of humeral head
8. Anterior superior labrum, superior and middle glenohumeral ligaments, and subscapularis tendon
9. Anterior inferior labrum
10. Anterior inferior glenohumeral ligament

TABLE 4-2   Second Part of 15-Point Anatomy Review—Visualizing from Anterior Portal

11. Posterior glenoid labrum
12. Posterior aspect of rotator cuff, including infraspinatus and supraspinatus tendons
13. Anterior glenoid labrum and inferior glenohumeral ligament attachments
14. Subscapularis tendon and recess, and middle glenohumeral ligament
15. Anterior surface of humeral head, with subscapularis attachment and biceps tendon passage

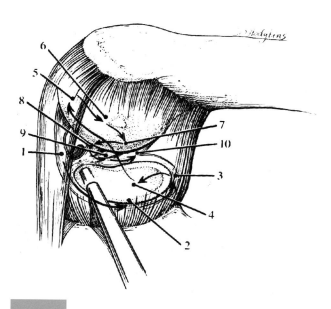

Figure 4-5
Ten important anatomical points are visualized through the posterior portal.

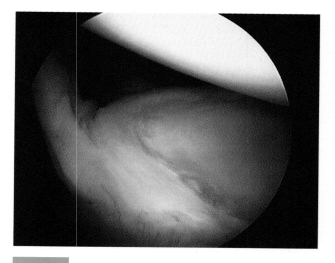

Figure 4-7
The superior labrum often appears loosely attached and may have a meniscoid-like appearance.

cate that a superior labrum anterior-posterior (SLAP) lesion is present (see Chap. 10).

There are several normal anatomical variants found in position 1. A meniscoid-type loosely attached superior labrum can be seen (Fig. 4-7). This type of superior labrum may appear pathological at first glance, but on

careful examination it is noted that the articular cartilage of the superior glenoid extends around the corner to the area where the labrum is attached. When this situation is present, no true pathology exists. The "vinculae biceps" are small strands of mesentery-like synovium that pass from the biceps tendon to the surrounding synovium and capsule. These should not be mistaken for scar tissue or tears of the biceps tendon. In addition, the biceps tendon may infrequently be completely ensheathed in capsule. This rare situation causes no symptoms and should not be disturbed (Fig. 4-8).

In position 2 the posterior labrum and capsular reflection are visualized (Fig. 4-9). The arthroscope is retracted and the bevel rotated inferiorly to visualize along the posterior labrum. It is helpful to elevate the arthroscope a few millimeters away from the labrum so that it is not resting on the posterior edge of the glenoid during this maneuver. The posterior labrum should be smooth, and usually is tightly attached to the glenoid surface. The posterior capsular recess normally appears redundant.

Position 3 includes the inferior axillary recess and the capsular attachment to the humeral head (Fig. 4-10). With the arthroscope in the axillary pouch, the bevel can be

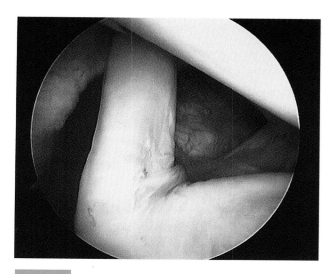

Figure 4-6
Position 1 includes the biceps tendon from its passage out of the rotator interval to its insertion on the superior labrum.

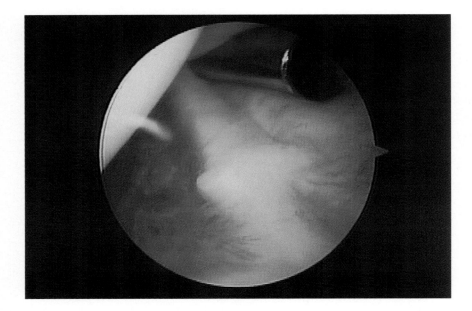

rotated to look superiorly at the insertion of the inferior capsule into the humeral head. Sometimes early chondromalacic lesions or osteophytes are seen in this location.

In position 4 the glenoid articular surface is visualized (Fig. 4-11). The inferiormost portion of the labrum is first evaluated; then the arthroscope is rotated to view the rest of the fossa. The articular cartilage of the glenoid has a relatively thin-appearing area about the midpoint of the glenoid. This normal variant can be confused with chondromalacia, but is

found in virtually all shoulders to some degree. Along the anterior edge of the glenoid there is an indentation, or dimple, which demarcates the superior two-fifths from the inferior three-fifths of the glenoid. This normal anatomical feature marks the point of fusion of the two ossific centers of the glenoid and can sometimes appear very deep, resembling an old fracture.

Position 5 includes the supraspinatus por-

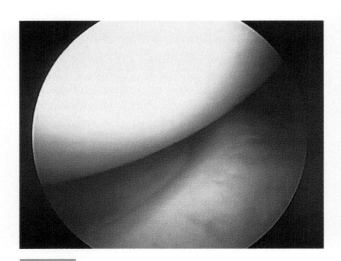

Figure 4-9
In position 2 the posterior labrum and posterior capsular reflection are seen.

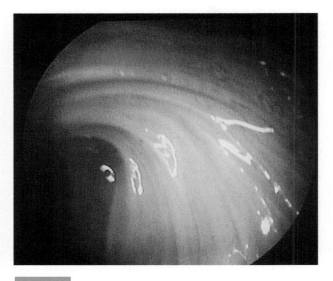

Figure 4-10
Position 3 includes the inferior axillary recess and the capsular attachment to the humeral head.

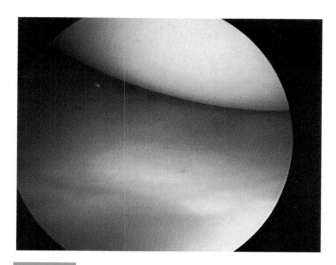

Figure 4-11
In position 4 the glenoid articular surface is evaluated from the inferior to the superior labra. Often, normally, the cartilage has a thin central depression that may appear pathological.

tion of the rotator cuff just posterior to the biceps tendon and its attachment to the humeral head adjacent to the articular cartilage (Fig. 4-12). The bevel of the arthroscope is rotated upward to the 11 and 12 o'clock positions in order to visualize this area most effectively. This portion of the rotator cuff usu-

ally has a firm attachment to the humeral head with no significant fraying or synovial reaction. It should be remembered that the rotator cuff tendon itself is covered, on the articular surface, with a layer of capsule as well as a layer of synovium. These two tissues can show some variations in the normal situation, which may be confusing. If the arthroscopic fluid pressure is low, the vascular pattern in the synovium covering the cuff can seem prominent. The normal vascularity is quite rich on the proximal portion of the cuff extending from the superior glenoid area and diminishes as it approaches the humeral head attachment. A thickening in the capsular tissue beneath the rotator cuff, passing perpendicular to the biceps tendon across the undersurface of the supraspinatus tendon, has been called "rotator cuff ridge" (Fig. 4-13). This normal, but sometimes unusual-appearing, fold frequently demarcates the boundary where the synovial vascularity tapers off. There is seldom a rich vascular supply above the upper border of the rotator cuff ridge. It has been suggested that this rotator cuff ridge formation corresponds to a transverse capsular band which is thought to reinforce the superior capsule and pass perpendicular to the coracohumeral ligament.

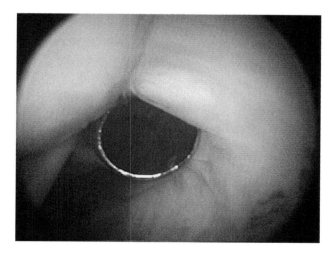

Figure 4-12
In position 5 the entire articular surface of the supraspinatus tendon is evaluated, from its passage over the glenoid to its insertion in the humeral head. A marker suture placed in this position is often used to help identify the corresponding area in the bursa.

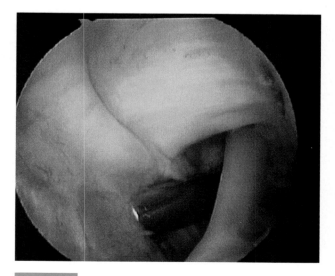

Figure 4-13
The "rotator cuff ridge" is a normal capsular thickening crossing the supraspinatus tendon from anterior to posterior on the articular surface.

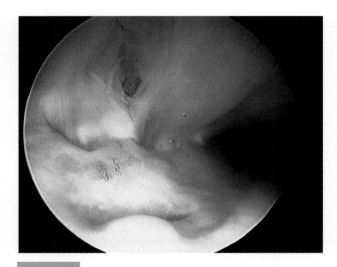

Figure 4-14
Position 6 includes the posterior attachment of the rotator cuff to the humeral head near the "bare area."

As the arthroscope is maneuvered around posteriorly, an area is often noted between the cuff attachment and the articular cartilage of the humeral head. This "transition zone" between the articular cartilage and cuff attachment is normal and leads to the "bare area" posteriorly.

Position 6 includes the posterior aspect of the rotator cuff and its attachment adjacent to the "bare area" of the humeral head (Fig. 4-14). This position is located by following the insertion of the cuff along the anatomical neck of the humerus posteriorly and superiorly. The arthroscope is carefully withdrawn, keeping the cuff attachment in view. The bevel of the arthroscope is then rotated to the 1 o'clock position as the tip is moved posteriorly. Care must be taken not to withdraw the arthroscope completely from the joint, since there are only a few millimeters of space available in this location for viewing. The insertion of the rotator cuff in this posterior area frequently appears somewhat loose, with openings in the superficial layers. The fibers do not normally appear fragmented or detached, but often do not have the solid, confluent appearance of the more anterior/superior supraspinatus portion. There is seldom a rich synovial vascular supply noted in this area of the cuff.

The "bare area" of the humeral head is seen adjacent to the posterior lateral rotator cuff attachment. A normal bare area can encompass a few millimeters of humeral head or can be very extensive, measuring up to 2 to 3 cm in size. It is recognized by the absence of the normal glistening-white articular cartilage that covers the rest of the humeral head. The margin of the bare area is usually smooth as it blends with the articular cartilage more medially. Within this area there are frequently indentations, and sometimes fairly deep holes, which are thought to be vascular access channels into the bone. Sometimes these have a very rough appearance under the arthroscopic magnification. This bare area should not be mistaken for a post-dislocation osteochondral fracture known as the Hill-Sachs lesion, which is usually located in the otherwise normal articular cartilage of the humeral head more medially. Occasionally the two areas overlap.

Position 7 includes the rest of the articular surface of the humeral head that can be viewed from the posterior portal (Fig. 4-15). The arthroscope is maneuvered more medially from its position near the bare area, and its bevel is rotated both clockwise and counterclockwise to allow visualization of the horizon of the humeral globe. The shoulder is then rotated in various directions while the

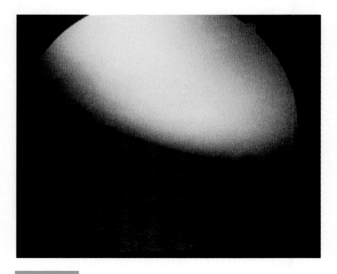

Figure 4-15
In position 7 the posterior and medial aspects of the globe of the humeral head are visualized.

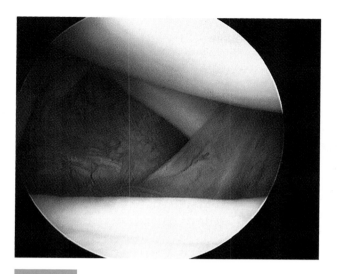

Figure 4-16
In position 8 the anterior superior labrum is visualized, along with the superior glenohumeral ligament, the subscapularis tendon, and the middle glenohumeral ligament.

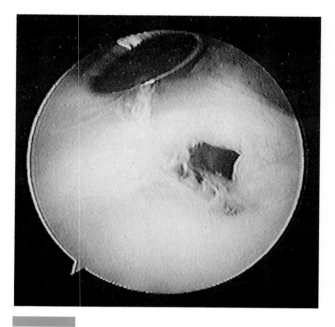

Figure 4-17
A sublabral hole is a normal variant beneath the anterior superior labrum seen in 11 percent of shoulders.

articular surface is viewed. An important area to evaluate is the central contact surface of the humeral head, which directly faces the glenoid. This is frequently the area where the articular cartilage first begins to break down in arthritis. Additionally, there can be early osteophytic formation inferiorly where the capsule-synovial reflection and humeral head unite.

Position 8 is the anterior superior triangle of the shoulder, including the anterior superior labrum, the superior glenohumeral ligament, the superior edge of the subscapularis tendon, and the middle glenohumeral ligament (Fig. 4-16). This position is visualized by placing the arthroscope on the glenoid surface and viewing just inferior to the biceps attachment. The anterior superior labrum is that portion below the biceps anchor and above the mid-glenoid notch. It is the most confusing area of the labrum and has several common normal variations that must be understood. In the most common situation, the anterior superior labrum attaches firmly to the glenoid rim (approximately 88 percent of cases).[1] There is seldom fraying or fragmentation in the normal situation. In approximately 11 percent of cases there is a normal opening

or sublabral foramen beneath the labral attachment (Fig. 4-17). The size of this hole can vary from a few millimeters to the size of the entire anterior superior quadrant. It is important to differentiate the normal sublabral hole from a Bankart-type traumatic labral detachment, a SLAP lesion[2] or an Andrews lesion.[3] The Bankart lesion must always occur below the anterior glenoid notch, but can extend more proximally. A SLAP lesion (injury to the superior labrum, from anterior to posterior) always includes the biceps anchor and extends posteriorly to it. With a SLAP lesion the tissues are frayed and fragmented; the traumatic or degenerative etiology should be obvious (see Chap. 10).

A very interesting and infrequent finding easily confused with a pathological anterior superior labral detachment is the so-called Buford complex.[4] This normal variant occurs in approximately 1.5 percent of shoulders. There are three factors included in the complex: (1) a thick cordlike middle glenohumeral ligament crosses the subscapularis tendon at a 45-degree angle; (2) the middle glenohumeral ligament attaches to the superior labrum just anterior to the base of the biceps anchor; and

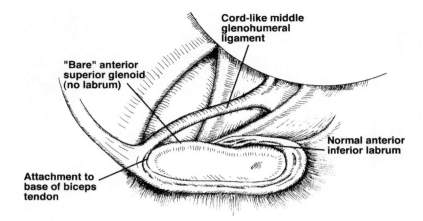

"Bare" anterior superior glenoid (no labrum)

Cord-like middle glenohumeral ligament

Normal anterior inferior labrum

Attachment to base of biceps tendon

Figure 4-18
The Buford complex is a rare but important anatomical formation to recognize in position 8. It is often mistaken for a pathological labral detachment.

(3) there is *no* labral tissue on the anterior superior labral edge. (See Fig. 4-18.) The appearance of this complex, at first glance, is quite striking, since there *appears* to be an avulsion of the anterior superior labrum and/or the middle glenohumeral ligament. On further inspection it is recognized that there is no significant fraying of the tissues and that the edges of the cordlike middle ligament are smooth and rolled. The Buford complex actually appears to give a hammock-like support to the anterior superior portion of the joint, and is seldom found in association with clinical instability (Fig. 4-19).

The superior glenohumeral ligament can of-

ten be seen in position 8 (Fig. 4-20). It usually appears as a small fold in the capsule located anterior and inferior to the biceps tendon. Its course parallels that of the biceps tendon, extending from the superior glenoid tubercle area to attach to the upper portion of the lesser tuberosity. Often the superior glenohumeral ligament has a common insertion with the most superior edge of the subscapularis tendon.

The subscapularis tendon is a very prominent landmark demarcating the inferior boundary of the anterior superior triangle. In most situations it has a rolled tendinous edge

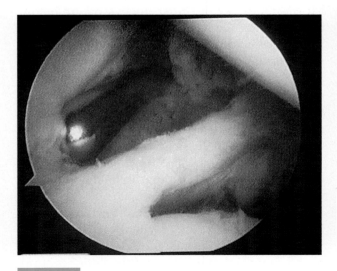

Figure 4-19
With the Buford complex the cordlike middle ligament attaches near the biceps tendon, with no superior labral tissue present on the anterior superior glenoid.

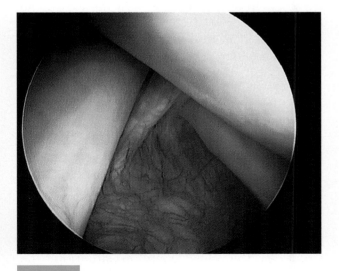

Figure 4-20
The superior glenohumeral ligament is seen as a thickening in the capsule just anterior to the biceps tendon, passing from the superior glenoid to the area of the lesser tuberosity near the subscapularis insertion.

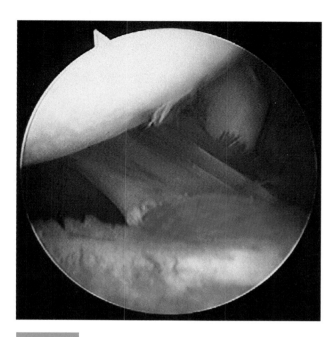

Figure 4-21
A cordlike middle glenohumeral ligament has an opening above and below into the subscapularis recess.

and passes vertically from its humeral head attachment, at the lesser tuberosity, to disappear below the glenoid rim. The middle glenohumeral ligament in the usual situation crosses between the midpoint and the lower third of the subscapularis tendon at an angle of approximately 45 degrees. There are several variations in the subscapularis tendon. The leading edge of the tendon may have a split appearance. This situation is rare; when it does occur, it appears as a smooth split in the tendon with no obvious fragmentation or synovial reaction around the tissues. In addition, there is no detachment of the tendon insertion. This situation is found in fewer than 0.5 percent of shoulders examined arthroscopically.

The middle glenohumeral ligament has the most variable appearance of all the anterior shoulder ligaments.[1] In the usual situation (approximately 66 percent of cases) it appears as a folded thickening in the anterior capsule that crosses the subscapularis tendon at a 45-degree angle to insert on the anterior superior neck of the glenoid on, or just medial to, the labrum. In this situation there is only one

opening into the subscapularis recess located superior to the leading edge of the middle ligament.

The most common variation in the middle ligament anatomy is the cordlike appearance (Fig. 4-21). As mentioned above, this variation is noted in approximately 19 percent of all shoulders. With a cordlike middle ligament, the appearance is of a smooth, cordlike structure rather than of a sheet of ligamentous tissue, as is seen more often. The cord may attach to the normal position of the middle ligament at the neck of the glenoid superiorly, or it may attach to the anterior superior labrum in association with the sublabral hole (Fig. 4-22). In either of these normal situations, access to the subscapularis recess is possible either above or below the cord.

A third variation of the middle ligament is that of a very attenuated appearance, or "thin veil," of ligament (Fig. 4-23). This is present in approximately 5 percent of shoulders. The middle ligament structure appears as a translucent fibrous sheet or a few flimsy fibrous bands. When present, this variation is usually accompanied by a very hypertrophic inferior glenohumeral ligament, which seems to be a compensatory mechanism. A final normal variant is the complete absence of the middle ligament, noted in approximately 1 percent of shoulders (Fig. 4-24). This situation is seen as a normal variant in patients

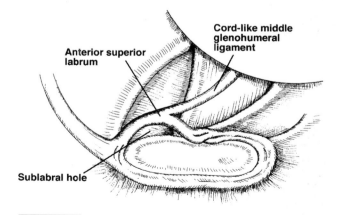

Figure 4-22
The cordlike middle glenohumeral ligament may attach to the superior labrum, often with an underlying sublabral hole.

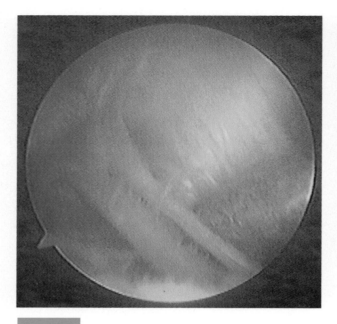

Figure 4-23
Sometimes the middle glenohumeral ligament appears as a "thin veil."

with a congenitally lax anterior capsule and may predispose them to recurrent atraumatic subluxation.

Position 9 includes the anterior inferior labrum (Fig. 4-25). By retracting the arthro-

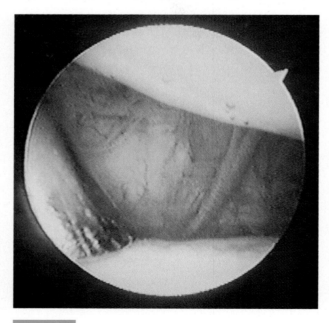

Figure 4-24
In 1 percent of patients the middle glenohumeral ligament is completely absent.

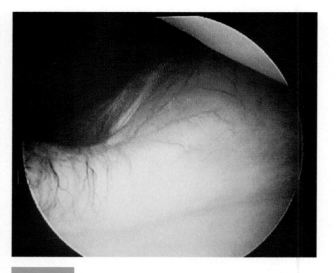

Figure 4-25
In position 9 the anterior middle and inferior labrum are seen. Most often the labrum attaches at the edge and blends with the articular cartilage.

scope to the level of the glenoid and rotating the bevel to the 3 o'clock position and viewing inferiorly, the entire anterior inferior labral attachment can be seen. There are two normal patterns of anterior labral attachments. In more than 90 percent of cases the labrum has a smooth attachment to the neck of the glenoid at the edge of the articular cartilage. This occurs from the mid-glenoid notch around the entire anterior and inferior portions of the glenoid. The second type of labral attachment is a "meniscoid type," in which the leading edge of the labrum is separated from the glenoid. In this type (approximately 10 percent of shoulders), a probe can be inserted between the articular surface of the glenoid and the overlying labrum. The capsular attachment to the labrum is still intact and will not separate from the glenoid when traction is applied. At the mid-glenoid notch there is frequently a tuft of synovium that overhangs the labrum. This synovial overgrowth can be quite prominent and can resemble fraying, but is normal (Fig. 4-26).

Position 10 includes the inferior glenohumeral ligament and anterior inferior capsule (Fig. 4-27). The tautness of these structures can be appreciated when the arthroscope is passed between the humeral

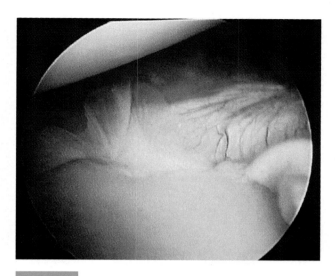

Figure 4-26
There is often a small feathery-appearing normal area of synovial overgrowth on the labrum near the anterior mid-glenoid notch.

head and the glenoid. Normally, with the arm in traction, the arthroscope can be maneuvered into the anterior recess with relative ease. If the ligaments are overly loose, it passes without any difficulty. Conversely, if

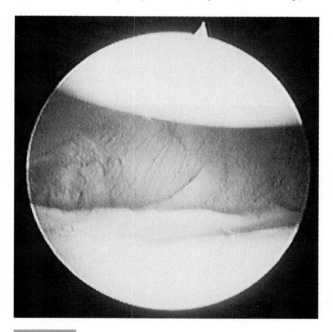

Figure 4-27
The anterior inferior capsule is visualized in position 10 by passing the arthroscope across the joint and viewing anteriorly past the labrum. In tight shoulders this may be difficult to see.

the ligaments are overly tight, as in adhesive capsulitis, the space between the head and glenoid is constricted, and the arthroscope passes with difficulty or not at all. The anterior capsular ligaments insert into the labrum and are firmly attached with it to the neck of the glenoid. The usually prominent superior band of the inferior ligament marks the uppermost extent and can attach as high as the anterior superior labrum. Except at the fold of the superior band of the inferior ligament, the capsular tissues are smooth and covered with thin synovial investment.

This completes the first 10 steps of the arthroscopic anatomy review, all of which have been performed through the posterior portal. Now the arthroscope is removed from the joint and inserted into the anterior cannula to complete the anatomy review of the glenohumeral joint. The outflow tubing is connected to the posterior cannula, and the pump activated (Fig. 4-28).

Position 11 includes visualization of the posterior labrum and the posterior capsule, looking across the joint from anterior to posterior (Fig. 4-29). The arthroscope is placed approximately in the center of the glenoid, and the posteriorly placed cannula is noted.

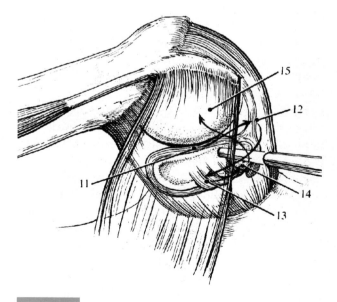

Figure 4-28
The five points of glenohumeral anatomy are visualized from the anterior portal (positions 11 through 15).

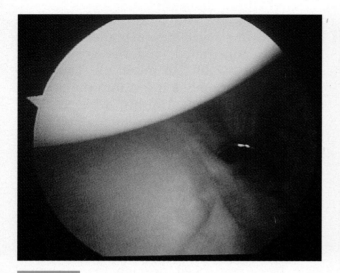

Figure 4-29
In position 11 the posterior labrum and posterior capsule are visualized.

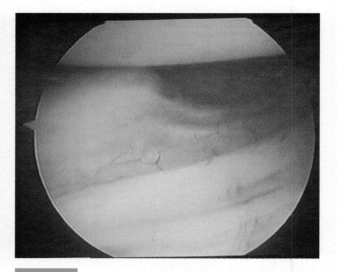

Figure 4-30
Sometimes the posterior band of the inferior capsular ligament can be seen.

The bevel of the arthroscope is rotated inferiorly, and the attachment of the posterior labrum and ligaments to the glenoid is visualized. The most common type of attachment of the posterior labrum is directly to the glenoid rim, with no separation between its attachment and articular cartilage. In a small percentage of shoulders (fewer than 5 percent) the normal posterior labrum is meniscoid in appearance. This finding should be suspected when a lip of labral material is seen overhanging the glenoid rim. Beneath the meniscoid-like labrum the articular cartilage should appear smooth, but sometimes it is thin. The labral edge should be firmly attached at the periphery. The attached posterior capsule ligamentous tissue is usually quite smooth except for the presence of a thickening, termed a *posterior band* of the inferior capsular ligament. This fold, when present, attaches to the midportion of the posterior labrum, and extends inferiorly and laterally at an angle of approximately 45 degrees (Fig. 4-30). This corresponds to the superior band of the anterior inferior glenohumeral ligament, mentioned above. There is a posterior capsular recess that cannot be well visualized from the anterior portal but has been noted previously from the posterior portal.

Position 12 includes the posterior superior capsule and the posterior aspect of the rotator cuff (Fig. 4-31). This area is visualized by noting again the position of the posterior cannula and then rotating the arthroscope bevel superiorly and retracting the arthroscope. The posterior cuff can be seen and palpated using the posterior cannula. The arthroscope can be retracted further so that the biceps tendon passes in front of it, and then the entire posterior and superior aspect of the rotator cuff

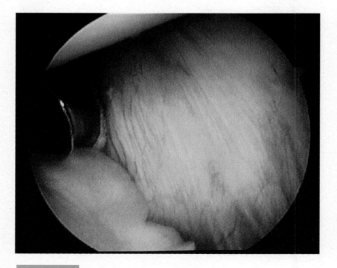

Figure 4-31
In position 12 the posterior aspect of the rotator cuff is visualized.

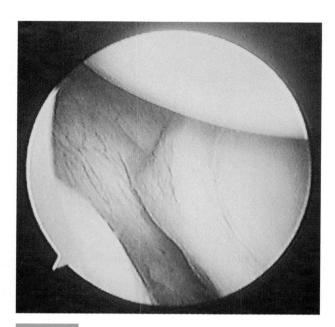

Figure 4-32
In position 13 the anterior labrum and the entire attachment of the inferior ligament, including the superior band, are visualized.

can be noted. The normal surface of the rotator cuff seen in this position is smooth; the vascularity should be regular. The arthroscope is then maneuvered around the superior part of the glenoid, past the root of the biceps tendon, and back into the glenoid fossa, and rotated anteriorly to visualize position 13.

Position 13 includes the anterior labrum and the attached anterior inferior ligament, particularly the superior band (Fig. 4-32). *Position 13 is the most important position in a surgeon's precise evaluation of the status and quality of the supporting ligamentous, labral, and capsular tissue for questions of instability.* When viewing from this position, the labrum can be palpated with a probe passed through a posterior portal, and any detachment can be demonstrated. The arm can be rotated internally and externally while noting the quality and security of the attachment of the ligamentous tissues and labrum. The important superior band of the inferior ligament appears as a thickened fold blending with the inferior capsular pouch distally and culminating in a thick band that attaches to

the labrum near, or slightly above, the mid-glenoid notch.

By internally rotating the arm, the anterior inferior ligament is seen to fold against the neck of the glenoid. External rotation causes the normal ligament to tighten up and stresses the labral attachment, which should remain snugly against the bone. On rare occasions, in the normal situation, a defined superior band is not visualized. This can occur in an atraumatic setting where the capsular ligaments are fused into a single solid sheet. Although it does not prove that instability is present, it seems to be associated with congenital laxity and may be a predisposing factor of atraumatic instability.

Position 14 is located by retracting the arthroscope further and rotating the tip anteriorly until the subscapularis tendon is found (Fig. 4-33). In this position the leading edge of the subscapularis tendon and the subscapularis recess, along with the middle glenoid humeral ligament, are seen. The arthroscope is then maneuvered into the subscapularis recess and rotated both anteriorly and posteriorly. The recess is variable in size but most of-

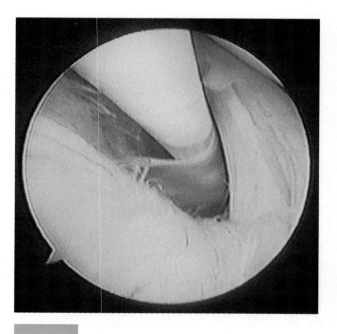

Figure 4-33
The subscapularis recess is evaluated in position 14. The arthroscope should be rotated 360 degrees to look for loose bodies.

ten can be entered and followed deep across the anterior aspect of the glenoid neck. Loose bodies, if present in the shoulder, most often are located in the subscapularis recess. Once the tip of the arthroscope is located within the recess it should be rotated 360 degrees to visualize the entire contents. The tip of the arthroscope is then oriented so that the leading edge of the subscapularis tendon is in view. This is followed back out to the middle glenohumeral ligament, which crosses the subscapularis tendon. The attachment of the middle ligament, either on the labrum or on the neck of the glenoid, is noted. Most commonly this attachment is a few millimeters below the glenoid margin, but it may be at the labrum proper, in the anterior superior quadrant.

Position 15 includes the attachment of the subscapularis tendon to the humeral head, the cartilage of the anterior surface of the humeral head, and the adjacent biceps tendon (Fig. 4-34). The tip of the arthroscope follows the leading edge of the subscapularis tendon up to its attachment into the humerus, at the lesser tuberosity. The superior glenohumeral ligament inserts into this area as well; often

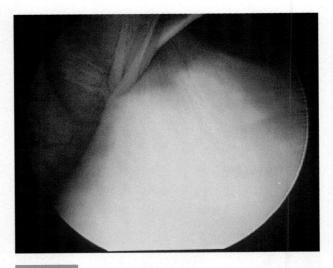

Figure 4-35
The anterior surface of the biceps tendon can be followed with the tip of the arthroscope out through the biceps tunnel.

there is a little irregularity of the synovium. The articular surface of the humeral head is then visualized anteriorly. Sometimes there is a normal "bare area" anteriorly as well. This appears as a thin area of anterior humeral head, devoid of articular cartilage, located superior to the attachment of the subscapularis tendon. This area should not be confused with an anterior humeral head defect found in conjunction with posterior instability. The arthroscope is rotated in a superior direction until the leading edge of the biceps tendon is encountered. After retracting the arthroscope a few millimeters and placing it directly on the biceps tendon, the surgeon can maneuver the scope along the surface of the tendon to a position just inside the biceps groove (Fig. 4-35). By rotating the arm, the stability of the biceps tendon and the quality of the investing synovium can be evaluated. Once this is completed, the arthroscopic cannula is positioned back into the joint; the arthroscopic surgical procedure can now proceed if it is needed.

References

1. Morgan C, Rames RD, Snyder SJ: Anatomical variations of the glenohumeral ligaments.

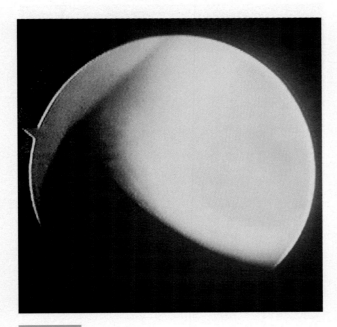

Figure 4-34
In position 15 the subscapularis tendon is seen attaching to the anterior surface of the humeral head.

Presented at the Annual Meeting of the American Academy of Orthopaedic Surgeons, Anaheim, CA, 1991.

2. Snyder SJ, Karzel RP, Del Pizzo W, et al: SLAP lesions of the shoulder. *Arthroscopy* 6:724, 1990.

3. Andrews JR, Carson WG Jr, McLeod WD: Glenoid labrum tears related to the long head of the biceps. *Am J Sports Med* 13:337, 1985.

4. Snyder SJ, Buford D, Wuh HCK: The Buford complex—the loose anterior superior labrum—middle glenohumeral ligament complex: A normal anatomical variant. Presented at the Annual Meeting of the American Academy of Orthopaedic Surgeons, Boston, MA, 1992

5

Diagnostic Bursoscopy with a Review of Normal Bursal Anatomy

Introduction

Like arthroscopy of the glenohumeral joint, bursoscopy, or endoscopy of the subacromial bursal space, requires a specialized technique for inserting the arthroscope into the appropriate location and recognizing the normal anatomy as well as common variations. This should be done in a simple, organized, and reproducible manner, with a minimum of iatrogenic tissue trauma. In addition, permanent records, both written and video-recorded, are important for documentation and review by the surgeon and also as a supplement to the medical record, for medical legal concerns.

Diagnostic Bursoscopy: Bursal Entry Technique

One of the most important maneuvers to master in shoulder arthroscopy is the technique for entering the subacromial bursa in an atraumatic manner so that the anatomy can be evaluated prior to any shaving. The subacromial bursa is a true and distinct space and is always present (Fig. 5-1). The anatomy of the bursa must be precisely understood in order for the surgeon to consistently and accurately gain entry into it. The bursa is an "anterior subacromial structure." Superiorly, the bursa covers, and is tightly adherent to, the periosteum and the coracoacromial ligament on the undersurface of the acromion. Inferiorly, the bursa covers the superior aspect of the rotator cuff tendon, the tuberosity of the humerus, and the rotator interval area. It is important to understand this anatomy when entering the bursa, since tunneling above or below this layer will result in arthroscopic placement outside the true bursal cavity. The posterior wall, or "posterior bursal curtain," is usually located beneath the midpoint of the acromion, approximately in line with the posterior edge of the AC joint. The bursa extends well anterior to the edge of the acromion beneath the deltoid and the coracoid processes. Its medial extent is near the undersurface of the AC joint. The lateral re-

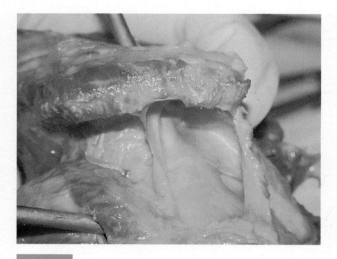

Figure 5-1
In this cadaver dissection the location of the subacromial bursa is seen. The posterior bursal curtain lies just below the midpoint of the acromion.

cess usually passes 7 to 8 cm lateral to the edge of the acromion. Frequently there is a fold of bursal tissue near the lateral acromial edge that separates the subacromial from the subdeltoid areas of the bursal cavity. This fold is usually incomplete; hence the arthroscopic designation of the "lateral subdeltoid bursal shelf." Occasionally the fold is complete and fuses with the bursal layer on the superior aspect of the rotator cuff tendon. In this situation, two separate bursal spaces are formed and do not interconnect. In order to evaluate

the subdeltoid portion of the space, it may be necessary to open the lateral shelf with an arthroscopic shaver.

Bursal Entry Technique

The technique used at SCOI to allow accurate, consistent bursal entry for evaluation of the subacromial space was developed only after considerable trial and error. Careful anatomical dissections in the cadaver lab helped to provide an understanding of the peculiar relationship of the bursal tissue to the surrounding structures.

Patient Positioning

The patient's body is maintained in the same position as used for glenohumeral arthroscopy; that is, in a lateral decubitus position, tilted 10 to 15 degrees posteriorly. The arm position is changed to approximately 10 to 15 degrees of abduction and a few degrees of forward flexion. This is accomplished either by turning the arm of the traction apparatus 180 degrees and lowering it an appropriate amount or, on some devices, by shortening the lever arm and changing the angle for less abduction. The traction weight used during bursoscopy averages 15 lb; it may be increased or decreased a few pounds if the arm is excessively over- or undersized. No draping changes are necessary for bursoscopy (Fig. 5-2).

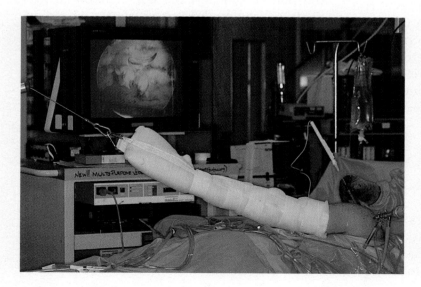

Figure 5-2
The arm is positioned in approximately 10 to 15 degrees of abduction, and a few degrees of forward flexion, for bursoscopy.

Subacromial Bursal Entry Technique

The technique for entering the subacromial bursa follows a five-step sequence to ensure proper instrument placement (Fig. 5-3):

1. The arthroscopic cannula, with a blunt-tipped obturator, is inserted through the posterior skin portal previously created for glenohumeral joint arthroscopy. The cannula is tunneled through the subcutaneous tissue until the posterior edge of the acromion is palpated.

2. The cannula is then redirected so that it passes through the deltoid muscle to palpate the posterior aspect of the humeral head.

3. The cannula is redirected again, to pass through the posterior bursal curtain at a midpoint between the undersurface of the acromion and the superior surface of the cuff. Usually a distinct "pop" can be felt as the posterior bursal curtain is penetrated at about the level of the midpoint of the subacromial space.

4. The cannula is then advanced to the anterior limit of the bursa, angling slightly inferiorly, and the obturator is removed. A tapered-tip guide rod is inserted through the cannula and passed out through the anterior bursal wall. It passes through the deltoid and out through the original anterior skin portal. It is helpful to try to avoid penetrating the coracoacromial ligament during this maneuver, because penetration of the ligament will limit the mobility of the scope and cannula in the anterior portal.

5. A second arthroscopic cannula is placed over the guide rod and gently worked through the anterior portal and deltoid muscle into the bursal space.

The final position of the two cannulae should be noted prior to removal of the guide rod. The tips of both cannulae should be located beneath the anterior *one-fifth* of the subacromial area. In this position the posterior cannula will probably be inserted to more than two-thirds of its length, and the anterior cannula to less than one-fourth of its length (Fig. 5-4). The assistant holds the anterior cannula while the guide rod is removed, to prevent it from backing out. The outflow drain is connected to the anterior cannula, if a pump is used, or to the inflow irrigation system, if a gravity inflow system is used. The arthroscope is inserted into the posterior cannula, and the pump activated to fill the bursa with fluid. Often it is helpful to pinch off the outflow for a few seconds to distend the bursal space. Immediately after inserting the arthroscope, the surgeon must determine if the arthroscope and anterior cannula are within the true bursal space. This will be obvious as the normal bursal cavity distends freely when

Figure 5-3

Entering the subacromial bursal space without tunneling above or below the bursal wall can usually be accomplished by following the five-step bursal entry technique (see text).

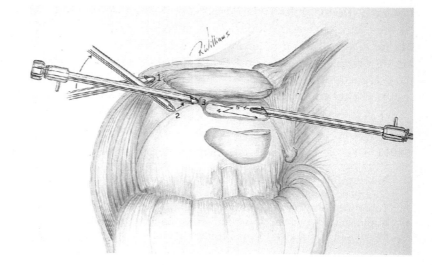

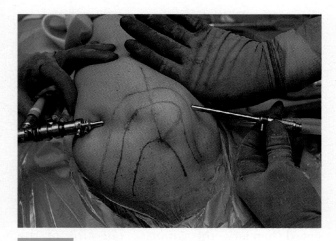

Figure 5-4
When both cannulae are properly positioned, the posterior cannula is inserted well past the midpoint of the undersurface of the acromion. The light from the arthroscope will transilluminate the fluid-filled bursa.

the inflow of fluid is begun. If a bursal walled cavity, or "room with a view," is not noted immediately, then the fluid flow should be discontinued and the five steps in the bursal entry repeated. If after two attempts a successful bursal placement is not achieved, a shaver can be used, via the anterior portal, to remove the obstructing bursal tissues.

Before any shaving commences, the surgeon must ascertain that the arthroscope and the shaver are in the general vicinity of the bursa and not mispositioned either too far laterally beneath the deltoid muscle, too far posteriorly behind the bursa, or too far medially beneath the clavicle. By shaving the obscuring tissues in the wrong location a surgeon can create a false bursal space, which may lead to an incorrect diagnosis and inappropriate surgical treatment.

Once the anterior and posterior portals are

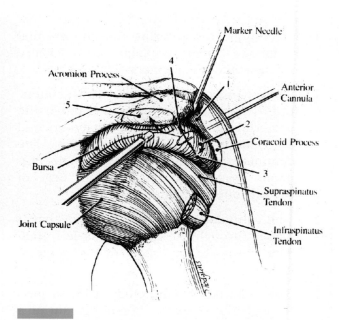

Figure 5-5
The bursal anatomy review begins with the arthroscope in the posterior portal, looking at five distinct anatomical features (see Table 5-1).

satisfactorily developed, a systematic anatomical review of the bursal contents is begun from the posterior portal (see Table 5-1 and Fig. 5-5).

For the entire evaluation and surgical procedure performed in the bursa, the video camera is oriented so that the acromion is located on the superior aspect of the video screen, and the rotator cuff on the inferior aspect. This position is one of convenience and convention; it is not anatomically correct relative to the patient's position on the table. The anatomy review is begun from the posterior portal.

Position 1 includes the inferior surface of the anterior acromion and coracoacromial lig-

---

TABLE 5-1   First Part of Bursal Anatomy Review—From Posterior Portal

1. Anterior/inferior aspect of acromion and coracoacromial ligament
2. Lateral acromial edge and subdeltoid bursal shelf
3. Tuberosity insertion of rotator cuff
4. Impingement area of rotator cuff (supraspinatus tendon)
5. Musculotendinous junction of rotator cuff and fat pad beneath AC joint

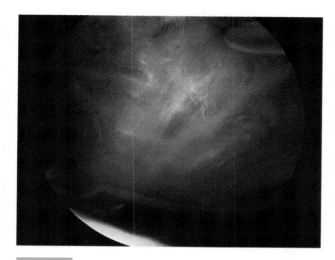

Figure 5-6
In position 1 the anterior undersurface of the acromion and the coracoacromial ligament are evaluated.

ament, as well as the anterior bursal wall (Fig. 5-6). To visualize this position the arthroscope is rotated with the bevel oriented superiorly, so that the glistening bursal covering of the acromial bone and the coracoacromial lig-

ament can be appreciated. The ligament appears as a thick fibrous band beneath the acromion, extending in an anterior and medial direction. The anterior edge of the acromion cannot be readily appreciated when the ligament is intact. Although the thickness and mass of the ligament may vary, there is never fraying or fragmentation of ligament fibers in the normal condition.

Position 2 includes the lateral acromial edge and the lateral subdeltoid bursal shelf (Fig. 5-7). The arthroscope is retracted slightly and rotated laterally to evaluate these structures. Sometimes the shelf is thickened or completely closed, obscuring the subdeltoid portion of the bursal cavity. Most often the shelf appears as a thin band of bursal tissue crossing from anterior to posterior, attached to the roof of the bursal space near the lateral border of the acromion. The remainder of the bursa should be smooth, with a regular vascular pattern.

Position 3 includes the greater tuberosity of the humerus and the insertion of the rotator cuff in that area (Fig. 5-8). This position is viewed by moving the arthroscope beneath the lateral bursal shelf and rotating the bevel to look directly at the humerus. The arm can then be rotated into internal and external ro-

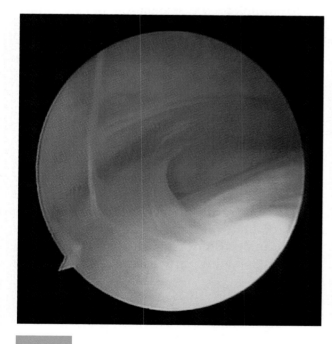

Figure 5-7
In position 2 the lateral edge of the acromion and the lateral subdeltoid bursal shelf are seen.

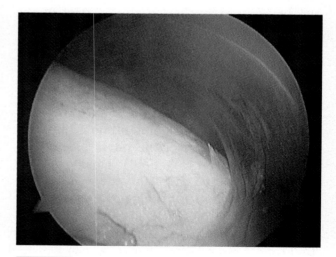

Figure 5-8
In position 3 the bursal covering of the greater tuberosity is seen, often with yellow deposits of adipose tissue and a fine vascular pattern.

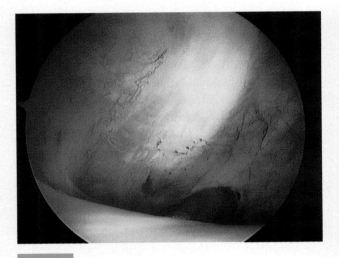

Figure 5-9
The critical zone of the rotator cuff is seen in position 4.
Calcium deposits, impingement, fraying, and early
rotator cuff failure are often seen in this area. The
lateral edge of the acromion is located just above.

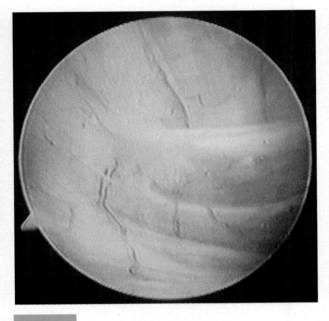

Figure 5-10
In position 5 the medial wall of the bursa is seen
beneath the AC joint.

tation to aid complete visualization. Sometimes small areas of fat and veins are noted
overlying the tuberosity in the synovial floor.

Position 4 includes the impingement area of
the rotator cuff, especially the supraspinatus
tendon and "critical zone" (Fig. 5-9). This position is viewed by moving the tip of the
arthroscope in a medial direction, medial to
the lateral subdeltoid bursal shelf, and turning
the bevel to view the superior aspect of the
cuff. The arm can be slowly rotated internally
and externally to achieve a complete view of
this area. The normal appearance of the rotator cuff is smooth, with no signs of inflammation or fiber fragmentation.

Position 5 is the medial aspect of the rotator cuff near the musculotendinous junction
and the medial wall of the bursa located beneath the AC joint (Fig. 5-10). This position is
viewed by rotating the arthroscope bevel medially. The smooth bursal appearance cover-

ing these tissues should be seen. Seldom is a
normal AC joint visible without removal of
bursal and capsular tissue.

To complete the evaluation of the bursal
anatomy, the arthroscope is changed to the
anterior portal and the posterior cannula connected to gravity drainage. (If a pump is not
used, an inflow system is connected to the
posterior cannula.) With the bursa redis-
tended, the anatomy review is completed (see
Table 5-2 and Fig. 5-11).

Position 6 includes the posterior aspect of
the acromion and posterior bursal curtain
(Fig. 5-12). To evaluate this area, locate the
cannula entering through the posterior bursal
curtain and turn the bevel of the arthroscope
upward. Like the anterior subacromial area,
the normal posterior inferior acromion has a
smooth glistening surface. The posterior bur-

TABLE 5-2   Second Part of Bursal Anatomy Review—From Anterior Portal

6. Posterior aspect of inferior acromion and posterior bursal curtain
7. Posterior aspect of rotator cuff
8. Rotator interval area covering biceps tendon and leading edge of subscapularis tendon

Figure 5-11
The last three areas of bursal anatomy are reviewed while viewing from the anterior portal (see Table 5-2).

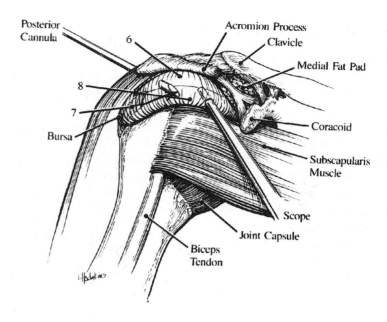

sal curtain attaches to the acromion above and to the cuff below. The posterior edge of the lateral subacromial bursal shelf attaches to the posterior bursal curtain.

Position 7 includes the posterior aspect of the rotator cuff that is located within the bursal cavity, including the leading edge of the infraspinatus and the posterior part of the supraspinatus tendon (Fig. 5-13). To view this

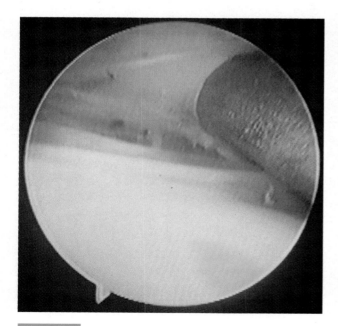

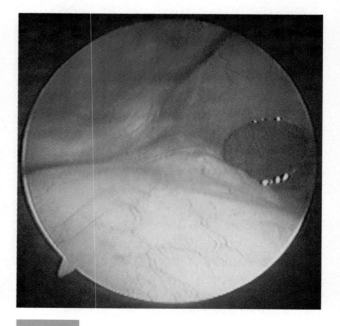

Figure 5-12
In position 6 the posterior bursal curtain is seen, with the posterior cannula penetrating it.

Figure 5-13
In position 7 the posterior aspect of the rotator cuff, and particularly the infraspinatus muscle insertion into the posterior cuff, can be seen.

area the arthroscope is retracted more anteriorly and the bevel rotated laterally. It is important to view the superior aspect of the cuff first and *then* pivot the arthroscope to allow visualization of the more lateral structures near the tuberosity attachment. The normal cuff surface appears smooth but with some small rugal-like folds, sometimes having small fatty deposits just beneath the synovial layer.

Position 8 includes the anterior structures of the bursa, located in the area of the rotator interval (Fig. 5-14). Beneath this area the biceps tendon, the coracohumeral ligament, the rotator cuff ridge, and the leading edge of the subscapularis tendon are located. The tip of the arthroscope is maneuvered around the front edge of the bursal space and rotated back and forth to visualize this area. (If the arthroscope has been placed through the coracoacromial ligament, it is difficult to perform this maneuver.) There are seldom any landmarks to identify this area in the normal situation. Palpation with a probe placed through the posterior or lateral portal can demonstrate the biceps tendon and, possibly, a thick rotator cuff ridge. Otherwise, the normal appearance of this area is smooth and relatively flat. A suture marker (see Chap. 11) placed in the rotator interval when viewing intra-articularly is a useful guide for orientation.

Several other areas are important in a thorough evaluation of the subacromial space. The anterior aspect of the bursal space may be closed off with an anterior curtain, or may be open, allowing visualization down the front of the shoulder to the lesser tuberosity. If it is necessary to view this area when the bursal space is closed, then shaving the anterior bursal tissue while following the coracoacromial ligament to the tip of the coracoid will allow a clear evaluation. Once this area is exposed, the biceps tendon, the lesser tuberosity, and the conjoined tendon, as well as the tip of the coracoid, may be seen.

The arch of the coracoid can also be followed by viewing with the arthroscope in the lateral portal. This may require shaving more

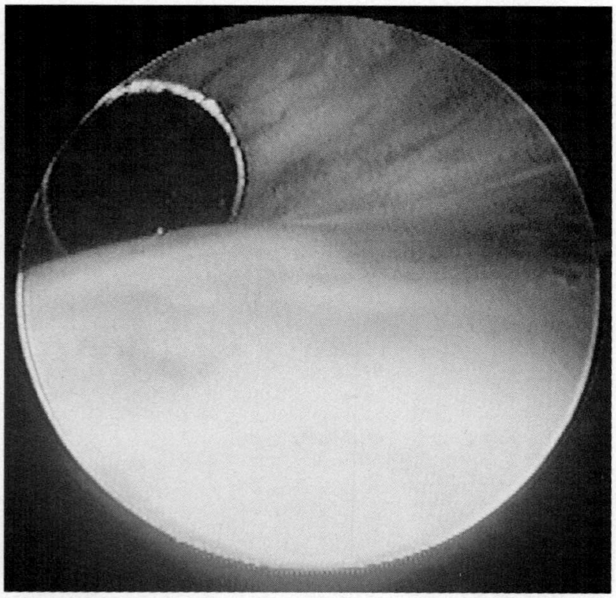

Figure 5-14
In position 8 the anterior bursal cavity is noted, including the area of the rotator interval and the leading edge of the subscapularis tendon. The erythematous area was found to be the biceps tunnel by passing a marker suture through a needle and viewing inside the glenohumeral joint.

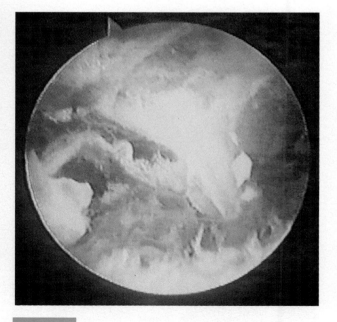

Figure 5-15
The spine of the scapula can be seen while viewing from the lateral portal once the medial bursal wall has been removed.

of the bursa, with the shaver entering through the anterior portal. The shaver and arthroscope progress along the arch of the coracoid from anterior to posterior, following from the tip to the base. The coracohumeral ligament and coracoclavicular ligaments may be evaluated with this maneuver. Additionally, if the coracoclavicular ligaments have been torn, the base of the coracoid can be located and debrided for refixation of the AC joint (see Chap. 9).

The posterior subacromial area is frequently considered to be outside the bursal cavity. If necessary, this area may be exposed by removing the posterior bursal curtain, with the shaver in the lateral portal and the arthroscope in the anterior portal. The undersurface of the posterior acromion can be evaluated, as well as the underside of the deltoid and the superior portion of the musculotendinous junction of the posterior rotator cuff mechanism.

The supraspinatus fossa can also be seen arthroscopically while working in the subacromial area. By following the superior aspect of the supraspinatus tendon of the rotator cuff medially to the musculotendinous junction, the spine of the scapula can be found (Fig. 5-15). By shaving some of the bursal wall in this area, the muscle belly can be followed into the supraspinatus fossa. This exposure may be needed for removing cysts, foreign bodies, etc. The neurovascular structures are avoided by remaining above the muscle.

Once the bursal anatomy review has been completed, a surgical procedure—either arthroscopic or open—may begin.

6

Arthroscopic Removal of Loose Bodies and Implants

Introduction

Loose bodies in the glenohumeral joint may often cause clinical symptoms. Mechanical symptoms, such as catching, locking, popping, and slipping of the joint, are the most obvious clinical manifestations of loose bodies. Symptoms such as aching, grinding, and irritation of the joint are also common. Not all loose bodies cause symptoms; but when an intra-articular loose body is suspected or diagnosed, and mechanical or inflammatory symptoms persist despite reasonable conservative care, arthroscopic removal of the loose body is prudent.

Diagnosis of Glenohumeral Loose Bodies

When a symptomatic loose body is present in the glenohumeral joint, the history and physical examination usually relate to the intermittent mechanical catching in the joint, or to the chronic inflammatory changes caused by the free-floating or tethered structure. There may have been a previous injury, such as a compression injury caused by a fall, or a dislocation. Either of these mechanisms can cause labral or osteocartilaginous free fragments, which, when nourished by the synovial fluid, can grow in size.

Previous surgical procedures—especially with implantation of metallic or plastic devices, including staples, screws, suture anchors, or wires—may also be responsible for the loose body (Figs. 6-1 through 6-4). Silicone or rubber parts from the diaphragm of the operating cannula, or insulation for electrode tips, may dislodge during surgery (Fig. 6-5). Penetrating injuries caused by bullet wounds or by knife or glass punctures, or other post-traumatic debris, may be the cause. A final, very dramatic, source of loose bodies is seen in cases of synovial inflammatory disease. Synovial osteochondromatosis or rheumatoid-type inflammatory arthritis can cause multiple cartilaginous or osteocartilaginous loose bodies.

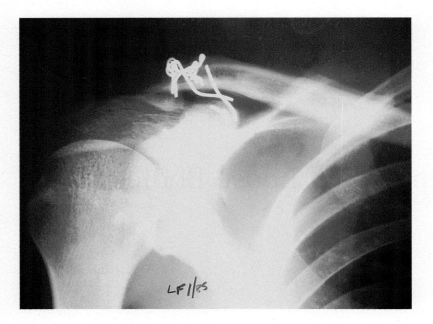

Figure 6-1
AP x-ray showing a wire fragment, apparently in the glenohumeral joint, from a previous AC joint reconstruction.

Radiologic Imaging Evaluation

In many cases the initial x-rays are all that is necessary to demonstrate loose bodies in the glenohumeral joint. It is important to have a complete x-ray profile of the joint, including AP, axillary, and supraspinatus outlet views. If the loose body is calcified or metallic it may be easily seen on standard radiographs, and its location determined by careful review of the standard views (Figs. 6-1 and 6-2). Sometimes additional exposures, such as internal and external rotation views and biceps tendon groove views, are helpful for precise

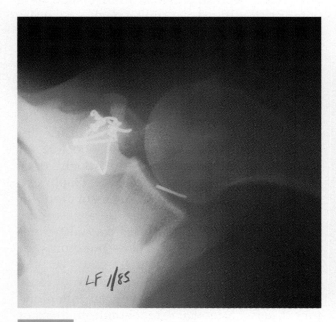

Figure 6-2
The axillary x-ray demonstrates conclusively that the fragment is within the glenohumeral joint.

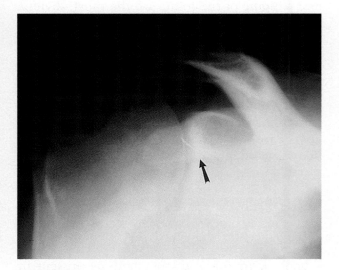

Figure 6-3
An AP x-ray demonstrates two small surgical needles in the shoulder, lost during a previous rotator cuff repair.

Figure 6-4
An axillary view demonstrates that one of the needles is most likely located in the anterior shoulder, and possibly in the subscapularis recess.

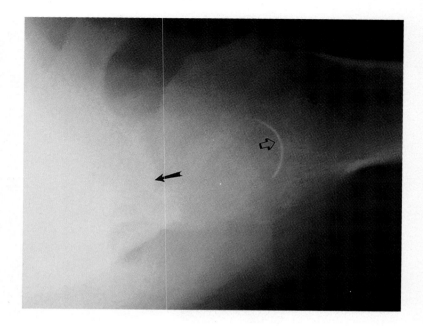

localization. Often it is impossible to be certain that an apparent loose body seen on an x-ray is truly within the glenohumeral joint; additional studies may be needed to confirm the intra-articular location. MRI scans are frequently helpful, since the multiplanar sequencing can give the precise localization of a loose body, and especially its relation to the surrounding soft tissues. For non-opaque loose bodies, the use of a contrast material such as gadolinium, or, infrequently, a standard arthrogram with CT, may give the final proof of the intra-articular location (Fig. 6-6). Sometimes, however, despite all imaging attempts, the exact location cannot be precisely determined, and direct arthroscopic visualization is necessary to confirm the diagnosis.

Arthroscopic Evaluation

The standard 15-point glenohumeral evaluation should be used in all arthroscopic procedures. It is especially important to understand and evaluate each anatomical location when a loose body is suspected. Having the inflow and outflow system functioning at all times is also very important. A free-floating loose body may evade arthroscopic visualization unless it is attracted toward an outflow suction source. From the posterior portal loose bodies may be noted infrequently in the posterior capsular recess and, more frequently, in the inferior axillary pouch. Sometimes a loose body may have a thin pedicle stalk tethering it in this location (Fig. 6-7). In that situation it functions as a loose body but is not completely free-

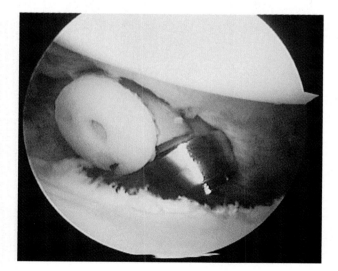

Figure 6-5
The silicone diaphragm from the plastic operating cannula has dislodged and caused a free-floating loose body.

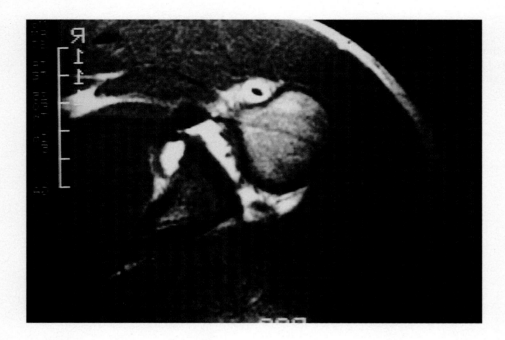

Figure 6-6
An MRI scan with gadolinium enhancement is helpful to demonstrate nonmetallic, non-opaque loose bodies in the posterior shoulder recess.

floating, and, hence, must be visually located, since it will not be attracted toward an outflow drainage cannula.

The most important location for loose bodies is the subscapularis recess. It is, therefore, extremely important to evaluate this area carefully with the arthroscope in the anterior portal. Position 14 in the standard glenohumeral evaluation includes insertion of the arthroscope into the subscapularis recess,

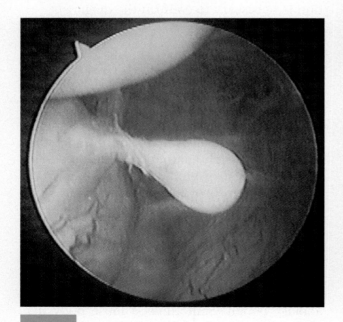

Figure 6-7
Loose bodies can be fixed on a pedicle in the inferior glenoid recess.

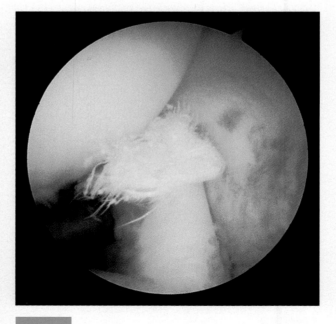

Figure 6-8
A flap of subscapularis tendon on a tethered pedicle was found trapped within the biceps groove, functioning as a loose body.

with rotation of the arthroscope to allow a panoramic view of the entire space. A final position where loose bodies can be noted is along the biceps tendon sheath, and out the biceps groove. Loose bodies infrequently are trapped in this area; more common here are "tethered" loose bodies (Fig. 6-8). In this situation, position 15 is very useful, since the arthroscope can actually be inserted into the biceps groove for direct visualization.

Removal of Loose Bodies

Depending on the location, the size, and the composition of the loose bodies, various techniques and instruments must be employed for successful and safe removal. The instruments commonly used for loose body removal include a large-bore (9- to 10-mm) operating cannula; an Arthrex grasping tool; a magnetic "Golden Retriever"; a large double-action pituitary rongeur; and a box of threaded K-wires. Whenever loose bodies are located in the subscapularis recess, it is helpful to create an additional anterior portal just above the subscapularis tendon. By viewing from the anterior superior portal and operating through the anterior inferior portal, most loose bodies in the subscapular bursa can be reached (Figs. 6-9 and 6-10).

Cartilaginous or Osteocartilaginous Loose Bodies

The most frequently encountered loose bodies in the shoulder joint are composed either of cartilage or of cartilage with a central bony nidus. Depending on the size of these loose bodies, they may sometimes be removed with a large outflow drainage cannula attached either to gravity drainage or to suction. If the diameter of the drainage tube is adequate, it may be used like a vacuum cleaner in conjunction with high-flow irrigation. More often, significant loose bodies are too large to be removed simply by a standard outflow cannula, and it is necessary to consider using either a larger-diameter tubing or a grasping clamp. The cannula systems available for arthroscopic stabilization procedures, such as stapling or suturing the labrum, have a larger diameter—around 9.5 mm. If these are available, they may be inserted over the ap-

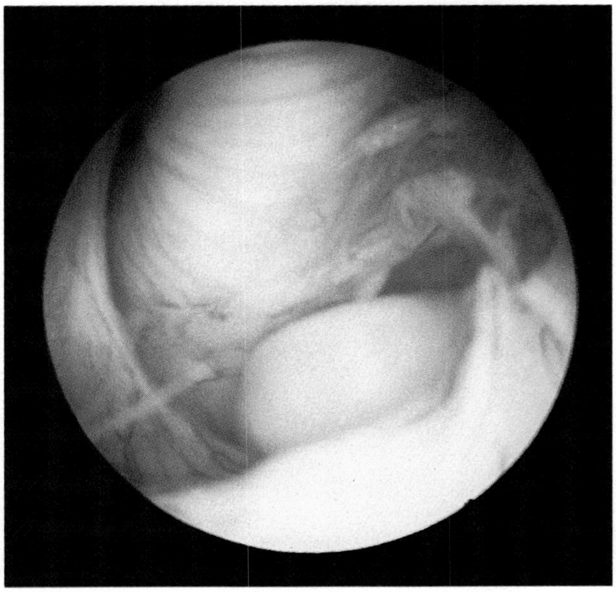

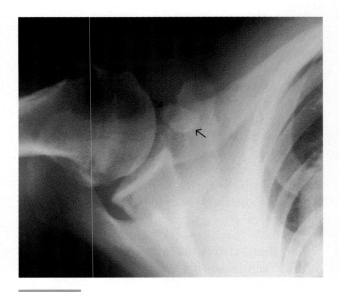

Figure 6-9
The most common location where loose bodies are found is the subscapularis recess.

Figure 6-10
The axillary x-ray is useful to diagnose calcific loose bodies in the subscapularis recess.

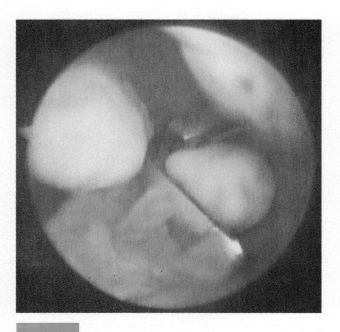

Figure 6-11
A double-action pituitary rongeur is helpful to morselize larger loose bodies for easier removal.

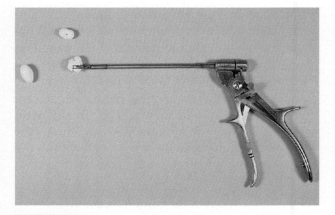

Figure 6-12
The Arthrex labral stitching tool is a handy device for removing loose bodies.

propriate guide rod and may be large enough to allow passage of the loose bodies.

If a large-diameter cannula is not available, or if the loose body is still too large, the loose body may be morselized to create smaller pieces. To morselize an osteochondral loose body, a large double-action pituitary rongeur is useful to grasp and cut it into smaller fragments (Fig. 6-11). Alternatively, the rongeur can hold a large loose body while an arthroscopic burr is used to abrade it into smaller pieces. The fragments can be either removed through the cannula or retrieved individually with a smaller grasping clamp.

Another instrument that has been helpful for removing large loose bodies is the cannulated labral suturing grasper sold by the Arthrex Company (Naples, Florida). The advantages of this grasper are many, including the small thickness of the grasping arms, which can surround a loose body without adding significantly to its outside diameter (Fig. 6-12). Additionally, suction can be applied to the central hole in the grasper (which is otherwise used for the suture pin placement); this will attract loose bodies (Figs. 6-13

and 6-14). Finally, once the loose body is secured in the clamp, a threaded Steinmann pin can be inserted through the center hole of the clamp and into the loose body. This "shish kebab" technique gives an additional fixation to the loose body. Further, if an osseous center is present in the loose body, the pin may give adequate purchase to allow simply sliding the

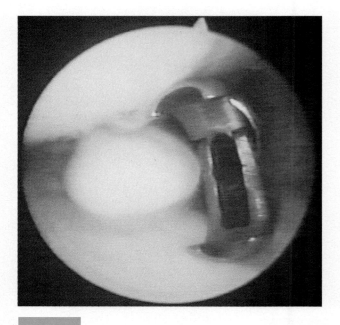

Figure 6-13
The Arthrex grasping cannula, with suction attached, will attract loose bodies into its jaws.

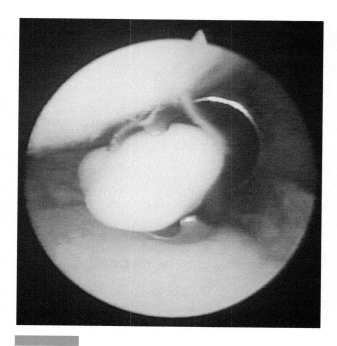

Figure 6-14
With the jaws closed, the loose body can be either pulled out through the cannula or extracted along with the cannula.

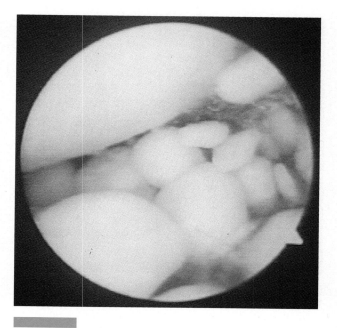

Figure 6-15
Multiple osteochondromatosis presents an extremely difficult arthroscopic challenge, and may require removal of a hundred or more loose bodies.

loose body out after removing the clamp and the cannula. It is important to test the security of the fixation once the pin is in place, by pushing the loose body against the glenoid (or another instrument) and observing to be certain that it cannot be easily dislodged. If it appears stable, the clamp can then be withdrawn, the loose body advanced to the inlet of the cannula, and the two removed together.

Multiple Loose Bodies

When there are multiple large loose bodies, such as found with synovial osteochondromatosis, their removal calls for techniques similar to those used for individual loose bodies, described above (Fig. 6-15). It is advisable, when this diagnosis is suspected from the preoperative x-rays, to have a large-bore (> 9 mm) cannula system available at surgery. Using this cannula, many of the loose bodies can be removed without need for frequent removal of the cannula. This lessens the chance of requiring multiple capsular punctures and subsequent extravasation of fluid into the soft

tissues anteriorly. As the soft tissue extravasation increases it becomes more difficult to locate the anterior portals, and the chance of losing loose bodies in the extra capsular soft tissues is increased.

Metallic and Other Loose Body Removal

It is not uncommon these days to encounter metallic loose bodies in the shoulder. These often follow surgical procedures, and include screws, staples, needles, fragments of wire, washers, and fragments of fixation pins. Additionally, metal debris from industrial and vehicular accidents, or from penetrating injuries from gunshot or knives, is sometimes found. The decision to attempt removal of these materials arthroscopically should be based not only on the size and location of the loose body, but also on the surgeon's skill and comfort level with these procedures. For metallic debris measuring larger than 1.5 cm, arthroscopic removal using standard techniques usually is not possible. (This does not include pins and screws, which can be

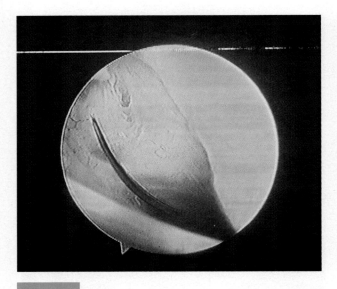

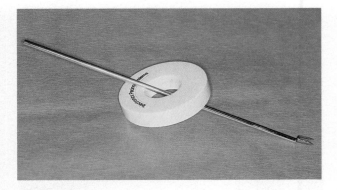

Figure 6-17
The magnetic "Golden Retriever" is useful for bringing metallic loose bodies out of the subscapularis recess to a position where they can be more easily grasped for removal.

Figure 6-16
A small surgical needle, lost during a previous rotator cuff repair, has migrated into the subscapularis bursa. It was removed with a "Golden Retriever."

grasped at one end.) The reason for this difficulty is the problem of morselizing metallic materials within the joint to allow removal of small pieces, as is done with softer materials.

To remove smaller metal or plastic loose bodies (screws, staples, anchors, etc.), the anterior mid-glenoid operating portal is most often used. Since these structures usually reside in the subscapularis recess, they are best visualized through the anterior superior portal (Fig. 6-16). Once they are located, extracting the metallic loose bodies from the subscapularis recess may be difficult. Since they are heavier than the osteocartilaginous or plastic loose bodies, most metallic loose bodies are not easily attracted by the suction technique. A magnetic instrument—such as the "Golden Retriever" (Fig. 6-17), from Instrument Makar, Inc. (Okemos, Michigan)—can be inserted through the operating cannula, and may be adequate to bring some metal loose bodies onto the more accessible glenoid surface. Once in this area, the magnet is removed and the loose body is deposited on the glenoid. The water flow is minimized, to prevent the currents from displacing the loose body; an appropriate grasping instrument is inserted

through an adequate-sized cannula and locked onto the loose body. If the object is a screw or pin fragment, it should be grasped at one or the other end rather than in the center. It can then be advanced to the mouth of the cannula and removed, either with or through the operating cannula.

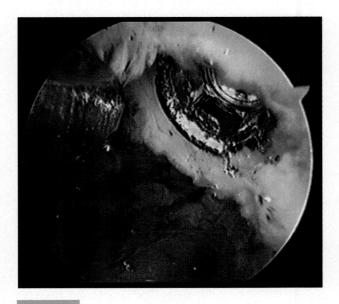

Figure 6-18
This arthroscopic screw, which was causing subscapularis irritation, could not be removed, because the hex head was stripped by the screwdriver.

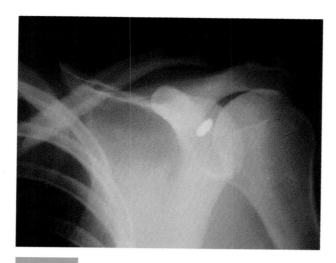

Figure 6-19
The head of an arthroscopically placed screw was causing irritation to the subscapularis tendon. During removal, the screw lag shank broke, leaving the threaded portion in the bone.

Removal of Fixed Implants (Screws, Staples, Pins, etc.)

When metallic implants are present in the bone and arthroscopic removal is desired, it is important to have the appropriate instruments available for the device that was used. The most common implants to date have been Instrument Makar staples, Dyonics arthroscopic screws, A.O. screws of various sizes, O.S.I. screws and washers, and Mitek titanium anchors. If the implant was not placed arthroscopically but rather by open techniques, then a myriad of devices are possible. The surgeon should be prepared in advance with various types of grasping instruments, including pituitary rongeurs and alligator clamps, as well as suction devices, large-bore cannulae, screwdrivers of various sizes, and magnetic extraction devices. Additionally, if the staple or screw used has a central slot or hole for the extractor, then a small-tipped curette or similar device may be needed to remove soft tissue before the extracting device can be employed. Sometimes a guide pin can be used as a drill to remove obstructing soft tissues. Once the central slot or hole is cleared, the appropriate extraction device—be it a cannulated screwdriver or a threaded device—can be inserted through the appropriate operating cannula, and the device removed.

Often the most difficult task is locating the implant, since it may be overgrown with soft tissues. Care must be taken to avoid iatrogenic damage to otherwise sound ligamentous and labral tissues. It is sometimes wise to abandon the procedure if significant difficulty arises in locating the device. An additional difficulty can occur if the metal of the device strips during attempted removal (Fig. 6-18). This can occur with the hex head of a screw, or the threads in a staple. When this occurs, if device removal is absolutely necessary, an open procedure will probably be needed. Further, if the screw or staple is firmly embedded in bone, the head may break off as a loose piece, leaving the remainder of the implant embedded in the bone. Seldom should heroic attempts be made to remove these fragments, unless infection is present (Fig. 6-19).

7

Arthroscope-Assisted Biceps Tendon Surgery

Introduction

The arthroscope is a valuable tool for evaluating and treating many types of biceps tendon pathology. The most common injuries to the biceps tendon include tendinitis, fraying, partial or complete rupture, instability, and spurring and stenosis of the biceps groove. In this chapter I will review our recommended techniques for evaluating the biceps tendon, using the history, physical examination, and imaging modalities as well as arthroscopy. I will also discuss the decision-making process we use to determine appropriate treatment for biceps tendon pathology. Finally, the various techniques for arthroscopic and mini-open surgical treatment of biceps problems will be presented.

History and Physical Examination Related to the Biceps Tendon

The biceps tendon is a common source of irritation in the anterior aspect of the shoulder.

Historically, injury to this tendon occurs with repetitive activities of pronation and supination, particularly with resistance or repetitive overhead activities, often at work. In addition, acute ruptures, either partial or complete, of the biceps tendon can occur with a lifting accident or a fall on the outstretched arm. When an acute complete rupture occurs, a lump of the detached muscle belly appears below the midpoint of the upper arm. Often there may be considerable pain and a large ecchymosis occurring immediately after the rupture (Fig. 7-1). Dislocation of the biceps tendon out of the intertubercular groove is a very *infrequent* occurrence. A forcefully resisted external rotation effort may produce a tear in the transverse humeral ligament, allowing the tendon to dislocate medially over the subscapularis tendon. More commonly, the dislocation occurs when either the subscapularis tendon or the supraspinatus tendon has suffered a tear extending to include the transverse humeral ligament, freeing the way for the biceps tendon to dislocate. Chronic degenerative changes also occur in the biceps as well as in the overlying rotator interval tissue, often secondarily to the repetitive trauma of subacromial impingement.

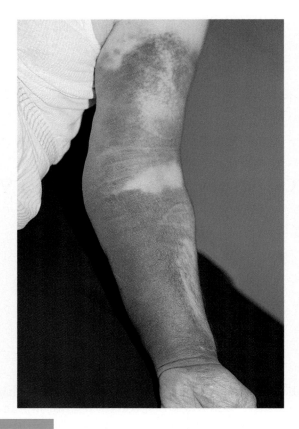

Figure 7-1
An acute biceps tendon rupture can cause very significant pain and ecchymosis.

Physical Examination

The biceps tendon is easily accessible for palpation in its position on the anterior aspect of the upper arm. To palpate the tendon, the index finger is placed over the upper arm approximately 4 to 6 cm below the anterolateral acromial angle. With gentle digital pressure in this area, the arm can be rotated while the patient is encouraged to relax the overlying deltoid muscle. This is best performed with the patient supine. A sharp, aching pain is felt if the biceps tendon is inflamed or has been injured. The examiner must be careful not to overinterpret this test, because even in the normal situation the biceps groove may be tender. Comparison with the opposite side is always helpful.

Speed's test is performed by applying manual resistance at the wrist against forward elevation while the patient holds the arm in approximately 45 degrees of forward flexion, with the elbow in extension and the hand in supination (Fig. 7-2). If pain occurs in the area of the biceps groove upon the examiner's application of resistance (or just upon the patient's assumption of this position), the test is considered positive. When the hand is changed to a pronated position, relaxing some tension on the biceps, and the test repeated, the pain is lessened. This test can be even more valuable if, after the finding of a positive result, a few mL of lidocaine injected into the biceps area negates the symptoms. Care must be taken to avoid inadvertent subacromial or intra-articular injection, which would confuse the test results by eliminating symptoms of impingement syndrome or intra-articular pathology.

Jurgensen's test—pain with resisted supination when the elbow is bent to 90 degrees and the arm is at the side—also stresses the biceps tendon. I have not found this test very helpful.

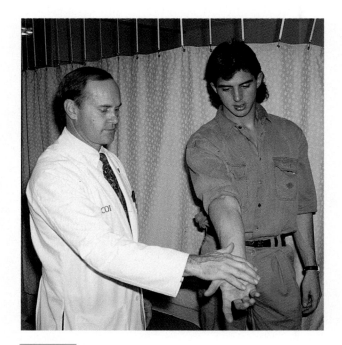

Figure 7-2
Speed's test, or biceps tendon stress test, is the most useful clinical sign to evaluate for biceps inflammation (see text).

Testing for subluxation of the biceps tendon in the groove can be performed by applying resistance to internal, and then external, rotation of the shoulder with the hand in supination and the elbow flexed at the side. Again, this is a very rare diagnosis, and, hence, the test is seldom positive. If the biceps tendon is unstable, a palpable or audible "snap" should occur as the tendon slips out of the groove when the arm is externally rotated. With internal rotation, it should then return to the groove. More often, if pain occurs with this maneuver before the biceps tendon is implicated, rotator cuff disease and glenohumeral pathology should be ruled out.

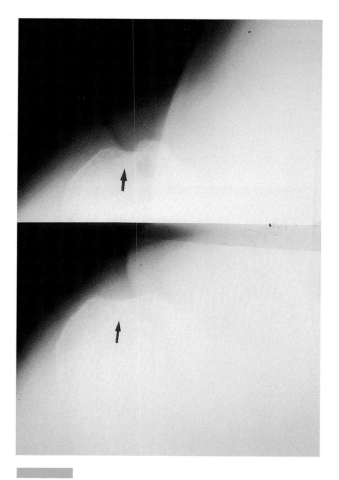

Figure 7-3
X-ray comparison of the right and left shoulders in a patient with a dysplastic biceps groove (bottom). At surgery, this patient had severe fraying of his biceps tendon and a large spur at the biceps outlet.

Imaging of the Biceps Tendon

Standard x-rays may be helpful in assessing potential biceps tendon pathology. Since anterior subacromial impingement may involve the biceps tendon as well as the rotator cuff tendon and bursa, an anterior subacromial spur, or type III acromion (Bigliani classification), may be associated with biceps tendon injuries (see Chap. 11). A special biceps tendon "groove view" may demonstrate a dysplastic biceps groove, which may be either too shallow or too steep or may have osteophytic formation or calcium deposition in or around the tendon (Fig. 7-3). On the AP view, cystic degenerative changes around the biceps groove may be present. The MRI scan is very suggestive of biceps pathology when excess "native" joint fluid is noted in the groove. This should not be overinterpreted without substantiation from clinical findings. In addition, the tendon may be absent from the groove or may be flattened, thickened, or deformed, especially when viewed in the axial cuts (Fig. 7-4). With gadolinium-enhanced images, the biceps tendon can be very well visualized, and the diagnosis of fraying or rupture of the tendon can be much more evident.

The diagnosis of biceps tendon instability can be readily made by an experienced examiner using ultrasound. Also, inflammation in and around the biceps tendon can be suggested. It has been my experience that this test can often be misleading in the general radiological community; the surgeon should be reluctant to accept a diagnosis based on ultrasound testing alone unless the radiologist has a proven record of reliable test results.

Arthroscopic Evaluation and Treatment of the Biceps Tendon

The biceps tendon is first visualized from the posterior portal. The anterior cannula is used

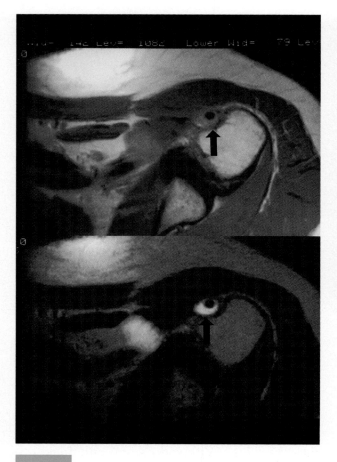

Figure 7-4
An MRI scan demonstrates excessive fluid around the biceps tendon in the lower part of the groove. This patient had severe biceps tendon fraying requiring tenodesis.

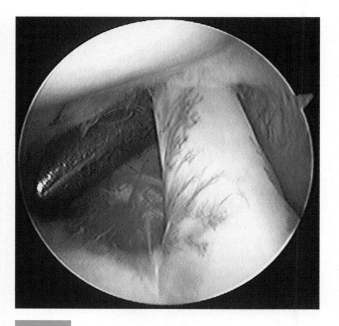

Figure 7-5
Inflammaton and erythema of the biceps tendon can be seen with biceps tendinitis.

to palpate it on both the superior and inferior surfaces. The elbow can be flexed to relax the tendon, which can then be pulled 1 cm or more into the joint by using the cannula. In chronic tendinitis without significant tendon fraying, there may be erythema and synovitis of the tendon and around the groove (Fig. 7-5).

The position of the biceps tendon in relation to the subscapularis tendon should be noted. When the tendon is unstable in the groove, it may sublux over the subscapularis tendon and be out of the normal position. Usually, the biceps tendon and the subscapularis tendon approach the humeral head at approximately 45 degrees to one another. There

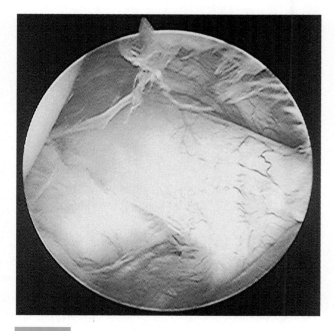

Figure 7-6
The biceps tendon is dislocated and is seen to cross in front of the subscapularis tendon, which has been partially torn.

is approximately a 1-cm space between the two tendons at the humeral head. If this relationship varies significantly, as when the biceps actually overlies the subscapularis tendon, then biceps tendon instability is present (Fig. 7-6). By placing the tip of the arthroscope in the biceps groove anteriorly—which requires refocusing the arthroscope, because of the proximity of the tendon—the instability can be directly observed with internal and external rotation of the arm. Additionally, when the subscapularis tendon has been avulsed from the lesser tuberosity, biceps tendon instability is more likely to occur.

A partial tear of the biceps presents as fraying of the intra-articular portion (Fig. 7-7). This injury ranges from minimal superficial abrasion to severe fragmentation and destruction. Treatment of these lesions arthroscopically includes very judicious debridement of the frayed fibers. Debridement is performed with the small full-radius-style shaver inserted through the anterior portal while visualizing from the posterior portal. Only after the tendon debridement is completed can one determine the extent of the tendon injury. If the bi-

ceps lesion is determined to be the only significant shoulder pathology, and if the tendon is significantly injured (with more than 30 to 40 percent of the fibers frayed), then the surgeon may choose to perform a biceps tenodesis.

In some cases of isolated biceps tendon fraying I have found that a spur or osteophyte located near the outlet of the biceps tendon groove into the joint was the cause of the injury (Fig. 7-8). In such cases a 4-mm ball burr inserted through the anterior superior portal can be used to remove the spur; this will avert further tendon damage (Fig. 7-9).

Following complete rupture of the long head of the biceps tendon, an intra-articular stump from the proximal tendon may be left in the joint. When the diagnosis is made, one should be suspicious of a remaining stump if clicking, catching, and grinding in the shoulder are persistent symptoms once the acute inflammation has resolved. When seen arthroscopically, the biceps tendon stump may initially be difficult to recognize. Since the stump is frequently very frayed and degenerative, it blocks the view through the arthroscope, making interpretation difficult. Severe

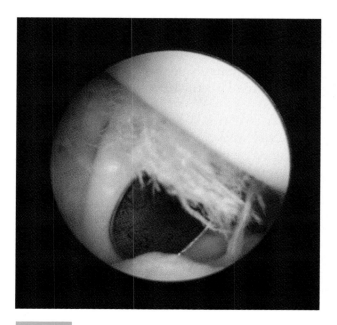

Figure 7-7
Traction on the biceps tendon with the anterior cannula may deliver a frayed portion of tendon from the groove.

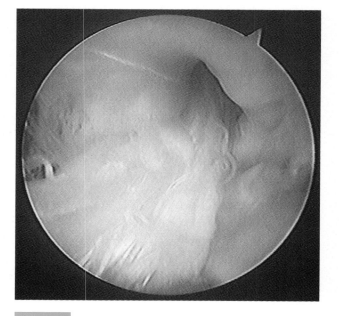

Figure 7-8
A spur or narrowing at the biceps groove can be seen arthroscopically, often with fraying of the biceps tendon.

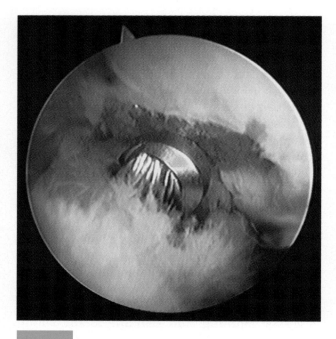

Figure 7-9
A 4-mm ball burr can be used to open the biceps groove and remove the offending bone spur.

glenohumeral synovitis is often associated with biceps rupture. The rotator cuff tendon, especially near the rotator interval, may likewise be injured. Treatment of the retained biceps stump is to remove the fragmented tendon remnant. A 5.5-mm shaving device is

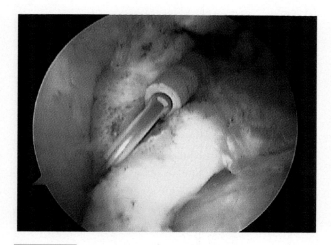

Figure 7-10
The Concept Subacromial Electrode is used to cleanly cut the stump of the biceps tendon just above the superior labrum.

inserted through the anterior portal to debride the fragments of tendon and allow more precise visualization. Once the diagnosis is confirmed, the stump is transected near the superior labrum attachment. An electrosurgical instrument, such as the "subacromial electrode," is very helpful in this situation, since it is difficult to cut an unstable tendon with standard arthroscopic tools such as knives or basket punches (Fig. 7-10). A suction punch may be useful. The superior labrum should be carefully preserved.

Arthroscope-Assisted Biceps Tenodesis (Table 7-1)

It has been my experience that isolated biceps disease is not so uncommon as used to be taught. Chronic biceps symptoms coupled with positive clinical findings and suggestive imaging tests frequently lead to diagnostic arthroscopy. When a severely degenerative tendon is visualized arthroscopically and the surgeon suspects this is the cause of the clinical problem, he or she should not hesitate to perform a tenodesis. The surgical procedure may be performed using conventional open surgery, completely arthroscopic techniques, or combined arthroscopic and mini-open methods.

There are two separate steps in a biceps tenodesis using the arthroscopic-assisted mini-open techniques: (1) the arthroscopic procedure, which involves arthroscopic evaluation, transection of the biceps tendon, and debridement, including subacromial decompression when impingement is present; and (2) the mini-open procedure, which involves secure fixation of the tendon to bone in the biceps groove. The arthroscopic procedure is performed with the arthroscope in the posterior portal and the operating cannula in the anterior superior portal. Prior to transecting the biceps tendon, it is advisable to insert a traction suture. This suture allows the surgeon to apply traction, facilitating tendon cut-

TABLE 7-1   Surgeon's Preference Card for Mini-Open Biceps Tenodesis

1. Standard arthroscopy set-up
2. Irrigating fluid—Synovisol
3. Electrosurgical pencil with standard tip and Concept Subacromial Electrode
4. 4.5-mm full-radius arthroscopic shaver blade
5. Standard mini-arthrotomy tray, including:
    2 small skin rakes
    3 Army-Navy retractors
6. High-speed burr with 6-mm ball tip
7. Yankauer-type suction tip
8. Right-angle clamp
9. 18-gauge wire or flexible wire suture passer
10. Power drill and assorted drill bits
11. Headlamp or spotlight
12. Suture:
    No. 2 Ethibond (2 packages, taper needle)—traction suture
    No. 1 Vicryl (1 package)—deltoid fascia
    3–0 Vicryl (1 package)—subcutaneous
    4–0 PDS (1 package)—skin
13. Postoperative support: sling or immobilizer with pillow spacer (Ultra Sling, Don Joy Inc.)

ting and ensuring that if the biceps tendon is completely transected, it will not be lost if it retracts down the arm. In addition, the traction suture may be used to serve as a guide to the location of the tendon in the biceps groove, since it is sometimes difficult to palpate when the arm is swollen and the landmarks are obscured.

To pass the traction/marker suture through the biceps tendon, an 18-gauge 2½-in spinal needle is first inserted percutaneously into the joint. The needle passes through the skin at a point just inferior to the anterolateral corner of the acromion. After penetrating the tendon with the needle, a no. 1 monofilament absorbable suture is inserted through the needle to pass through the biceps tendon and into the joint. A grasping clamp inserted through the operating cannula into the anterior portal grasps the suture and pulls it out (Fig. 7-11). A large "mulberry" knot is tied in the monofilament suture; the knot is then pulled back down the cannula and into the joint. This knot prevents the traction suture from pulling out of the biceps tendon (Fig. 7-12). By placing traction on the suture externally, tension is applied to the tendon, facilitating its transection.

I prefer to use an electrosurgical tool with

the Concept Subacromial Electrode in a plastic operating cannula to release the biceps tendon. The tendon is carefully transected under direct vision at its base, taking care to

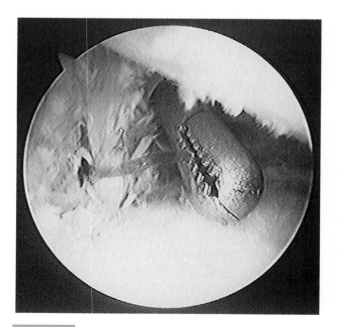

Figure 7-11
A no. 1 PDS suture has been passed through the frayed biceps tendon via a 17-gauge epidural needle and retrieved out the anterior cannula with a grasping clamp

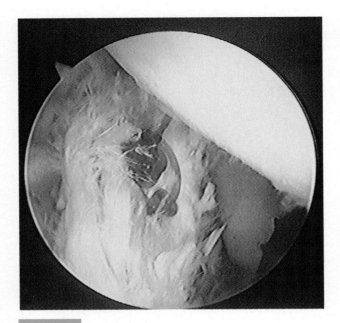

Figure 7-12
A large interference knot tied in the suture prevents it from passing through the tendon when traction is applied.

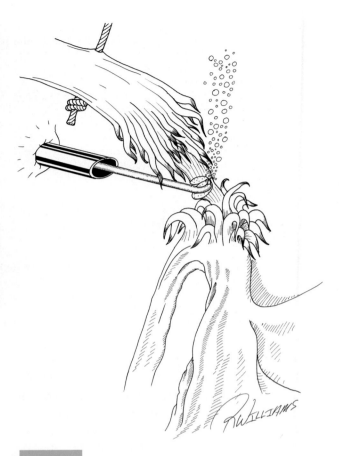

Figure 7-13
The biceps tendon is transected approximately 90 percent at its base using an electrosurgical cutter.

protect the superior labral tissues (Fig. 7-13). The transection should stop before cutting completely through the tendon, leaving a few fibers uncut to hold the tendon at its normal resting length. When the base of the tendon has been cut about 90 percent, the tenodesis, either mini-open or arthroscopic, is performed.

The SCOI technique for biceps tenodesis is very stable, allowing rapid postoperative mobilization. The arm is held in the arthroscopy traction apparatus in the bursoscopy position, but the traction weight is reduced to 5 lb. The operating table is tilted posteriorly about 20 degrees to place the anterior side of the shoulder more upright. The biceps groove is located with digital palpation and marked with a pencil. If the deltoid muscle is swollen or hypertrophic and the groove cannot be palpated, then its location can be estimated quite easily. The appropriate location for the incision is usually midway between the anterior and lateral arthroscopy portals, approximately 4 cm below the anterior lateral acromial angle (Fig. 7-14). The 4-cm incision is made only through

the skin, so as to avoid any potential damage to the underlying soft tissues. Small subcutaneous flaps are developed to help with exposure. The deltoid fascia is opened sharply in line with the muscle fibers. The muscle is then opened, using blunt techniques, for the length of the incision. I prefer to use my finger to perform this dissection. Once the humerus is palpated, two blunt-tipped Army-Navy retractors are positioned to maintain exposure.

The arm is rotated. Now, with fingertip palpation on the humerus, the biceps tendon can be felt. The arm is positioned so that the groove lies directly below the skin incision. A scrub technician or second assistant is instructed to maintain the arm in that position. It is helpful if the necessary instruments are placed on a Mayo stand located within easy reach of the surgeon.

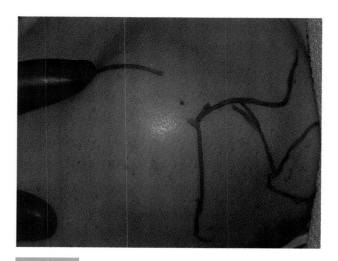

Figure 7-14
The incision for the biceps tenodesis should be marked before the joint is distended. It is placed approximately 4 cm below the anterolateral acromial angle, directly over the biceps groove.

The transverse humeral ligament is opened to expose the biceps tendon. A figure-of-eight marker suture is passed through the tendon near the upper end of the incision to serve as a traction suture and also to mark a point where the tendon normally lies in the groove. An electrosurgical burn mark is made adjacent to the marker suture to serve as a guide

in setting the tension in the tendon during implantation (Fig. 7-15). The proximal tendon is delivered into the surgical field after passing a right angle clamp beneath it and pulling sharply to avulse the last few fibers from the attachment in the joint.

Three Army-Navy retractors are very helpful at this point. One retractor is placed on the anterior, and one on the posterior, side of the incision; the third holds the biceps tendon distally so that the entire groove is exposed. Hemostasis should be meticulously achieved, since it can be difficult to view in the depths of the small incision with any significant bleeding. A headlamp or spotlight is useful. The transected end of the tendon is prepared by first excising the proximal 1.5 cm. This is necessary to ensure that the resting tension will be proper after the tendon is implanted.

A suture of no. 2 braided nonabsorbable material is woven, using a double baseball stitch through the distal 1 cm of the tendon, with both ends of the suture exiting the end of the stump (Fig. 7-16). A burr hole is made in the center of the biceps groove at the location previously marked by the electrosurgical burn. The hole is of the same diameter as the biceps tendon. The burr is angled inferiorly to undercut the cortex distally approximately 3

Figure 7-15
The electrosurgical tool is used to mark a spot near the midpoint of the biceps groove where the burr hole will be made.

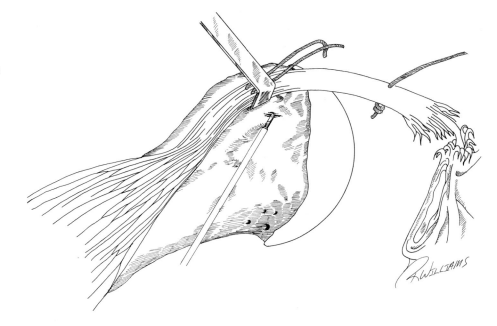

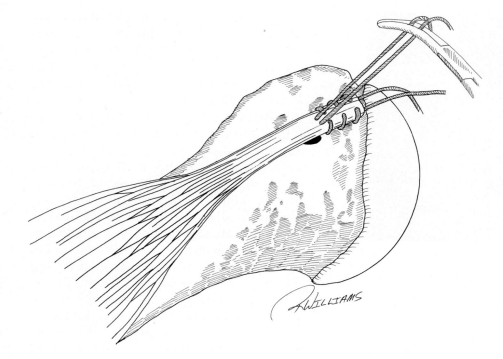

cm (Fig. 7-17). Two holes are drilled, one on
either side of the biceps groove, approximately 1.5 cm distal from the central hole. A
wire loop is inserted into one of the distal drill
holes and retrieved with a clamp from the
central hole (Fig. 7-18). The no. 2 sutures are

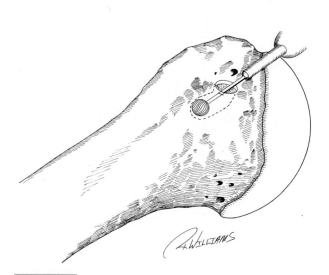

Figure 7-17
A high-speed burr with the guard removed is used to
create an L-shaped tunnel, beginning in the center of
the groove and extending distally about 3 cm.

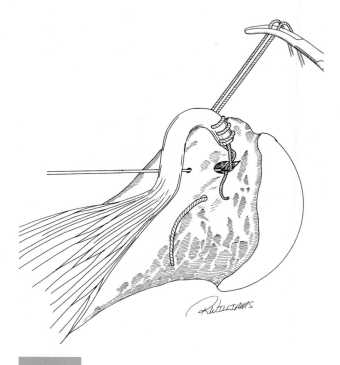

Figure 7-18
A flexible wire suture retriever is passed through the
inferior drill holes and out through the central burr hole
to retrieve the biceps tendon lead sutures.

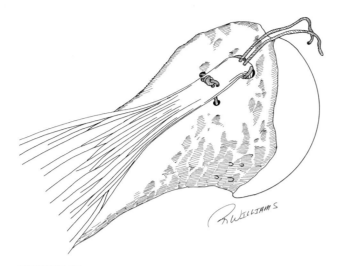

tendon using a free needle and are tied together, securing the tendon in its position within the bony trough (Fig. 7-19). The traction suture can be used to back up the repair by passing both limbs through adjacent soft tissues and tying them together.

Wound closure is performed using no. 0 absorbable suture for the deltoid fascia, no. 3–0 absorbable suture for the subcutaneous tissue, and no. 4–0 clear monofilament suture for the skin. Steri-strips are applied, followed by an absorbative dressing, and the arm is placed in an Ultra Sling (Don Joy Inc.).

Figure 7-19
The biceps tendon is seated in the burr hole and the tension adjusted until the marker suture is located at the opening of the central burr hole. The sutures are then passed through the biceps tendon using a free needle and tied together.

Technique for Complete Arthroscopic Biceps Tenodesis (Articular Side) (Table 7-2)

When significant biceps fraying is noted during the glenohumeral arthroscopy but no bursal pathology is discovered, the surgeon may elect to perform the biceps tenodesis using the completely arthroscopic intra-articular technique. This procedure requires three arthroscopic portals. The arthroscope is held in the posterior superior portal, and two operating cannulas with rubber diaphragms are inserted into the anterior superior and anterior mid-glenoid portal positions. A spinal needle

pulled through the central burr hole and out the anterior and posterior holes with the wire suture passer. Traction applied to the leading sutures pulls the proximal end of the tendon into the central drill hole and down the medullary canal of the humerus. The tension can be adjusted until the marker suture placed in the tendon is at the level of the central burr hole. One or both of the ends of the no. 2 sutures are passed through the biceps

TABLE 7-2   Surgeon's Preference Card for Biceps Tenodesis—Completely Arthroscopic

1. Standard arthroscopy set-up
2. Irrigating fluid—Synovisol
3. Electrosurgical pencil with Concept Subacromial Electrode
4. 4.5-mm full-radius arthroscopic shaver blade and 4.0-mm acrominoplasty burr
5. Suture anchor set (Mitek G4 suture anchors or Concept Revo 4-mm suture anchor screws)
6. Suture:
   No. 2 Ethibond (2-colored, 2 packages)
   3–0 Vicryl (undyed, 1 package)—subcutaneous
7. Arthroscopic operating cannulas: No. 2 (5.5-mm with fluid diaphragm)
8. Arthroscopic knot-pusher
9. 17-gauge, 6-in epidural needle
10. Suture Shuttle Relay no. 3 (Concept, Inc.)
11. Immobilization: Ultra Sling (Don Joy Inc.) immobilizer, preferably with small pillow spacer

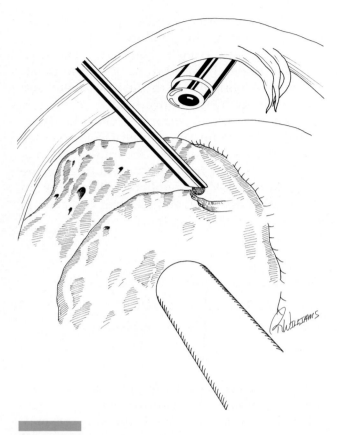

Figure 7-20
The 4-mm ball burr is used to decorticate the biceps groove through the anterior superior portal.

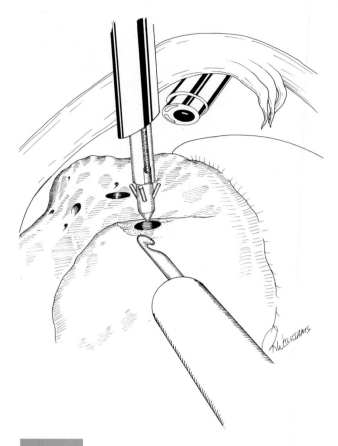

Figure 7-21
A suture anchor, preloaded with no. 2 nonabsorbable braided suture, is passed through the anterior superior cannula into the drill hole in the biceps groove.

is helpful in assessing various angles to the biceps groove to determine the best location for the anterior superior portal. The best location for direct access to the biceps tendon and its groove is usually below the anterolateral corner of the acromion. After the biceps tendon is debrided, a 4.0-mm ball burr is inserted through the anterior superior portal to decorticate the floor of the biceps groove as far distally as possible (Fig. 7-20).

A smooth-shafted drill or bone punch is used through the anterior superior cannula to make two holes in the biceps groove: one slightly more proximal and anterior, the second slightly more distal and posterior. A suture anchor preloaded with no. 2 nonabsorbable braided suture is inserted via the superior cannula into the prepared drill holes (Figs. 7-21 and 7-22). After implanting the first anchor, the crochet hook retrieves one

limb of the suture out the anterior mid-glenoid portal. A 17-gauge 6-in epidural needle is then inserted through the anterior superior cannula and directed to pass through the biceps tendon at about its midpoint, just above the anchor. A suture Shuttle Relay (Concept, Inc.) is sent through the epi-dural needle and retrieved with the grasping clamp out the anterior mid-glenoid portal (Fig. 7-23). Before pulling the suture Shuttle Relay out of the portal, the needle is removed to prevent damage to the shuttle casing. One limb of the nonabsorbable suture material, which has been previously positioned in the lateral portal, is threaded through the eyelet of the shuttle. By pulling on the opposite limb of the shuttle, which is still exiting the anterior superior cannula, the shuttle and the first limb of the su-

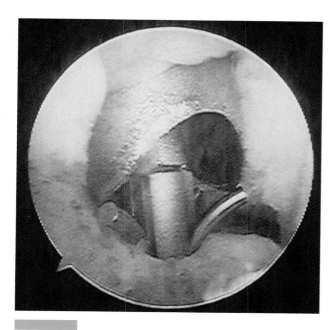

Figure 7-22
A cannula must be used with Mitek anchors to prevent snagging on the soft tissues.

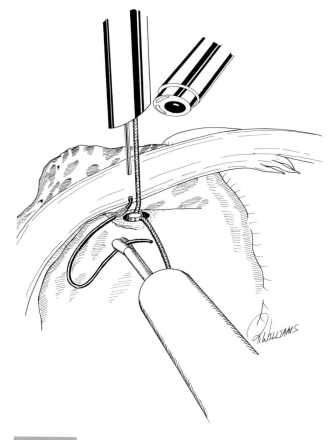

Figure 7-23
The Shuttle Relay is passed through the epidural needle and retrieved with a grasper from the anterior portal.

ture are carried through the joint and through the biceps tendon and out the anterior superior portal.

If a mattress suture is desired, the epidural needle is reinserted to pass through the biceps tendon again, near the implantation site of the suture anchor. Again the suture Shuttle Relay is sent through the tendon and retrieved anteriorly after the needle is removed. The second limb of the nonabsorbable suture, previously retrieved with a crochet hook out the anterior mid-glenoid portal, is loaded into the eyelet of the shuttle and pulled out through the tendon and the anterior portal (Fig. 7-24). The sutures are tied together using multiple stacked simple knots (Fig. 7-25). The repair is tested for security with a palpating probe. Usually additional fixation is desired, and a second anchor can be implanted into the second pre-drilled hole and the entire process repeated.

Once the tenodesis is completed, the biceps stump can be removed with an electrosurgical tool with a subacromial electrode tip. First, the proximal biceps tendon is excised just medial to the tenodesis knot. The long remaining stump of the tendon is transected, also with

the electrosurgical cutter, and removed with a large grasping instrument or the mechanical shaver (Figs. 7-26 and 7-27). Any residual rough edges are smoothed with the shaver. An x-ray is taken in the recovery room to document the location of the suture anchors (Fig. 7-28).

Technique for Complete Arthroscopic Biceps Tenodesis (Bursal Side)

While viewing the biceps tendon with the arthroscope posteriorly, a traction suture is inserted percutaneously through the biceps tendon just proximal to the superior labral an-

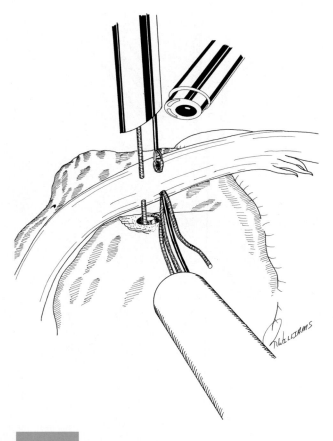

Figure 7-24
A mattress suture is made by passing the shuttle again through the biceps tendon to retrieve the second limb of the original suture.

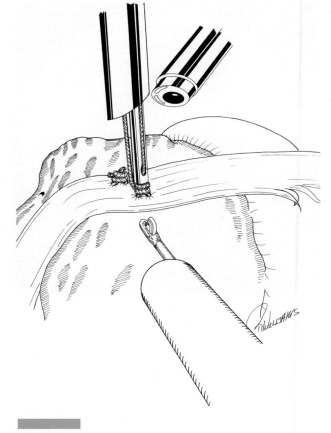

Figure 7-25
The sutures are tied using an arthroscopic knot pusher; the tails are cut with a basket punch.

chor. Using a "subacromial electrode" and a nonconductive irrigating solution, the biceps tendon attachment is transected approximately 90 percent, just above its superior labral attachment (Fig. 7-13). The arm is changed to the bursoscopy position. The bursal anatomy is reviewed and the shaver is used to remove any obstructing bursal bands. The marker/traction suture is located; if the rotator cuff tendon is torn in the neighborhood of the biceps tendon, it is usually easy to locate the biceps tendon by visualizing beneath the tear in the rotator interval.

The arthroscope is placed in the posterior portal and the shaver and burr in the lateral portal to prepare the biceps groove. A 4-mm ball-shaped burr is used to lightly decorticate and debride the floor of the biceps groove for

approximately 1 to 1.5 cm. A small hook or grasping clamp is helpful to retract the biceps via the anterior cannula, to allow better visualization of the groove. Through the anterior operating cannula, an appropriate-sized drill is inserted. One or two anchor holes are made in the biceps groove, approximately 0.5 cm below the outlet. A suture anchor is inserted into one hole, preloaded with no. 2 nonabsorbable braided suture. A crochet hook retrieves one limb of the suture out the lateral portal.

A 6-in 17-gauge epidural needle is inserted through the anterior operating cannula and directed to pierce the tissues of the rotator interval and pass through the biceps tendon just above the area of the suture anchor. The tip of the needle is rotated posteriorly, and a suture

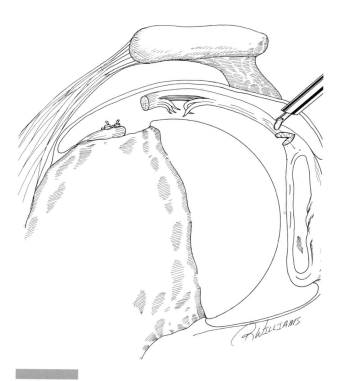

Figure 7-26
The electrosurgical cutter is used to transect the biceps stump, which is then removed with a grasping clamp.

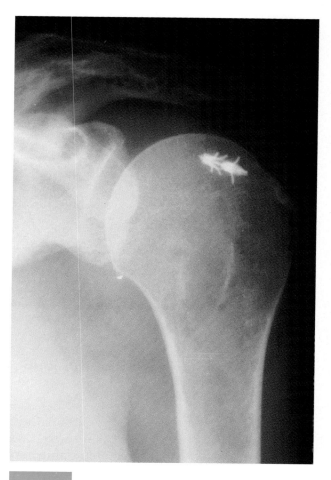

Figure 7-28
This x-ray shows two Mitek anchors well fixed in the biceps groove after an arthroscopic tenodesis.

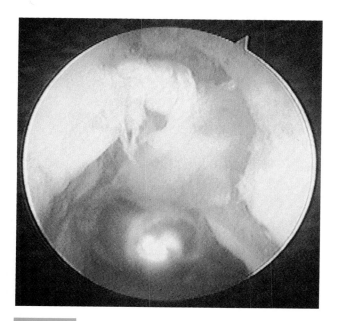

Figure 7-27
The fixation is tested with a palpating probe to ascertain that it is sound.

Shuttle Relay is passed through it and into the bursa. A grasping clamp holds the shuttle while the needle is removed. The shuttle is pulled through and out the lateral cannula. The first limb of the no. 2 Ethibond suture is inserted into the eyelet of the Shuttle and carried with the Shuttle down the lateral cannula, through the bottom and out the top of the biceps tendon, through the rotator interval tissues, and back out the anterior cannula.

The crochet hook is used to retrieve the second limb of the suture by grasping it near the anchor and pulling it out the lateral operating portal. The epidural needle is reinserted through the anterior cannula and passed through the rotator interval tissue and biceps tendon a second time, leaving a good soft-tis-

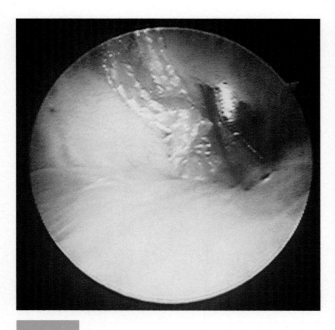

Figure 7-29
The knot pusher is used to secure the suture over the biceps tendon and rotator interval tissue on the bursal side of the biceps groove.

sue bridge between it and the first suture limb. The suture Shuttle Relay is inserted and again retrieved with the grasping clamp out the lateral cannula. The remaining limb of the suture is loaded into the eyelet of the shuttle and carried through the biceps tendon and rotator interval tissues and out the anterior cannula. The sutures are then tied together very securely, using five individual knot passes locked in place with a knot pusher (Fig. 7-29).

The tenodesis is tested for security using the palpating probe. If the fixation is not sufficient, a second anchor may be inserted a little more distal in the groove.

The remaining stump of the biceps tendon is transected just medial to the suture knots. A grasping clamp can remove the biceps stump after first avulsing the small fragment of tendon left attached to the superior labrum. The small full-thickness rotator cuff tear should be repaired arthroscopically (see Chap. 11).

Postoperative Care

An Ultra Sling and ice are used for the first few days postoperatively, until the acute surgical pain subsides. This is seldom more than 2 to 3 days. On the evening of the operative day the patient begins using therapy putty to exercise the grip and forearm muscles, and begins gentle active range-of-motion exercises of the elbow, wrist, and hand. Pendulum exercises are added as soon as symptoms allow—usually 2 to 3 days post-operation. Overhead pulley, range-of-motion, and gentle rubber band exercises begin at approximately 1 week. The patient can progress as the symptoms allow, but should avoid all heavy biceps resistance exercises for 3 months. Sporting activities, particularly with throwing or climbing, should also be avoided for 3 months.

8

Use of the Arthroscope in Evaluation and Treatment of Arthritis and Synovitis of the Shoulder

Introduction

The glenohumeral joint may be the site for a variety of types of synovitis and arthritis. Posttraumatic degenerative changes leading to classic osteoarthritis are the most common. Rheumatoid arthritis, gout, infections, synovial chondromatosis and osteochondromatosis, hemophiliac arthritis, pigmented villonodular synovitis, and chondrocalcinosis can also occur. The rate of these inflammatory conditions affecting the shoulder is low compared to that found in the weight-bearing joints of the lower extremities. In this chapter I will discuss the use of the arthroscope for evaluating, diagnosing, and, in certain instances, treating these inflammatory and degenerative conditions.

Degenerative Arthritis

In most instances a patient with degenerative arthritis of the glenohumeral joint presents with a complaint of grinding, aching, stiffness, decreased mobility, and limited function of the shoulder. Usually the symptoms begin insidiously, and the patient reports a progression over several months or years. Frequently there is no clear-cut traumatic event antedating the onset of symptoms. There may have been an event, such as a fall, a motor vehicle accident, or a throwing episode, giving rise to the acute onset of the clinical symptoms and the disability. Grinding with shoulder movement may or may not be painful. There may be other joints involved if this is a poly-articular degenerative arthritic condition, but more often it is confined to one or both shoulders.

On physical examination the classic findings with degenerative arthritis include wasting and atrophy of the muscles around the shoulder girdle. Limitation in the range of motion, both active and passive, is variable. Internal rotation contracture is common in advanced cases. Depending on the severity of the condition, the pain associated with the ac-

Figure 8-1
The AP x-ray in degenerative arthritis often shows an osteophyte on the inferior aspect of the humeral head, with early flattening and sclerosis of the glenoid.

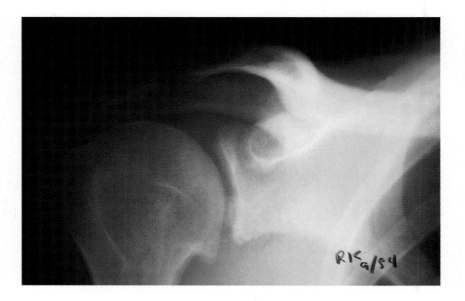

tive or passive motion may be mild or severe. Very frequently there is crepitus, and sometimes popping and snapping with active and passive range of motion. Seldom is there significant point tenderness around the shoulder. Resisted rotator cuff and biceps motion may not be painful with mild stress, but with heavier resistance the pain usually increases secondarily to joint-compression forces. Direct rotator cuff testing usually demonstrates good cuff function. Joint stability is usually intact.

Standard x-ray examination of the shoulder usually reveals the diagnosis. In the early stages of degenerative arthritis the x-ray changes may lag behind clinical symptoms. Helpful radiological clues include spur formation near the inferior capsular insertion on the humeral head, flattening of the glenoid with peripheral osteophytes, intraosseous cyst formation near the biceps tendon groove and greater tuberosity (Fig. 8-1). Additionally, and most important, the thickness of the articular cartilage space between the humeral head and the glenoid can be estimated on the AP and axillary projections; narrowing of this space is a very important finding (Fig. 8-2). Unless the rotator cuff tendon has been chronically torn, the humeral-acromial interval will be normal. MRI examination of the degenerative shoulder

joint does not help significantly, except to demonstrate the status of the rotator cuff tendon. A bone scan is extremely helpful to demonstrate the bony reaction related to arthritis around the shoulder, especially when compared to the opposite, normal, shoulder. CT scans and tomograms probably do not add

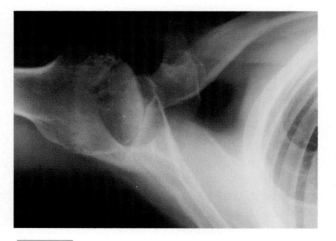

Figure 8-2
The axillary lateral x-ray is the best exposure for evaluation of the thickness of the remaining articular cartilage interval.

much to the diagnosis except to more precisely locate loose bodies.

Arthroscopic Evaluation

Arthroscopic evaluation for degenerative arthritis is performed infrequently and only for very specific indications. Debridement of the arthritic shoulder joint has been minimally helpful. In the young patient whose main complaints are catching and snapping, arthroscopic debridement may be of some benefit. In my opinion one cannot expect to improve shoulder motion much with arthroscopy alone, and manipulation of the shoulder joint as a therapeutic adjunct is seldom helpful. When the articular surfaces are degenerated, and the joint space narrowed, it is often extremely difficult to insert the arthroscope into the joint even enough for lavage and visualization. In this situation arthroscopy should *not* be considered a viable treatment option. Earlier in the course of the disease, if debridement is performed, the

shaver is utilized through an operating cannula placed initially in the anterior superior portal. The loose fragments of articular cartilage are selectively removed with care taken to protect any remaining viable articular surfaces (Fig. 8-3). Although it has never been proved that abrasion arthroplasty is beneficial in the shoulder, I have observed on a few occasions, with second-look arthroscopy, that the previously sclerotic subchondral bone may be re-covered by a type of fibrocartilage after abrasion (Fig. 8-4).

The glenoid labrum is usually degenerative as well, particularly in the superior portion, where a type I SLAP lesion (degeneration and fraying of the superior labrum from anterior to posterior below the biceps anchor) is commonly found. This area, as well as the rest of the labral tissues, can be carefully and selectively debrided, with utmost care taken not to damage the ligamentous attachments, particularly of the anterior inferior quadrant (Fig. 8-5). Biceps tendon and rotator cuff fraying is also commonly associated with this condition;

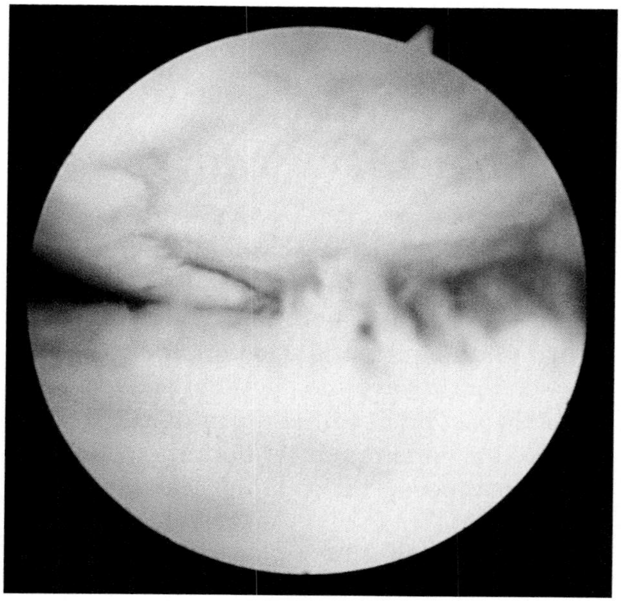

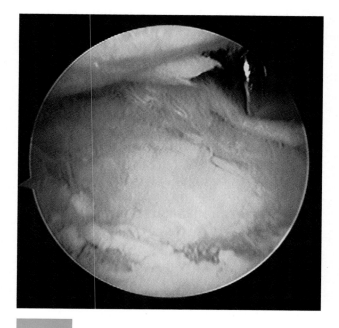

Figure 8-4

An abrasion arthroplasty was performed 6 years ago on this degenerative glenoid. A fibrocartilage patch is still present in the area of the abrasion, but the surrounding articular cartilage has degenerated.

Figure 8-3

Loose degenerative articular cartilage flaps are carefully debrided in degenerative arthritis.

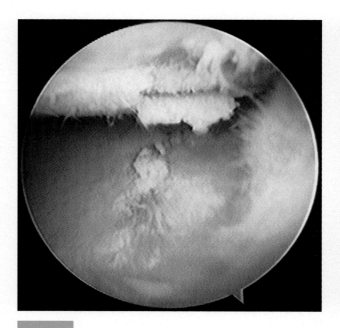

Figure 8-5
Fraying and fragmentation of the glenoid labrum often accompanies degenerative joint disease. It should be selectively debrided.

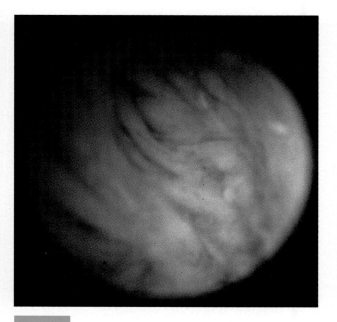

Figure 8-6
Often the reactive synovitis in degenerative joint disease is quite severe. Symptoms can often be improved with careful selective debridement.

these should be debrided judiciously. A search for loose bodies in the subscapularis recess and axillary pouch should be performed, removing all free-floating or tethered loose bodies, which may cause catching in the joint. The last step of debridement is to perform a synovectomy. The reactive synovium forming fronds and pedunculated polyps should be removed (Fig. 8-6). This portion of the operation is performed last, because bleeding is frequently encountered. The anesthesiologist can help with bleeding control by keeping the systolic blood pressure at or below 90 mmHg, provided that the patient is stable. Additionally, the pressure on the arthroscopic pump or fluid inflow system can be adjusted upward to maintain a clear visual field. Electrosurgery is often helpful to coagulate the larger bleeding vessels, but it should always be used with a nonconductive fluid, such as Synovisol (Baxter Travenol, Inc.), to enhance safety and efficacy.

It is extremely important, before performing arthroscopic surgery in a patient with degenerative arthritis, that realistic goals are set and understood by the surgeon and the pa-

tient. Temporary relief of mechanical, and some inflammatory, symptoms may be a benefit of this technique, but no long-term cure should be expected.

Rheumatoid-Type Inflammatory Arthritis

Rheumatoid arthritis commonly affects the shoulder joint, but the other forms of inflammatory arthritis—such as gout, psoriatic arthritis, and pigmented villonodular synovitis—seldom involve the shoulder. The value of the arthroscope lies in confirming the diagnosis of the inflammatory condition and, in some instances, in treating the associated synovitis.

The history of a patient with inflammatory arthritis is usually one of a chronic disease process, often involving other joints besides the shoulder. The hips, knees, and ankle joints are most often involved. Depending on the severity and chronicity of the shoulder involvement, there may be considerable atrophy around the shoulder. Sometimes, very significant swelling may be obvious anteriorly and laterally. In addition, the degree of pain, weakness, and limited motion depends on the chronicity and severity of the inflammatory and destructive changes. The rotator cuff tendon is frequently involved, limiting abduction and rotation power. Crepitation is often present with active and passive range of motion. Limitations of joint mobility also depend on the severity of the disease process. Often there are other joint manifestations of the disease in the hands, elbows, knees, ankles, and feet. For the more rare inflammatory conditions, such as pigmented villonodular synovitis, gout, pseudogout, and Reiter's disease, there may be no other joint changes.

Radiological Changes

The x-ray may demonstrate classic changes associated with inflammatory synovial diseases of the shoulder. The bones often appear osteopenic, especially when compared to the uninvolved joints. The classic changes associated with cystic bony resorption are located adjacent to the capsular attachment areas, especially below the rotator cuff tendon (Fig. 8-7). Seldom is the bone sclerotic, and seldom

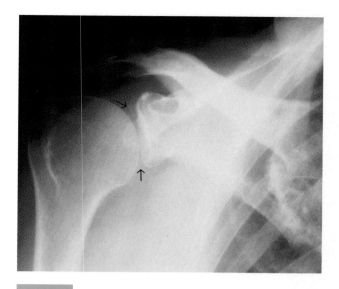

Figure 8-8
A moderate case of chondrocalcinosis, or pseudogout, demonstrates a thin layer of calcium on the glenoid surface.

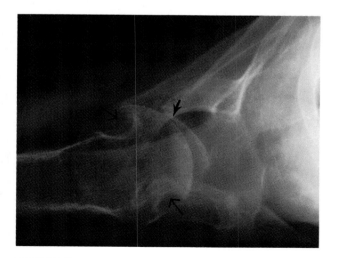

Figure 8-7
The x-ray in rheumatoid arthritis often shows osteopenia with resorption cysts around the humeral head and narrowing of the articular cartilage interval.

are spurs or significant loose bodies present except in cases of osteochondromatosis. The articular cartilage interval may be narrowed. If the rotator cuff tendon is torn there may be proximal humeral migration with narrowing of the humeral-acromial space. Additionally, there may be calcific deposits in the soft tissues—especially in the labrum and articular cartilage—if chondrocalcinosis, or pseudogout, is present (Fig. 8-8). When synovial osteochondromatosis is the active disease process, a collection of osteochondral loose bodies, most often residing in the subscapularis bursal area, can be seen (Fig. 8-9). MRI imaging frequently reveals a large joint effusion, sometimes extending to the bursal area. In addition, resorption cysts and synovial overgrowth are readily apparent. The soft tissues around the shoulder can also be evaluated, especially the rotator cuff tendon.

Arthroscopic Evaluation and Treatment

The standard arthroscopic examination is performed, beginning, as always, with a full 15-point evaluation from the anterior and poste-

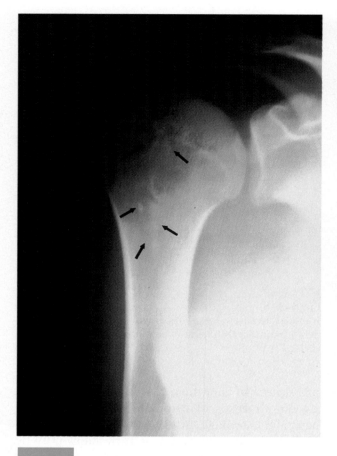

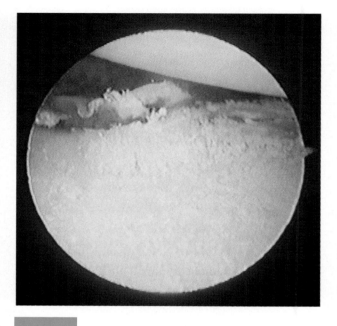

Figure 8-10
The synovitis associated with pseudogout usually is not as dramatic as that seen in the true gouty condition. The calcium pyrophosphate deposits may be seen not only in the labrum and in certain areas in the synovium, but also on the articular cartilage surface, especially the glenoid.

Figure 8-9
Synovial osteochondromatosis typically demonstrates a large collection of loose bodies in the subscapularis recess and axillary pouch and biceps groove. If the cartilaginous loose bodies have not ossified (synovial chondromatosis), then the x-ray is usually normal.

rior portals. A synovial biopsy can be sent for microscopic pathological evaluation to confirm a questionable diagnosis. If crystals are present, a synovial tissue sample that includes crystal formation can be sent in absolute alcohol for evaluation under a polarized microscope (Fig. 8-10). Uric acid crystals and calcium pyrophosphate crystals found in gout and pseudogout have variable birefringent properties (Fig. 8-11). Rheumatoid arthritis and pigmented villonodular synovitis have very characteristic cellular patterns, which can usually be recognized by the pathologist to confirm a diagnosis. Infected synovium will often reveal cellular necrosis as well as bacteria and macrophage cells, while degenerative

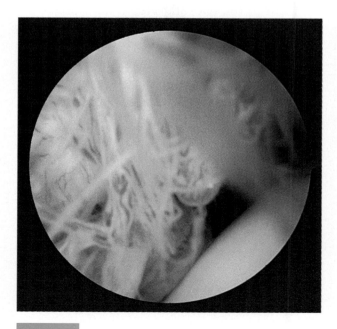

Figure 8-11
The diagnosis of gouty arthritis can usually be made on synovial biopsy, but the tissues must be handled properly so that the crystals are not dissolved.

arthritis shows non-specific inflammatory changes.

Arthroscopic Debridement and Synovectomy

Although it has not been shown to cure the synovitis of rheumatoid arthritis or the other inflammatory arthritides, arthroscopic synovectomy in these conditions does afford the patient a certain degree of symptom relief and palliation. The synovectomy is performed using a blunt-ended synovial resector, as opposed to an aggressive end-cutting tool. Since all of the joint areas have been inspected prior to the synovial debridement, the surgeon is aware of the areas of major involvement and can concentrate on those areas. The superior glenoid recess frequently has pockets of synovial material, as do the subscapularis recess and the posterior and inferior capsular folds (Fig. 8-12). Sometimes it is necessary to create a third portal anteriorly, just above the subscapularis tendon, to permit visualization

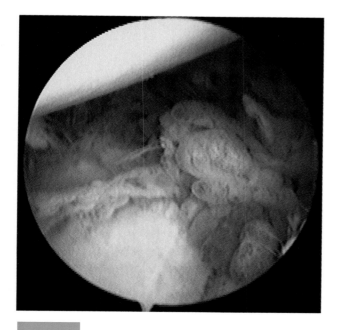

Figure 8-12
A pocket of rheumatoid synovium is visible in the posterior inferior aspect of the axillary pouch.

from the anterior superior portal while operating in the subscapularis recess and along the anterior capsular folds. Since bleeding is always a problem, the anesthesiologist should be encouraged to maintain the blood pressure at the lowest level that is safe for the patient's cardiovascular system. An arthroscopic pump system is invaluable; the pressure setting should be maintained at the lowest level that will control bleeding. The use of electrocautery via an insulated operating cannula is often helpful. The irrigation fluid used should be a nonconductive solution, such as Synovisol (Baxter Travenol, Inc.), to permit the safe application of electrocautery at the lowest possible setting.

I must re-emphasize that when one is performing the synovectomy, just the *superficial surface* of the synovium is removed. This is why a nonaggressive synovectomy shaver is recommended, and why careful visualization during the resection is mandatory. Damage to the underlying ligamentous and capsular tissues and rotator cuff tendon can complicate the postoperative recovery. Care should also be taken when operating around the articular surfaces, since the subchondral bone supporting the remaining articular cartilage may be quite soft. The cystic areas located on the posterior humeral head can be debrided as well, with the resecting tool in the posterior portal.

Synovial Chondromatosis and Osteochondromatosis

Debridement in synovial chondromatosis or osteochondromatosis most often involves removal of the multiple loose bodies in addition to the synovectomy (Fig. 8-13). The loose bodies are located in all areas of the joint, but are most difficult to remove from the subscapularis recess. A technique for this procedure is found in Chap. 6.

Hemophilia

Synovectomy in the shoulder joint in hemophiliacs is a very infrequently performed pro-

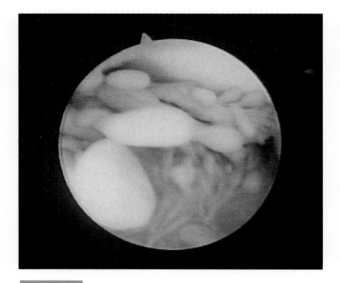

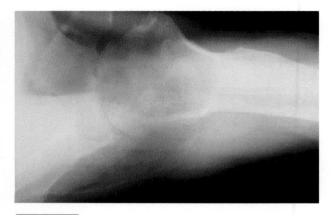

Figure 8-14

The x-ray may be very dramatic when infection is present, showing severe bony destruction.

Figure 8-13

Treatment of synovial chondromatosis requires removal not only of the multiple loose bodies, but also of the budding synovium that is forming the cartilage bodies.

cedure. It should be undertaken only by a surgeon who has special training not only in arthroscopy, but in the management of complications of hemophilia. A team approach is best for this difficult task. The team should include a hematologist, an internist and/or pediatrician, and a rehabilitation team, all of them familiar with the treatment of this condition. With concentrated factor VIII now available, the patient should be pretreated to a level of 100 percent. This level must be maintained for at least 2 weeks postoperatively. One significant problem that has been seen following synovectomy of the knee is that a clot forms, becomes thick and rubbery, and cannot be evacuated with a needle. For this reason, in the knee at least, it is often necessary to return the patient to surgery and evacuate the clot through a suprapatellar incision, using a grasping instrument followed by lavage. This may cause additional bleeding and result in a secondary clot formation requiring a similar procedure. In the shoulder I do not have first-hand experience with this postoperative situation, but I expect it would be the same as in the knee. For this reason I suggest that the surgeon be prepared to return the patient to

surgery at 7 to 10 days if the shoulder is tense and stiff, and expect that clot removal will be needed. Additionally, since the HIV contamination of transfusion material has sharply increased, the surgical team must be well educated in the important safety precautions to be used during surgical procedures on hemophiliacs. Postoperative rehabilitation in the hemophiliac is extremely important and, again, requires the devotion of a specially trained therapist.

Infection

Fortunately, infection in the glenohumeral joint is quite rare. Symptoms of glenohumeral infection may range from severe overwhelming sepsis to minor but progressive discomfort and disability. The x-ray is often very dramatic, showing rapid massive bone destruction (Fig. 8-14). When the diagnosis is made and the workup has been completed, arthroscopy can be of significant therapeutic benefit. The arthroscopic procedure includes synovectomy and debridement. Often, if the infection is severe, multiple bony and cartilaginous fragments are present in the joint (Fig. 8-15). The 5.5-mm synovial resector is helpful to remove these larger fragments, but

Rehabilitation

Following synovectomy and debridement of the shoulder in degenerative or inflammatory arthritis, the postoperative treatment is geared toward regaining early motion or preventing scarring and stiffness. The arm is supported in an Ultra Sling for the first week; but elbow, wrist, and hand exercises are begun on the first postoperative day. Pendulum exercises can be instituted as soon as the patient is comfortable. Rapid progression to elevation (both forward and in abduction), assisted with a pulley, begins within the first week. When symptoms allow, the physical therapist encourages active assisted motion and progresses to resisted exercises. The therapy should progress until maximum improvement is reached, both in range of motion and in muscle strengthening. The goals set for the patient should be reasonable, based on the surgeon's evaluation of the rehabilitation potential. The patient should not be forced by the surgeon or therapist to work toward impossible goals. It is important, when the diagnosis is confirmed, that an appropriate rheumatologic specialist be consulted to help with patient management. The optimal medical therapy available for management of these conditions changes continually; unless the physician is up to date in this field, he or she cannot expect to provide the best possible long-term patient care.

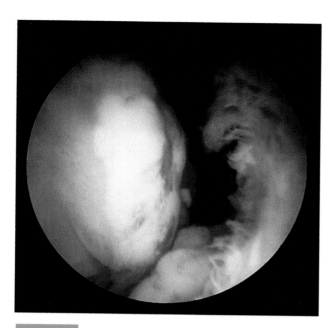

Figure 8-15
When an infected shoulder is treated arthroscopically, it is often necessary to remove free-floating fragments of articular cartilage and bone as well as to perform the synovectomy.

sometimes a pituitary rongeur or a suction punch is needed. An excellent debridement and joint lavage can be performed with these techniques. If desired, ingress and egress tubes can be inserted through the arthroscopic portals to allow continued joint irrigation for a few days in the postoperative period.

9

Arthroscopic Surgery of the Acromioclavicular Joint

Introduction

The acromioclavicular (AC) joint is a common site for pathology in the shoulder causing symptoms of pain, either directly related to the joint injury or indirectly related to the irritation and compression of the rotator cuff muscle-tendon unit below. Because it is located superficially and therefore vulnerable to direct violent trauma, the AC joint is frequently sprained or dislocated in sporting activities and motor vehicle collisions. There is controversy about the optimal treatment for complete type III and IV dislocations. Although recent literature indicates a trend toward the favoring of nonoperative treatment,[1,2] many respected authors still favor open surgical repair in high-demand situations, such as athletics and industry,[3,4] or when the cosmetic appearance of a high-riding clavicle is unacceptable.

Most authors agree that the proper treatment for type I and II AC joint sprains is con-servative. A sling to support the arm, or perhaps a figure-of-eight clavicular brace, is usually adequate, followed by strengthening and range-of-motion exercises when acute symptoms subside. Full activities are usually allowed when the symptoms resolve and strength and motion are restored.

Although in most patients minor AC joint sprains heal without further problems, a small percentage of cases eventually progress to painful degenerative AC joint arthralgia. In addition, the chronic compressive forces placed on the joint with weight-lifting, both on the job and in recreational exercise programs, can cause progressive deterioration of the joint leading to a condition called "weight-lifter's shoulder," or distal clavicle osteolysis (DCO). This condition was first described by Dupas et al.,[5] in 1936; however, the definitive report by Cahill,[6] in 1982, reviewed the clinical histories of 46 males with this affliction. Patients with DCO are generally muscular; frequently they are athletic and are involved in heavy weight-lifting activities.

88

The natural aging process also seems to lead to joint deterioration in some individuals. This deterioration may be related to the peculiar and variable anatomy of the AC joint, or to small injuries in earlier life. When this occurs, the joint space becomes narrow and osteophytes form around the periphery. Cystic degeneration may also occur. This process may lead to pain within and around the AC joint. Impingement syndrome in the shoulder frequently includes AC joint pathology, when inferior acromial and clavicular spurs compress the underlying bursa, biceps tendon, and rotator cuff.

This chapter will present the techniques used at SCOI for evaluation of the AC joint historically, clinically, and radiologically, and will outline a treatment plan that includes both medical and surgical approaches. Arthroscopic techniques for performing the "mini-Mumford" and complete Mumford procedures will be described. We will also review a new technique for arthroscopic reconstruction of the AC joint after a complete dislocation. This technique uses the transferred coracoacromial ligament after resecting the distal clavicle and reinforces the repair with heavy sutures between the coracoid process and the clavicle (arthroscopic Weaver-Dunn-type procedure).

Anatomy of the AC Joint

Since the AC joint is a true synovial articulation, it is completely enclosed by a fibrous joint capsule that attaches to the edges of the articular cartilaginous surfaces. The inner surface of the capsule is lined with the synovial membrane. The capsule is reinforced both superiorly and inferiorly by thickenings called *acromioclavicular ligaments.* The clavicular and acromial surfaces are separated by a variable wedge-shaped articular disk composed of fibrocartilage. The main blood supply for the AC joint is from the acromial branch of the suprascapular artery posteriorly and the acromial branch of the thoracoacromial artery anteriorly. Joint stability is provided by the strong coracoclavicular ligaments, designated the *conoid* and the *trapezoid.* These ligaments connect the clavicle to the coracoid process, beginning at the conoid tubercle on the inferior aspect of the distal third of the clavicle and extending to the coracoid process. Lateral, posterior, and superior displacement, as well as excess rotation of the clavicle, are therefore resisted by these ligaments (Fig. 9-1).[7]

The articular facet of the acromion on the clavicle is variable but is usually small and ovoid in shape. The inclination of the joint is

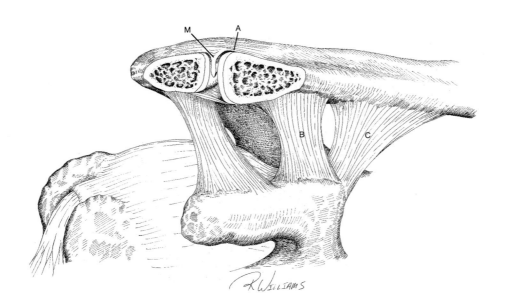

Figure 9-1
The AC joint is stabilized by the strong coracoclavicular ligaments (conoid and trapezoid) as well as by the AC joint capsule. Sometimes a small incomplete disk of meniscal type cartilage is present between the hyaline cartilage of the acromial and clavicular facets.

variable too; it can be perpendicular or oblique. DePalma[8] has recorded the natural degenerative process of the AC joint that includes degeneration of the articular disk, joint space narrowing, and erosion of the articular cartilage. These changes often parallel the natural aging process and degeneration in the glenohumeral joint of the shoulder.

History

AC Joint Sprains and Dislocations

Trauma is perhaps the leading cause of injury to the AC joint. Depending on the severity of the injury, the joint may sustain a direct compression injury, damaging the articular surface, or may be torn apart, as with a sprain or a possibly complete dislocation. The history usually is of a fall—either directly compressing the shoulder or indirectly, on the outstretched arm, also causing compression of the AC joint. The force of the fall drives the scapula and humerus downward and forward relative to the clavicle and can rupture the AC joint and the coracoclavicular ligaments. In the most severe situation the deltoid and trapezius muscle attachments to the distal clavicle rupture. The severity and direction of the trauma dictate the degree of the sprain or dislocation. A type I injury causes no actual displacement, but merely partial tearing of the ligamentous tissues (Fig. 9-2). The articular cartilage may be damaged in the AC joint with a type I sprain. A type II injury causes partial rupture of the coracoclavicular ligaments and the AC joint capsule, with partial displacement (subluxation) of the joint (Fig. 9-3). A type III or IV injury occurs when both the AC and coracoclavicular ligaments are completely disrupted. In this injury the lateral end of the clavicle is dislocated above the articular facet of the acromion (Fig. 9-4). When the displacement of the clavicle tends to override the superior acromion, the injury is of type IV (Fig. 9-5). Often the tip of the clavicle may pene-

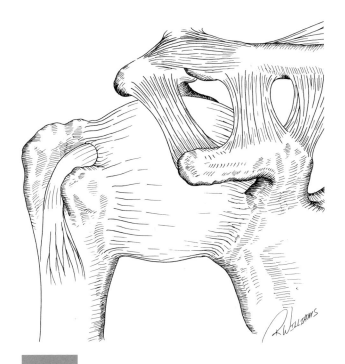

Figure 9-2
In a type I AC joint sprain the supporting ligaments are slightly stretched, but no joint displacement occurs.

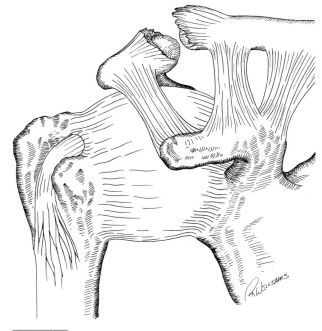

Figure 9-3
In a type II AC joint sprain the AC joint capsule is partly torn and the distal clavicle is partly displaced.

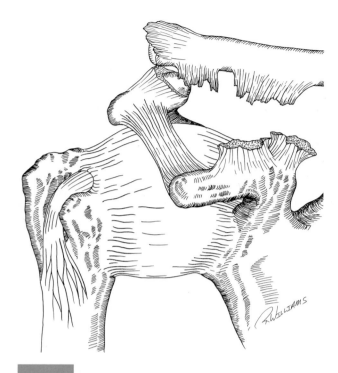

Figure 9-4
In a type III AC joint dislocation the joint capsule and the conoid and trapezoid ligaments are completely ruptured, and the clavicular facet completely dislocates above the acromial facet.

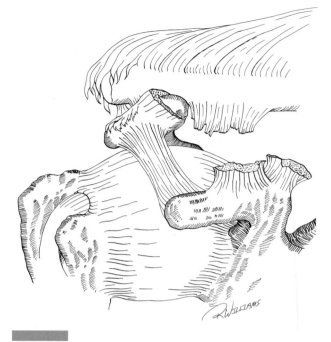

Figure 9-5
A type IV AC joint dislocation includes rupture of the coracoclavicular and AC ligaments; in addition, the deltoid and trapezial muscles and fascia are torn, and the clavicle usually displaces above the acromion.

trate the trapezius muscle, causing a button-hole effect that magnifies the deformity and impedes reduction (Fig. 9-6). Other classes of dislocations have also been reported, including posterior, high superior, and inferior dislocations; but these are rare and usually not amenable to arthroscopic repair.

AC Joint Degenerative Arthritis

Degenerative arthritis of the AC joint commonly presents as chronic shoulder pain of uncertain etiology. Most patients are middle-aged males. The dominant arm is most often affected. The pain may be insidious in onset or may be related to a specific traumatic event; in either case the chronic nature of the pain brings the patient in for evaluation. The patient will point to the AC joint area as the source of the problem, but often also reports symptoms referred to the deltoid, biceps, and impingement areas. The symptoms are most often exacerbated by lifting and by sleeping

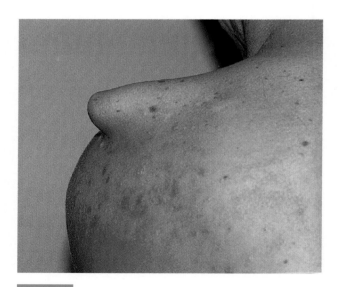

Figure 9-6
A type IV AC joint dislocation can be very disfiguring and is often uncomfortable.

on the affected side at night. There may be grinding, popping, and crepitus in that area as well. The patient may notice progressive swelling over the joint in comparison to the opposite side.

Distal Clavicle Osteolysis

A unique pathological situation occurs in some recreational and competitive weight-lifters, as well as in heavy manual laborers. These patients develop a very debilitating pain in the AC joint area related to certain types of weight-lifting. The bench press exercise is usually the most troublesome and is often eliminated from the workout schedule because of the pain it causes. These patients are very frustrated and anxious to get back to their activities; often they have sought consultation with a family doctor or with a paramedical healer, such as a chiropractor, athletic trainer, or physical therapist. Very frequently the problem defies diagnosis, because the x-ray is frequently unremarkable early in the course of the disease. In a workers' compensation situation, the patient often is labeled as a malingerer. The usual tests have been negative, yet the patient complains of persistent symptoms when attempting to return to work.

Physical Examination of the AC Joint

Inspection of the AC joint can demonstrate displacement of the distal end of the clavicle when significant instability is present. This should be compared to the opposite side, since a normal bulbous distal clavicle may appear at first glance to be subluxed or dislocated. Swelling around the AC joint may occur; infrequently, a degenerative cyst, or "ganglion," may be noted. Skin abrasions are often present when a bicycle accident or similar trauma is the cause of the injury.

Palpation of the AC joint with ongoing inflammation will demonstrate localized pain in that area. The tenderness may be localized to the anterior or posterior aspect, especially if a

degenerative intraclavicular cyst is located there. Crepitation in the joint can be appreciated when palpating the joint while the shoulder is moved. With AC joint dislocation, displacement of the joint can be detected; frequently the distal clavicle can be reduced by applying pressure to the superior surface. In the acute situation this is very painful. Careful palpation of the sternoclavicular area, the acromion, and the ribs must rule out injury to these structures. In the chronic situation of a type III or IV dislocation it is normally not possible to reduce the AC joint, since the fibrous healing response has usually obliterated the previous joint space, stabilizing the clavicle in its dislocated position.

A specific test for AC joint inflammation is the *horizontal adduction compression test*. The patient places the hand of the painful shoulder on the posterior aspect of the opposite shoulder, thereby placing the shoulder in a forward-flexed and adducted position. The examiner then gently presses the elbow, forcing the shoulder into more adduction, compressing the AC joint (Fig. 9-7). Pain in the AC joint caused by this maneuver is considered a positive test. Pushup-type exercises

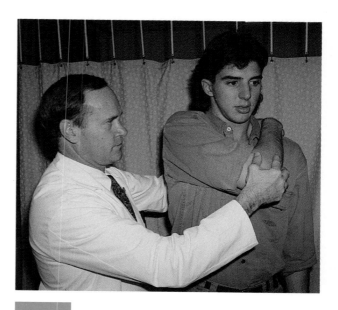

Figure 9-7
The AC joint adduction compression test is often the only positive clinical test, aside from local tenderness to direct palpation over the joint.

can serve as a provocative test for AC joint pain and inflammation as well.

Additional related tests—including supraspinatus muscle resistance, impingement I and II, and biceps tension tests—are sometimes positive, particularly if there is a spur beneath the AC joint causing bursitis, tendinitis, or the "impingement" phenomenon.

A useful test in evaluating AC joint symptoms is to inject the joint with lidocaine. If the pain previously noted with the adduction AC joint compression test is improved after the injection, the diagnosis of AC joint arthralgia is confirmed.

Imaging Techniques in the AC Joint

X-Ray Evaluation

The standard shoulder x-ray series should include a view of the AC joint. The most reliable view is performed by centering the x-ray beam on the AC joint with an angle of 15 to 20 degrees cephalad. Sometimes it is necessary, after reviewing the film, to change the angle to a slightly more medial or lateral direction, depending on the inclination of the joint. The joint should be inspected carefully, with a bright spotlight and sometimes a magnifying glass, for narrowing, intraosseous cystic formation, and peripheral osteophytes. Rarefaction (osteolysis) of the distal 1 cm of clavicle can be seen as well (Fig. 9-8). Increased subchondral sclerosis and peripheral spurs may indicate a degenerative process. An axillary lateral view is helpful in differentiating type III from type IV dislocations. When a type IV injury is present the clavicle will be displaced posteriorly, and/or override the acromion, when seen on the axillary view.

When instability of the AC joint is suspected, standard AP views of both shoulders are taken and the coracoclavicular distances measured and compared. If instability is not obvious as indicated by widening of the coracoclavicular space, then a stress view can be performed. The patient holds a 10-lb weight in each hand during the x-ray exposure. He or she is instructed to relax the shoulder mus-

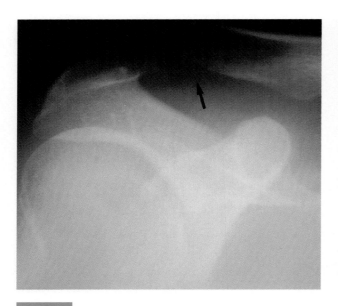

Figure 9-8
In distal clavicle osteolysis, there is cystic resorption of the distal clavicle with poor visualization of the subchondral pla

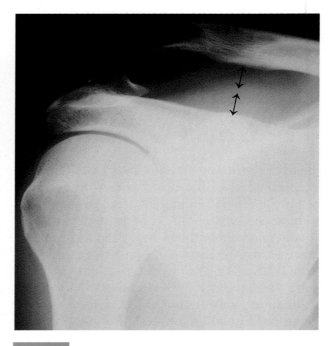

Figure 9-9
A stress view of the AC joint demonstrates widening of the coracoclavicular space in comparison to the normal side.

Figure 9-10
A technetium bone scan is a very sensitive test for inflammation in and around the AC joint, and should be compared to the opposite side.

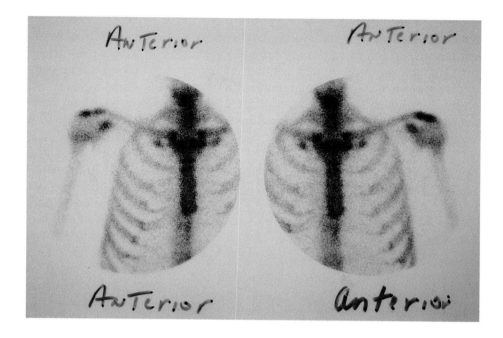

cles and allow the shoulder to "droop." If the clavicle is noted to be displaced proximally and the coracoclavicular space is widened compared to the opposite shoulder, then AC joint instability is diagnosed (Fig. 9-9).

A technetium phosphate bone scan is frequently used to document hyperemia in the AC joint area associated with inflammatory or posttraumatic conditions. In osteolysis of the distal clavicle the bone scan may be the only positive objective test to confirm a clinical suspicion (Fig. 9-10). MR imaging of the AC joint is often confusing. Frequently the radiological report indicates encroachment on the musculotendinous area of the rotator cuff below the AC joint by a spur. This situation may be interpreted by the radiologist as "impingement" and may lead the orthopaedic surgeon to a false diagnosis of the clinical situation. Since the contour of the inferior aspect of the AC joint is usually slightly convex and covered by a relatively thick capsule that has an MRI signal similar to bone, it may appear to indent the supraspinatus muscle (Fig. 9-11). This appearance should not be construed as proof that a pathological condition of clinical impingement exists.

Arthritic changes, particularly with cystic degeneration of the AC joint, may appear somewhat exaggerated on the MRI scan and, again, are easily overdiagnosed. It can be helpful to note large fluid collections around the joint; such findings can aid in the clinical

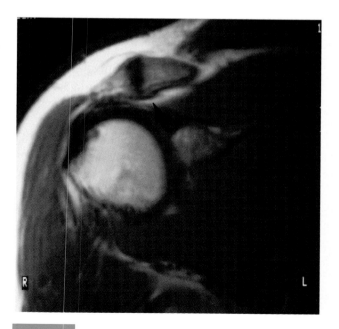

Figure 9-11
MRI scan is sometimes helpful with the AC joint, but is often misinterpreted as showing "impingement" of the supraspinatus muscle (arrow).

workup. The surgeon must carefully interpret the MRI data in light of the history and clinical examination, rather than accept the diagnosis from the radiological report. All shoulder surgeons who routinely order MRI scans should strive to become as skillful at interpreting them as they are at reading standard x-rays of the shoulder.[9,10]

Arthroscopic Evaluation and Treatment of AC Joint Pathology

Direct arthroscopic visual examination of the AC joint usually is not practical, especially when arthritic changes are present or the joint has been dislocated. Although it is possible to insert a small-diameter arthroscope into the joint when no narrowing is present, the articular surfaces may be easily damaged. We do not advocate this for routine diagnostic testing.

The arthroscope is extremely valuable for partial resection of the inferior aspect of the AC joint (mini-Mumford procedure) and for complete resection of the AC joint (Mumford procedure).[11] It is also useful when reconstructing a severe AC joint dislocation. It may also be helpful for harvesting the coracoacromial ligament, or may be used throughout the reconstruction to perform a complete arthroscopic Weaver-Dunn procedure.

Arthroscopic Mini-Mumford Procedure, or Resection of the Inferior Aspect of the AC Joint

The most common arthroscopic approach to the AC joint is through the subacromial space. The acromial facet of the AC joint is frequently hypertrophic when impingement syndrome or degenerative arthritis is present, and it is usually resected during subacromial decompression surgery. Leaving a hyper-

trophic inferior AC joint spur may cause failure of the decompression procedure or progression of the symptoms after an otherwise adequate surgery. At the time of preoperative planning for a subacromial decompression, the surgeon should pay careful attention to the radiological appearance of the inferior aspect of the AC joint (Fig. 9-12). If during surgery it is found necessary to perform a mini-Mumford, the following technique is used once the decompression is completed.

A nonconductive solution, such as Synovisol (isosmolar glycerol, Baxter Travenol, Deerfield, Illinois) is used as the irrigating fluid. The electrosurgical instrument is inserted through an insulated cannula via the lateral subacromial portal or the posterior portal to cross-hatch and resect the capsule of the inferior aspect of the AC joint. A motorized shaver and a 5-mm suction punch are used to remove capsular debris, exposing the undersurface of the joint. The acromionizer burr is next used to flatten the acromial facet of the joint until it is flush with the remainder of the acromial undersurface. The burr may be used from either the posterior or lateral

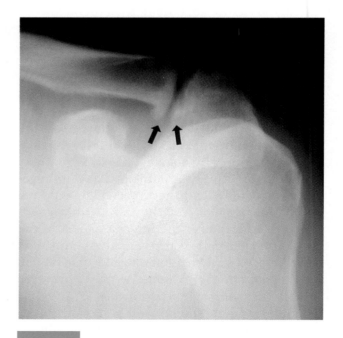

Figure 9-12
Large spurs may be present on both the acromial and clavicular sides of the AC joint when arthritis is present.

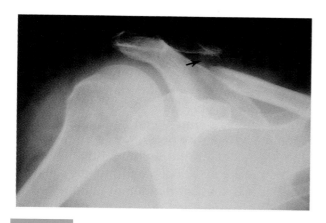

Figure 9-13
Care must be taken when performing a mini-Mumford procedure to prevent postoperative fracture.

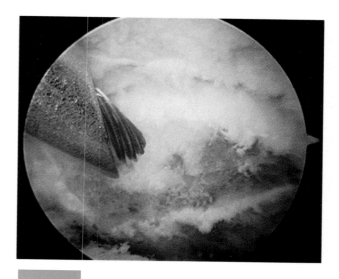

Figure 9-14
When the mini-Mumford procedure is completed, the undersurface of the AC joint is completely flat on both the acromial and clavicular sides.

portal. The inferior aspect of the distal clavicle is thus exposed for inspection. Since degenerative changes are difficult to appreciate and no standard classification system is useful, the decision to proceed with complete or partial distal clavicle resection should be made prior to the beginning of the surgical procedure. When complete subacromial decompression is the surgical goal, resecting the acromial facet, as well as the underhanging lip of the distal clavicular facet, may be necessary.

With the arthroscope viewing from the posterior portal, the 4.0-mm acromionizer burr is inserted through a cannula via the lateral subacromial portal, and the underhanging portion of the distal clavicle is carefully flattened. It is important to recognize that *just* the underhanging facet of the joint should be excised, and no attempt should be made to flatten the entire undersurface of the clavicle. The clavicle angles in a medial and caudal direction away from the acromion; if the surgeon attempts to flatten it completely, a significant divot may be created on the undersurface of the distal tip of the bone, creating a stress riser or perhaps even a fracture (Fig. 9-13). Careful surgical orientation and recognition of this fact will prevent overzealous resection. The operation is complete when the burring instrument can be laid flat beneath the acromion and the AC joint with no underhanging bone present (Fig. 9-14).

Complete Arthroscopic Resection of the Distal Clavicle (Mumford Procedure)

There are three commonly used approaches for performing the arthroscopic Mumford procedure: (1) superior, (2) anterior, and (3) the lateral "Claviculizer" approach.

Superior Approach[12]

The superior approach to distal clavicle resection is often very useful when degenerative arthritis is present. Following arthroscopic subacromial decompression and excision of the inferior capsule and the AC joint facet, the arthroscope is placed in either the lateral or the posterior portal with the bevel turned upward toward the AC joint for better visualization. With the room lights dimmed, the AC joint space will be transilluminated. A spinal needle can be placed percutaneously through the joint and into the subacromial space. When arthritis is present this may be somewhat difficult; the needle can be alternatively placed just anterior to the joint and angled posteriorly into the subacromial space.

A small stab wound is made in the midpoint of the joint superiorly, and a small-diameter shaving tool, such as a 3.0-mm full-radius shaver, is inserted directly into the AC joint without a cannula. The shaver is used to begin the soft tissue resection, removing cartilaginous and capsular debris and widening the joint. The progressive resection is viewed from the lateral portal with the bevel of the arthroscope rotated superiorly. When the soft tissues are removed and visualization is improved, the small-diameter high-speed motorized burr is inserted superiorly, and the acromial and clavicular facets can be resected. Although the resection is tedious, it is quite straightforward when good visualization is available. Sometimes the superior edge of the clavicle is difficult to see, and a 70-degree-angled arthroscope is useful. The resection continues medially until approximately 1.5 cm of bone has been removed. A larger-diameter burr may be employed when adequate room is available. It is often necessary to use the electrosurgical tool to coagulate capsular bleeders and resect additional soft tissues.

Attempts are made to leave the superior capsule intact as much as possible to help preserve the stability of the joint, although this is difficult with the superior approach.

The arthroscope can be transferred to the anterior subacromial portal for a more direct view of the AC joint when adequate room is available. From this portal the acromial facet of the AC joint can be seen, and the resection can be completed. The AC joint gap is measured using the parallel pin technique (Fig. 9-15). With the arthroscope viewing from the anterior portal, two pins are placed percutaneously through the resected joint, one at the end of the clavicle and one at the acromial facet. With the pins parallel, the gap between them is measured with a ruler. A 1.5-cm space is adequate in the average-sized individual (Fig. 9-16). After completion of the resection and evacuation of the debris from the subacromial space, the superior portal should be closed with an inverted absorbable suture to prevent communication of the bone ends with the skin.

Anterior Subacromial Portal Technique

The anterior subacromial portal technique, although more tedious than the superior approach, allows sparing of the superior AC joint capsule. Since the surgeon stands on the posterior aspect of the patient and operates in the anterior portal, it can be visually confus-

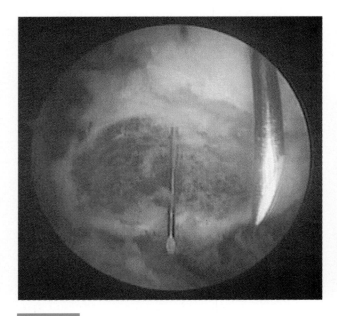

Figure 9-15
Two pins placed at either end of the resected AC joint can be used to measure the width of the resection.

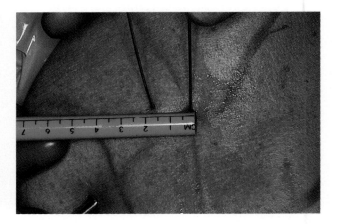

Figure 9-16
A ruler is used to measure the space between the two parallel pins. A 1.5-cm gap is usually acceptable.

ing and physically fatiguing to perform this operation properly. The technique for AC joint resection from the anterior portal is as follows:

An arthroscopic subacromial decompression is usually performed first, unless absolutely no sign of a subacromial spur or impingement is noted. The electrosurgical tool is used to open and morselize the AC joint capsule, and the mechanical shaver is used to debride the entire space below the AC joint. The arthroscope is then placed in the lateral portal and the operating cannula changed to the anterior portal directly adjacent to the anterior edge of the AC joint. (The position of this portal should be planned prior to the creation of the anterior portal, during the glenohumeral portion of the arthroscopic examination.) A drainage cannula is inserted through the posterior portal and connected to gravity drainage tubing. The 4.0-mm acromionizer burr is inserted into the anterior portal, and the resection begins with the removal of a segment of anterior clavicle approximately 1 cm deep (Fig. 9-17). The appropriate depth of the resection is gauged by noting that the thick-

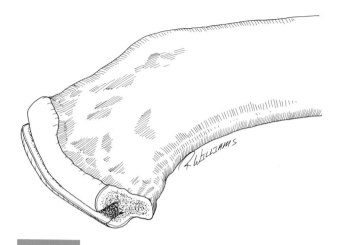

Figure 9-18
The second step of the anterior-portal Mumford procedure is to create a midline trough from anterior to posterior across the end of the clavicle.

ness of the burring instrument is approximately 4 mm. Two burr thicknesses for the initial cut will approximate the depth needed for the initial clavicular resection.

Once this initial anterior cortical segment has been removed, a midline trough is made directly across the center of the distal clavicle from the anterior to the posterior cortex (Fig. 9-18). This trough divides the remaining bone into superior and inferior portions. The acromionizer is then used to remove the inferior portion of the distal clavicle, progressing from anterior to posterior (Fig. 9-19). By segmenting the bone in this fashion it is much easier to maintain a correct orientation concerning the depth of resection. Once the inferior segment is removed, the superior portion is approached with the arthroscopic bevel rotated upward to allow visualization into the joint (Fig. 9-20). This is begun at the anterior edge where the initial trough was created, and progresses across the superior margin to the posterior border. Care must be taken to avoid amputating any superior osteophyte during this resection (Fig. 9-21).

If difficulty is encountered in visualizing the superior border of the clavicle, several alternative techniques can be used. The arthroscope can be changed to the posterior portal,

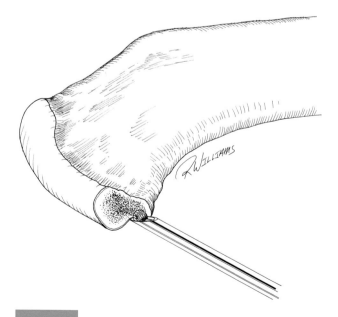

Figure 9-17
The first step in the Mumford procedure from the anterior portal is to cut off the anterior edge of the clavicle.

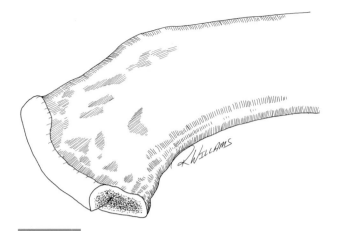

Figure 9-19

The third step of the anterior-portal Mumford procedure is to remove the inferior segment of the distal clavicle below the midline trough.

which sometimes aids in visualizing this area. Additionally, by compressing the superior border of the distal clavicle, it may be delivered a few millimeters farther into the subacromial space for better visualization. Finally, the acromial facet of the AC joint can be beveled via the anterior portal, allowing better visualization from either the lateral or the posterior portal.

When the resection of the distal clavicle is

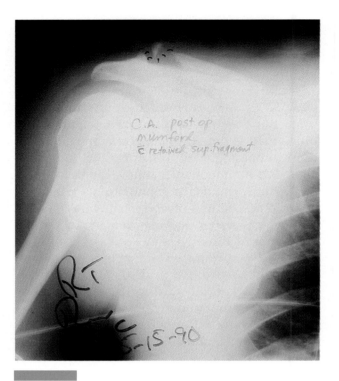

Figure 9-21

The superior osteophyte can be amputated if care is not taken when advancing the burr across the superior portion of the clavicle.

completed, the two-parallel-pin measuring technique can be employed to evaluate the adequacy of the resection (Figs. 9-15 and 9-16). If additional bone removal is needed, the four steps used for the initial resection are repeated: (1) the anterior vertical cortex resection, (2) the midline anterior-to-posterior trough, (3) excision of the inferior segment, and (4) excision of the superior segment.

The last portion of the operation includes beveling the inferior edge of the distal clavicle. This is performed while viewing from the posterior portal and passing the burr through the lateral portal. The cortex on the lower end of the clavicle is beveled just slightly to remove the sharp cortical edge. Care is taken not to advance the burr medially, which might endanger the coracoclavicular ligaments (Fig. 9-22). After the debris is washed from the subacromial space, the skin wounds are closed with subcutaneous sutures and Steri-strips.

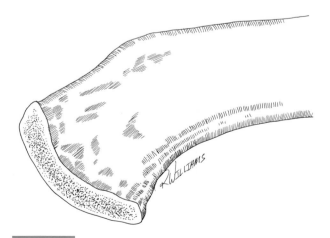

Figure 9-20

The fourth step of the anterior-portal Mumford procedure is excision of the superior segment of the distal clavicle. Care must be taken not to leave a superior osteophyte.

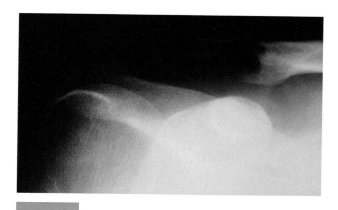

Figure 9-22
If too much clavicle is resected, the coracoclavicular ligaments can be injured.

Distal Clavicle Resection from the Lateral Portal (Claviculizer Technique) (Table 9-1)

The preferred method of distal clavicle resection at SCOI employs an end-cutting router-type tool called the Claviculizer (Dyonics Inc., Andover, Massachusetts) (Fig. 9-23). This tool, developed especially for the arthroscopic Mumford procedure, utilizes an aggressive end- and side-cutting burr, the Stone Cutter Burr. The Claviculizer utilizes a short sheath that functions as a depth-stop collar to prevent excessively deep penetration of the burr tip into the clavicle. The system is available in two sizes, 4.0 and 5.5 mm, and includes a Claviculizer short sheath and an acromionizer hooded sheath with the appropriate-sized obturators. By using the Claviculizer, the bony resection for the complete arthroscopic Mumford procedure can usually be performed in approximately 10 min.

The subacromial decompression is performed first, with special attention paid to resection and upward beveling of the acromial facet of the AC joint; this allows maximum exposure of the distal clavicle. The sheath of the Claviculizer functions as its own cannula, so no separate operating cannula is needed. The arthroscope views from the posterior portal. The outflow cannula, connected to a gravity drain tube, is inserted into the anterior portal. The Claviculizer is inserted through the lateral portal to allow an end-on approach to the distal clavicle. The speed of the power system is set to 5000 rpm or as high as possible. The tip of the Claviculizer burr is placed in the center of the exposed clavicle and drills into the bone until the depth-stop collar is reached. This creates a central clavicular socket of a premeasured depth (usually 1.25 to 1.5 cm) (Fig. 9-24). Since bone resection is very rapid, the arthroscopic pump is always

TABLE 9-1   Surgeon's Preference Card for Arthroscopic AC Joint Resection (Mumford Procedure)

Patient position: Standard lateral bursoscopy position
Draping: Shoulder arthroscopy drape
Electrocautery: Subacromial electrode tip
Traction: Standard shoulder arthroscopy 2-lb, 5-lb, & 10-lb weights
Special Equipment:
    Standard arthroscopy set-up
    18-gauge spinal needle (no. 2)
    Ruler
    Acromionizer burr (4.0 mm), full-radius shaver (4.5 mm)
    Arthroscopic pump
    Large outflow cannula with gravity drain connection
    Claviculizer system with 1.25-cm depth stop (Dyonics, Inc.)
    Large suction punch
Arthroscopic Solution: Synovisol (2.6% glycerol)
Wound Closure: 3-0 undyed Vicryl and Steri-strips
Dressing: 4 × 4s, ABDs, 3-in Micropore tape
Immobilization: Ultra Sling (DonJoy, Inc.)
Other: Polar Care ice water pad

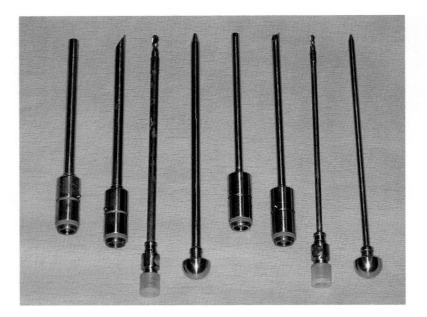

Figure 9-23
The Claviculizer set from Dyonics, Inc., includes large and small Stone Cutter burrs, each with a Claviculizer short sheath and an acromionizer hooded sheath, along with appropriate obturators.

used and adjusted for its maximum flow to clear bony debris. The initial central hole is progressively enlarged using circular motions of the Claviculizer, taking care to avoid medial penetration deeper than the depth-stop collar. The remaining clavicular cortex is used with the collar to judge the depth of resection (Fig. 9-25). On the anterior surface it is common to perforate the cortex, but this does not create a problem. Once the entire central portion of the clavicle has been hollowed, the edge of the

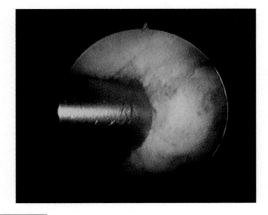

Figure 9-24
The first step in the Mumford procedure using the Claviculizer is to create a central hole in the clavicle to the depth of the Claviculizer sheath.

Claviculizer burr is used to remove the remaining cortex from the inside out, leaving only periosteum. A suction punch or an aggressive shaver inserted via the lateral portal removes the remaining soft tissue (Fig. 9-26).

It is often *not* possible to remove the superior cortex with the Claviculizer from the lateral portal, especially when a narrow joint is present with degenerative arthritis. Once the maximum possible amount of inferior clavicle has been removed, the resection is completed through the anterior portal. The Stone Cutter Burr is removed from the Claviculizer short sheath and placed in the acromionizer hooded sheath, which is included in the set. The acromionizer is then inserted through the anterior portal. The remaining superior portion is resected, beginning anterolaterally and extending posteriorly to a depth similar to that attained in the previously resected inferior clavicle (Fig. 9-27). Care should be taken to avoid amputating the superior segment medially before resecting the most lateral portion; this would create a free fragment of bone that would be more difficult to remove with the burr without damage to the superior capsule. At the completion of the resection, the entire end of the clavicle should be visible from the posterior and lateral portals (Fig. 9-28).

Finally, the inferior border of the clavicle

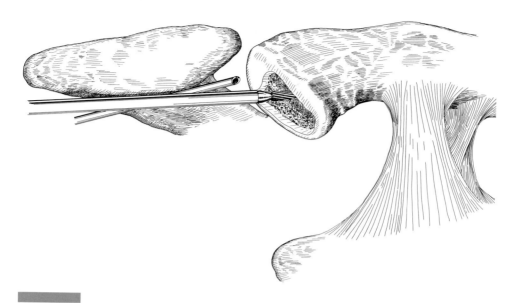

Figure 9-25
The clavicle is then hollowed out using a rotary motion of the Claviculizer

may be beveled from the lateral portal to prevent a sharp edge above the supraspinatus muscle. The final visualization via the anterior portal confirms the completeness of the resection, on both the acromial and clavicular sides, from anterior to posterior. Any spicules of cortex or rough edges can be noted and corrected using the acromionizer burr via the anterior portal while viewing from either posterior or lateral.

Several points of caution must be stressed about the use of the Claviculizer technique:

1. Since the instrument is very aggressive, it should be started in the center of the clavicle and advanced no farther than the depth-stop collar indicates.

2. Attempts should be made to keep the tip of the instrument perpendicular to the face of the clavicle.

Figure 9-26
The soft tissues remaining around the clavicle can be removed with a suction punch or a shaver.

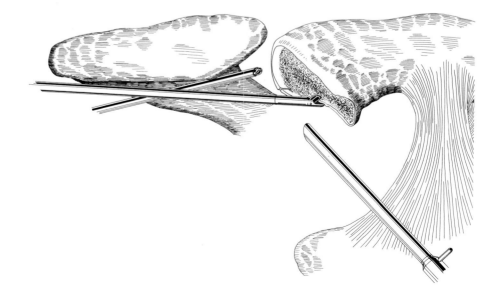

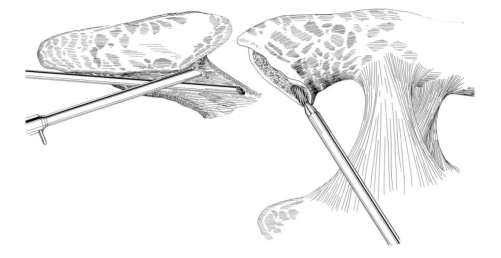

Figure 9-27
The superior rim of the
clavicle is removed using the
acromionizer sheath through
the anterior portal.

3. Penetration of the cortex by the tip of the instrument does not present a problem except on the superior surface, where a free fragment may be difficult to remove.

4. It is important to have a high-flow irrigation system to clean out the fragments of bone; the surgeon should allow adequate time to ensure clear visualization. A gravity outflow cannula is best for this purpose, along with a high-flow arthroscopic pump system.

5. We recommend *not* using suction on the Claviculizer or acromionizer blades during the resection, since it will often cause soft tissues to be wound around the burr. This requires frequent delays for cleaning.

Postoperative Treatment

After completing distal clavicle resection, at least for the first several cases, an x-ray

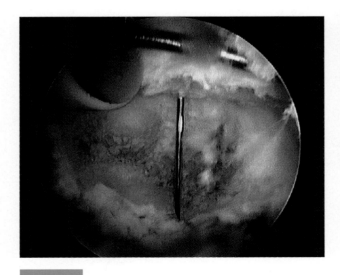

Figure 9-28
At the completion of the Mumford resection, the entire end of the distal clavicle should be easily seen from the posterior or lateral portal.

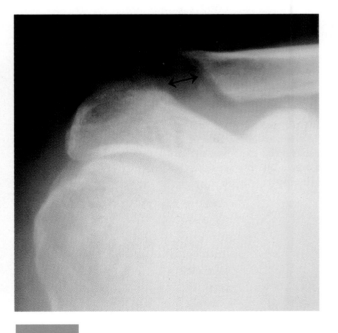

Figure 9-29
An x-ray should be taken in the operating room for the first few cases to assess the quality of the resection.

Figure 9-30
The Shoulder Therapy Kit (STK, from Breg, Inc.) contains an assortment of exercise equipment that the patient can use both at home and in physical therapy, along with an instruction booklet.

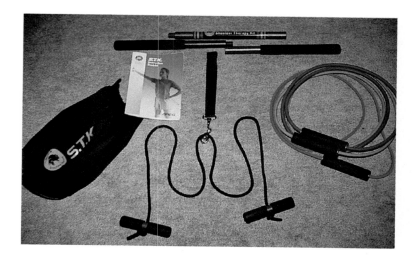

should be taken in the operating room prior to awakening the patient, to assess the completeness of the bony excision (Fig. 9-29). Once the technique has been mastered, a postoperative x-ray in the office is acceptable. The most frequent problem noted on the postoperative x-ray is a deficient resection of the superior cortex. Extra attention should be directed to this area during surgery. The wounds can be closed with subcutaneous sutures and Steri-strips and a padded compression dressing applied. Often we apply an ice water dispersion pad (Polar Care, Breg, Inc., Carlsbad, California) over a thin sterile cotton dressing. This greatly reduces the postoperative discomfort and is helpful especially if an interscalene block has not been used before surgery. An absorptive compression dressing is then applied over the Polar Care pad, and the arm is supported in a sling for comfort.

When the patient is alert, exercises are begun, using therapy putty for the grip along with elbow, wrist, and hand motion. Pendulum exercises are instituted within the first 24 h; after a dressing change the following day, gentle range-of-motion activities with an overhead pulley are begun. Our patients are given a shoulder therapy kit (STK, Breg, Inc.), with instructions, before surgery, to encourage early gentle mobilization of the shoulder even before a physical therapist is seen (Fig. 9-30). At 1 week after surgery the patient is seen in the office and usually sent to physical therapy to continue a shoulder mobiliza-

tion program. At 3 to 4 weeks, the patient usually has resumed most normal daily activities; but heavy shoulder activities are delayed until 2 to 3 months after surgery. A check x-ray is taken about 3 months after surgery to ensure that no regrowth of clavicle has occurred. Although a few small flakes of bone seem to occur postoperatively in some of our patients, we have never encountered any significant regrowth of the clavicle after the use of arthroscopic techniques.

Arthroscopic Reconstruction for a Complete AC Joint Dislocation (Modified Weaver-Dunn Procedure) (Table 9-2)

The decision whether to reconstruct the AC joint after a type III or IV dislocation may be difficult. The deformity may be quite significant but the surgeon and patient are often unwilling to risk the potential surgical complications and scar to alleviate the bony deformity (Fig. 9-31). Because the shoulder is suspended by the AC joint and the coracoclavicular ligaments, the shoulder will often droop, causing additional problems with upper extremity function. If the distal clavicle has buttonholed

TABLE 9-2   Surgeon's Preference Card for Modified Arthroscopic Weaver-Dunn Procedure

Patient position: Standard lateral bursoscopy position
Draping: Shoulder arthroscopy drape
Electrocautery: Subacromial electrode tip
Traction: Standard shoulder arthroscopy 2-lb, 5-lb, and 10-lb weights
Special Equipment:
    Standard arthroscopy set-up
    18-gauge spinal needle, 17-gauge epidural needle
    Ruler
    Acromionizer burr (4.5 mm)
    Arthroscopic pump
    Large outflow cannula with gravity drain connection
    Claviculizer system with 1.25-cm depth stop
    Large suction punch
    Shuttle Relay suture passing device (no. 4)
    Titanium Clavicular Washer Set (Mitek, Inc.) (optional)
    Suture anchor set (Mitek Super Anchors)
    Suture material for fixation (surgeon's preference: no. 8 Ethibond vs. no. 5 Ethibond)
    Arthroscopic suture punch (modified Caspari, Concept Inc., or Concept suture hooks)
Arthroscopic Solution: Synovisol (2.6% glycerol)
Wound Closure: 3-0 undyed Vicryl and Steri-strips
Dressing: 4 × 4s, ABDs, 3-in Micropore tape
Immobilization: Shoulder immobilizer with small abduction pillow (Ultra Sling, DonJoy, Inc.)
Other: Polar Care ice water pad

through the trapezius (type IV dislocation), pain and limited function are often present.

The surgeon faced with selecting a procedure to reconstruct a joint may choose from

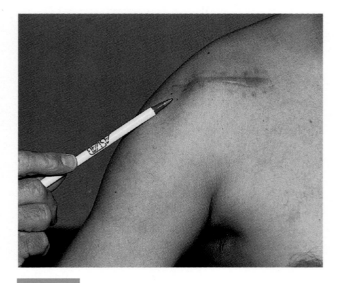

Figure 9-31
Sometimes the scar from an open distal clavicle stabilization can be unsightly.

myriad surgical procedures. Many of these procedures advocate reducing the joint and transfixing the AC articulation with pins. A long-term study by Smith and Steward demonstrated that 24 percent of patients who *did not* have distal clavicle excision with their AC joint reconstruction developed degenerative arthritis, versus 4.5 percent of patients who did have concomitant distal clavicle resection.[13] Other significant surgical complications include infections and hardware problems, particularly with fracture and migration of pins, wires, and screws. The use of a heavy clavicular-coracoid fixation screw has its proponents as well, but a second procedure is always necessary to remove this fixation, for fear of late complications of hardware failure and/or fracture[14] (Fig. 9-32).

In 1972, Weaver and Dunn first reported their procedure for treatment of acute and chronic complete AC joint dislocations. They advocated resecting the distal 2 cm of the clavicle and transferring the acromial end of the coracoacromial ligament into the resected end of the clavicle.[3] Later, because of a few

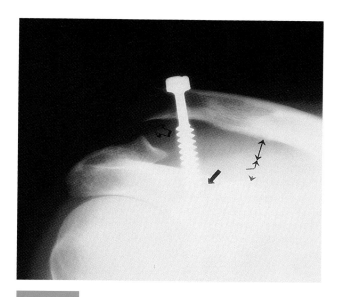

Figure 9-32
Many complications can occur with coracoclavicular screws that are not perfectly placed or that remain too long. This x-ray demonstrates the second unsuccessful trial for fixation using this technique.

cases of late loss of reduction, the procedure was modified to include a noose of three strands of braided PDS suture around the coracoid and through a clavicular drill hole.[15] Other authors favor this technique as well, reporting excellent results with no significant late complications[16,17] (Fig. 9-33). Although this operation seems to greatly improve the surgical results of AC joint reconstruction by eliminating the potential for arthritis and postoperative hardware complications, it requires a 3- to 4-in incision on the superior-anterior aspect of the shoulder, with removal of a portion of anterior deltoid and trapezius muscle for exposure. Thus the potential for postoperative problems with deltoid tendon reattachment, infection, and unsightly scar formation is present. We believe that if the Weaver-Dunn procedure can be performed arthroscopically, these potential problems will be eliminated. We have developed our technique in a step-by-step fashion.

The first step was to perfect the arthroscopic Mumford procedure. We have used all three of the arthroscopic techniques described in this chapter in more than 50 cases,

but prefer the speed and accuracy of the Claviculizer system.

The second step was harvesting the coracoacromial ligament from the undersurface of the acromion. Since we use the Subacromial Electrode (Concept, Inc.) to transect the coracoacromial ligament during subacromial decompression surgery, it seemed logical to use it to harvest the ligament too. We found that we could remove a large segment of the coracoacromial ligament from the undersurface of the acromion intact and dissect the remainder of the ligament carefully off the undersurface of the deltoid with a combination of the electrical cutter and a Liberator Elevator (Concept, Inc.) all the way to the tip of the coracoid process. We have used this technique as an adjunct to our open Weaver-Dunn procedure in 10 cases, obviating the need for releasing any deltoid from the acromion to harvest the ligament.

We believed it was necessary to be able to visualize the superior aspect of the coracoid process to allow placing a suture anchor to hold the coracoid and the acromion together while the transferred coracoacromial ligament was healing. After following the coracoacro-

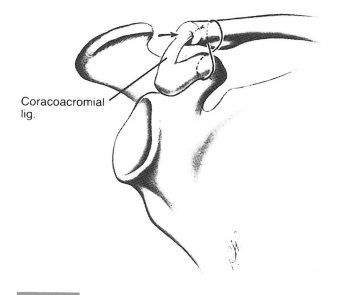

Figure 9-33
The Weaver-Dunn procedure is a well-accepted stabilization procedure for chronic, and sometimes acute, type III and IV AC joint dislocations.

mial ligament to the tip of the coracoid process, we proceeded to view along the superior lateral portion of the coracoid in a posteriomedial direction. We found that we were able to visualize the superior surface of the base of the coracoid. When the coracoclavicular ligaments were torn, a broad expanse of strong cortical bone was present that would easily accommodate our implantable fixation device. Since it would be extremely difficult to pass a loop of suture around the coracoid arthroscopically, it was necessary to deploy a device to anchor the sutures directly into the coracoid bone at the previous site of origin of the coracoclavicular ligament. In this way the tether effect of the fixation could be aligned in an anatomical manner in an inferior-to-superior direction, avoiding the anteriorly directed vector forces that occur with the usual coracoid loop techniques. When the four-arc suture anchor (Super Anchor, Mitek, Inc.) became available, we had the necessary fixation devices to complete our repair.

The strength of the coracoclavicular fixation was tested in the biomechanics lab at DonJoy Inc. (Carlsbad, California). Using cadaver shoulders with ruptured AC and CC ligaments, the anchors were inserted into the coracoid, and two strands of no. 5 Ethibond suture were passed through a clavicle drill hole, replicating the SCOI technique. The repair was tested to failure using an MTS machine. The system failed, with suture breakage near the knots, at an average force of 120 lb.

The final step was to solve the problem of passing a strong, permanent suture in a weave fashion, using multiple passes, through the tip of the coracoacromial ligament. This became possible when the Shuttle Relay (Concept, Inc.) was developed (see Chap. 12). This device permits us to make multiple passes of a strong permanent suture through the end of the coracoacromial ligament, thereby ensuring a firm hold on the ligament without sacrificing length or requiring multiple individual sutures. The Shuttle Relay can be passed through a modified Caspari Suture Punch (Concept, Inc.) or a straight or curved suture-

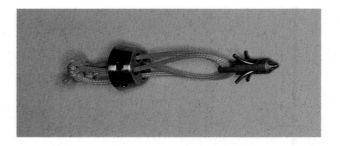

Figure 9-34
The Titanium Clavicular Washer (Mitek, Inc.) is an experimental device for fixing the coracoclavicular sutures to maintain the AC joint reduction when used in conjunction with a strong suture anchor in the coracoid process.

passing needle. The Shuttle Relay also serves as a leader, allowing us to pull the coracoacromial sutures through the end of the clavicle and out through the superior drill hole.

A final development to simplify the operation was the Titanium Clavicular Washer (Mitek, Inc.). This is a saucer-shaped titanium button that allows the surgeon to perform the entire operation using a transclavicular approach through a single drill hole (Fig. 9-34). The washer/anchor is then used as a central fixation point in the clavicle, allowing all sutures to be securely tied below the superior clavicular cortical surface while still avoiding undue stress concentrations, which later might lead to clavicular fracture. At the time of this writing, the Titanium Clavicular Washer is still experimental and available only for trial and testing purposes.

Technique for the Arthroscopic Modified Weaver-Dunn Procedure

The patient is positioned in the standard lateral position with the arm in the bursoscopy position, using 12 to 15 lb of distraction weight. A diagnostic arthroscopy and bursoscopy, and any necessary arthroscopic surgery, are performed.

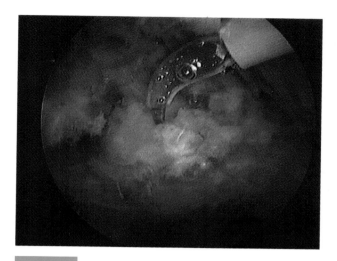

Figure 9-35
The Subacromial Electrode (Concept, Inc.) is used to harvest the coracoacromial ligament from the undersurface of the acromion and deltoid.

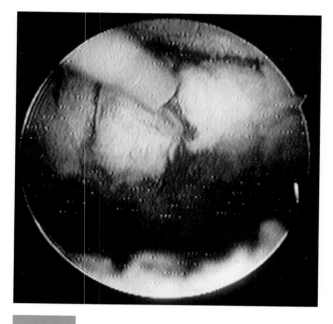

Figure 9-36
The electrosurgical tool is used to cut and morselize the scar tissue filling the previous AC joint.

Coracoacromial Ligament Resection and Decompression

The irrigating fluid should be nonconductive, like Synovisol (isosmolar glycerol from Baxter Travenol, Inc.). The Subacromial Electrode on the Concept electrosurgical pencil is inserted into the lateral insulated cannula to harvest the coracoacromial ligament. The tip of the electrode outlines the acromial attachment on the undersurface of the acromion, and the ligament is carefully resected off the bone (Fig. 9-35). At the anterior edge of the acromion, a small portion of the ligament is dissected from the undersurface of the deltoid. If a subacromial decompression is desired, it is performed at this point. It is important to bevel the acromial facet of the AC joint to allow excellent visualization of the distal clavicle. No sutures are placed in the coracoacromial ligament until later, to avoid their obstructing visualization during the early portions of the procedure.

Arthroscopic Mumford Procedure

Using the electrosurgical tool, again from the lateral portal, the scar tissue in the area of the previous AC joint is morselized (Fig. 9-36). An aggressive shaver is used through the lateral and anterior portals to remove the scar tissue and expose the end of the clavicle. Since the clavicle is in a dislocated position, it will be more difficult to expose than when performing the standard Mumford procedure. An assortment of instruments, including the electrosurgical cutter, an aggressive large-diameter shaver, and a large suction punch, are used as necessary. Once the fibrous scar is removed, the clavicular tip is exposed and can be easily visualized. Sometimes depressing the clavicle from above is helpful, but usually it is not necessary.

The standard arthroscopic Mumford procedure is performed using the surgeon's preferred method (see Mumford procedure, above). It is important to excise the clavicle in full-thickness fashion with the bone beveled inferiorly. The Claviculizer is also helpful to core out the center portion of the distal clavicle for an additional 1.5 cm once the resection has been completed (Fig. 9-37). This socket can be deepened a little more, or widened, as needed to accommodate the transferred coracoacromial ligament.

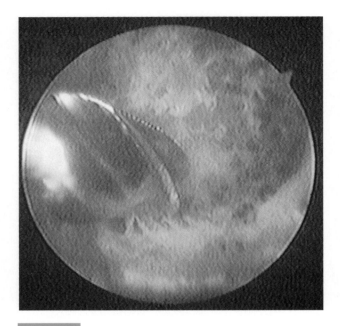

Figure 9-37
The Claviculizer is used to core out a socket 1.5 cm into the end of the resected clavicle.

Preparing the Coracoid

With the arthroscope in the posterior portal and the shaver in the lateral portal, the coracoacromial ligament is followed to the tip of the coracoid process. Often, but not always, this requires removing a portion of the anterior wall of the bursa. Once the tip of the coracoid is located, the arthroscope and shaver together follow the arc of the coracoid back to the base. The fragments of the torn coracoclavicular ligaments are easily recognized at the superior base of the coracoid process. Portions of these ligaments are removed from the bone to allow visualization for implantation of the suture anchors.

Insertion of Suture Anchors

A 1.5-cm incision is made from anterior to posterior over the superior aspect of the clavicle, approximately 4 cm medial from the excised tip. The electrosurgical tool is used to cut an X in the soft tissue on the midpoint of the superior clavicle, and an elevator is used to peel back the periosteum for exposure of the bone. The exact position for this incision can be judged by measuring the preoperative

x-ray to locate the site of the conoid tubercle on the clavicle. This position can then be located by measuring from either the acromial or the sternal end of the clavicle, whichever is easier to palpate. It is often better to expose the clavicle prior to beginning the arthroscopy, before significant swelling occurs.

A 4-mm drill hole is made in the center of the clavicle from superior to inferior through the full thickness, exiting near the conoid tubercle (Fig. 9-38). The appropriate drill chosen for the anchor is then passed through the 4-mm clavicular drill hole and down to the coracoid near the base. One or two holes are drilled in the coracoid directly beneath the clavicle while observing with the arthroscope (Fig. 9-39). If two holes are drilled, there should be a gap of at least 1 cm between them. Next, the cone-shaped reamer is used to contour the superior clavicular hole until it seats flush with the superior surface of the clavicle. If the Titanium Clavicular Washer is used, it should be inserted into the drill hole to test for a perfect fit. When the washer is seated, its upper edge should be flush with the

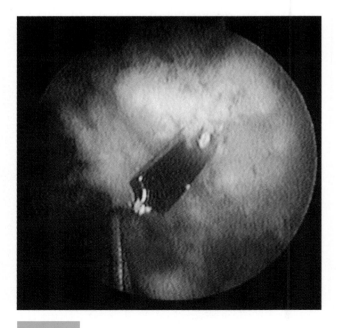

Figure 9-38
The first drill hold through the clavicle is made approximately 4 cm medial from the resected end of the clavicle.

The sutures are then threaded through the appropriate holes in the titanium washer. Suture pairs should pass through adjacent holes so that they do not criss-cross one another when tied.

Suturing the Coracoacromial Ligament

Since the end of the coracoacromial ligament has previously been released from the bone, it remains partially fixed to the deltoid muscle. Using a modified Caspari Punch or a 17-gauge epidural needle, a suture Shuttle Relay is passed through the tip of the ligament and removed using a grasper through a cannula in the anterior portal. A strand of no. 2 Ethibond suture placed in the eyelet of the Shuttle Relay is carried through the end of the ligament and out the anterior cannula (Fig. 9-41). This process is repeated two or three times, passing the tails of the original Ethibond suture with the shuttle. In this way, a strong woven stitch is formed that will resist pullout when traction is applied. Both tails of the suture are then pulled out the lateral portal.

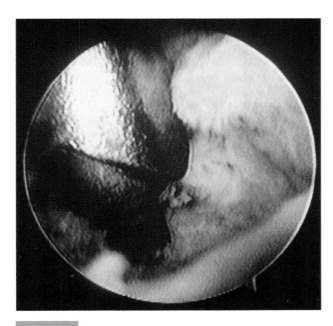

Figure 9-39
The coracoid drill hole or holes are made by using a long drill, with a depth stop, that passes directly through the initial hole in the clavicle.

superior cortex of the clavicle. After removing the washer, the Mitek Super Anchors (Fig. 9-40) are inserted. These should be preloaded with either one or two no. 5 permanent braided sutures. After seating the anchors, the suture is left passing out through the clavicular drill hole.

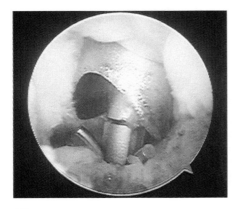

Figure 9-40
Suture anchors are preloaded with the fixation suture and then implanted into the coracoid under direct vision.

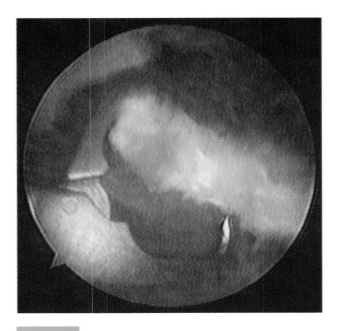

Figure 9-41
The Shuttle Relay suture-passing device is used with the Caspari punch to pass a no. 2 nonabsorbable braided suture through the coracoacromial ligament.

With the arthroscope posteriorly and the Liberator Elevator laterally, the coracoacromial ligament is carefully dissected off the inferior aspect of the deltoid muscle down to the coracoid attachment. The sutures in the end of the coracoacromial ligament help apply traction through the lateral portal which aids in this dissection. Often a few of the anteriormost fibers of the ligament must be released to achieve a straighter pull from the midpoint of the coracoid base to the inferior aspect of the distal clavicle.

When the ligament has been completely mobilized, a 17-gauge epidural needle is inserted through the drill hole in the superior aspect of the clavicle, exiting through the hollowed-out socket in the end of the clavicle. It will be necessary to use a small drill or K-wire first to create a hole for passage of the needle. A Shuttle Relay is passed through the epidural needle and retrieved with a grasper through the lateral cannula. Both ends of the coracoacromial ligament suture are placed in the eyelet of the Shuttle Relay, which is then pulled back out the superior clavicle, carrying

the end of the ligament into the clavicular socket and the suture tails out through the conical drill hole on the superior aspect of the clavicle (Fig. 9-40). The sutures are then passed through the appropriate holes of the titanium clavicular washer.

Reduction and Fixation of the Clavicle

The traction weight is removed from the patient's arm, and the sutures carefully pulled upward while the washer is seated into the clavicle. The washer should not be completely seated until the sutures are taut as visualized from below (Fig. 9-42). Also, the coracoclavicular ligament should be pulled snugly into the hole prepared in the tip of the clavicle. Finally, as the washer is seated, pressure is applied to the clavicle to hold it in a slightly overreduced position, so that the undersurface is about 6 to 7 mm away from the coracoid. The first suture is then tied securely, seating the knot within the concavity in the washer. The suture is palpated while visualizing it arthroscopically above the coracoid. The second suture is then tied in a similar fashion. The tension and security of the su-

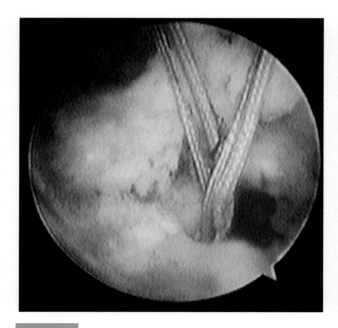

Figure 9-42
Four strands of no. 5 permanent Ethibond suture are fixed to the coracoid with an implantable anchor and passed through a drill hole in the bottom of the clavicle.

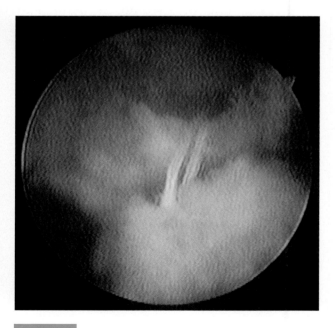

Figure 9-43
The coracoacromial ligament is pulled into the socket in the end of the clavicle.

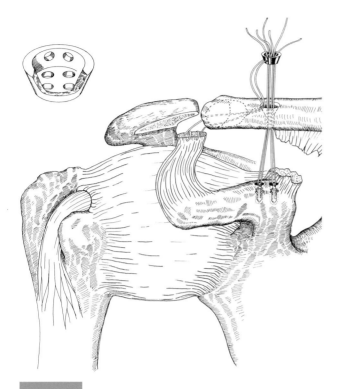

Figure 9-44
The arthroscopic Weaver-Dunn procedure reconstructs the torn coracoclavicular ligament using the transferred coracoacromial ligament and stabilizes the repair with strong, nonabsorbable sutures between the coracoid and the clavicle.

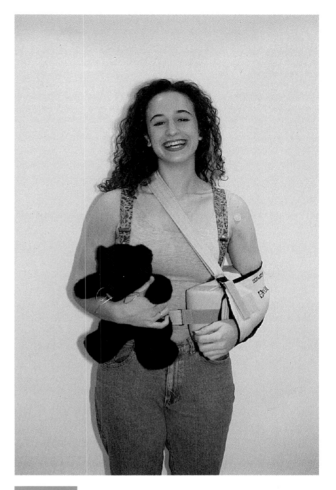

Figure 9-45
Postoperatively, the arm is supported in a pillow immobilizer which opens to allow exercise of the elbow, wrist, and hand, while still offering excellent comfortable support. (Ultra Sling, DonJoy, Inc., Carlsbad, California). The arm is held in neutral rotation, avoiding an internal rotation contracture, and the axilla is slightly open for air circulation.

tures are tested with a palpating probe. Traction is placed back on the arm to ensure that the fixation is solid. Lastly, the sutures holding the coracoacromial ligament are tensioned and tied, leading the ligament into the end of the clavicle (Figs. 9-43 and 9-44). The tension of the ligament is tested with a palpating probe. The suture tails are then cut and the skin closed with inverted subcutaneous sutures and Steri-strips.

An Alternative Technique
If a Titanium Clavicular Washer Set is not available, the preceding steps can still be used; but instead of reaming and inserting the washer superiorly, the sutures can be divided and one limb of each passed around the anterior clavicle. The sutures are then tied so that the knots are resting below the bone anteriorly. The coracoacromial ligament sutures are passed through the end of the clavicle using two drill holes rather than one, and the suture tails are tied over the intervening bony bridge.

Postoperative Care

A Polar Care (Berg, Inc., Carlsbad, California) portable ice pad is placed just outside a thin sterile cotton dressing and covered with absorptive cotton padding. The arm is supported in an immobilizer sling, preferably with a

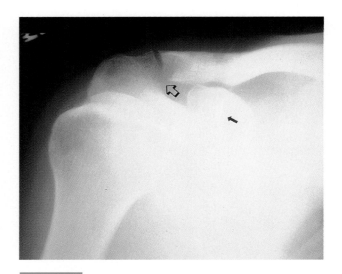

Figure 9-46
A postoperative x-ray following an arthroscopic Weaver-Dunn procedure shows the suture anchor to be in good position in the coracoid and the superior surface of the clavicle to be well reduced and in line with the top of the acromion.

small pillow to prevent immobilization of the arm in excess internal rotation (Ultra Sling, DonJoy, Inc., Carlsbad, California)(Fig. 9-45). Usually no abduction brace is needed. An x-ray should be taken postoperatively to document the coracoclavicular distance and assess and record the positions of the anchors (Fig. 9-46).

Elbow, wrist, and hand exercises are started immediately, but the Ultra Sling is maintained for 3 weeks to allow the soft tissues to heal. At 3 weeks passive elevation is begun; after that, progressive active exercises are begun by 6 weeks. No strenuous exercise is allowed for approximately 4 months. A check x-ray should be made about 3 months after surgery.

Discussion

Since there have been no long-term follow-ups of this modified arthroscopic Weaver-Dunn procedure, either with or without the titanium washer, it should be considered an experimental operation. The potential problems of this procedure include premature suture failure or anchor pullout, coracoid or clavicular fracture, and foreign body reaction or infection to the implants. This procedure is extremely demanding technically; any surgeon intending to attempt it should first practice it in a laboratory setting.

References

1. Taft TN, Wilson FC, Oglesby JW: Dislocation of the acromioclavicular joint. *J Bone Joint Surg* 69A:1045, 1987.

2. Tibone J, Sellers R, Tonino P: Strength testing after third-degree acromioclavicular dislocations. *Am J Sports Med* 20:328, 1992.

3. Weaver JK, Dunn HK: Treatment of acromioclavicular injuries, especially complete acromioclavicular separation. *J Bone Joint Surg* 54A:1187, 1972.

4. Rockwood CA, Matsen MA: *The Shoulder.* Philadelphia, Saunders, 1990.

5. Dupas J, Badelon P, Dayae G: Aspects radiologiques d'un osteolyse essentielle progressive de la main gauche. *J Radiol* 20:383, 1936.

6. Cahill BR: Osteolysis of the distal part of the clavicle in male athletes. *J Bone Joint Surg* 64:1053, 1982.

7. Fukuda K, Craig EV, Kai-Nan A, et al: Biomechanical study of the ligamentous system of the acromioclavicular joint. *J Bone Joint Surg* 68A:434, 1986.

8. DePalma AF: *Surgery of the Shoulder.* Philadelphia, Lippincott, 1983, 3rd ed.

9. Mink JH, Deutsch AL: *MRI of the Musculoskeletal System: A Teaching File.* Raven Press, New York, 1990.

10. Hodler J, Kursunoglu-Brahme S, Snyder S, et al: Rotator cuff disease: Assessment with MR arthrography versus standard MR imaging in 36 patients with arthroscopic confirmation. *J Radiol* 182:431, 1992.

11. Gartsman GM, Combs AH, Davis PF, Tullos HS: Arthroscopic acromioclavicular joint resection: An anatomic study. *Am J Sports Med* 19:2, 1991.

12. Snyder SJ: Arthroscopic acromioclavicular joint debridement and distal clavicle resection. *Tech Orthop* 3:41, 1988.

13. Smith MJ, Steward MJ: Acute acromioclavicular separations. A 20-year study. *Am J Sports Med* 7:52, 1979.

14. Rockwood CA, Williams JR, Young DC: Injuries to the acromioclavicular joint, in Rockwood CA, Green DP, Bucholz RW (eds): *Fractures in Adults.* Philadelphia, Lippincott, 1991, pp 1181–1251.

15. Weaver JK: Grade III coracoclavicular separation. Orthop Consultation, Oct. 1984, p 7.

16. Neer CS: Cuff tears, biceps lesions and impingement, in *Shoulder Reconstruction.* Philadelphia, Saunders, 1990, pp 41–142.

17. Rauschning W, Nordesjo L, Nordgren B et al: Resection arthroscopy for repair of complete acromioclavicular separations. *Arch Orthop Traumat Surg* 97:161, 1980.

10

Labral Lesions (Non-Instability) and SLAP Lesions

Introduction

The anatomy and function of the glenoid labrum has been a source of considerable confusion for arthroscopic shoulder surgeons. The labrum consists of a ring of fibrous tissue with interposed elastic fibers that encircle the articular face of the glenoid (Fig. 10-1). The attachment of the labrum centrally blends with the articular cartilage surface, while peripherally it is joined by the fibrous tissue of the capsule and capsular ligaments. A fibrocartilage "intra zone" can be seen variably in the posterior, superior, and anterior labrum, but is rarely seen inferiorly. A free inner edge of the labrum, which may or may not be present, may give it a "meniscoid" appearance, which can be confused with pathological detachment (Fig. 10-2). This meniscus-like appearance most commonly occurs superiorly, but may also be seen anteriorly and posteriorly, and infrequently along the inferior labral

Figure 10-1
The glenoid labrum usually forms a complete circle attached peripherally to the rim of the glenoid cavity. The capsule and ligaments attach directly to the labrum; in some instances the middle ligament attaches just medial to the labrum on the neck of the glenoid.

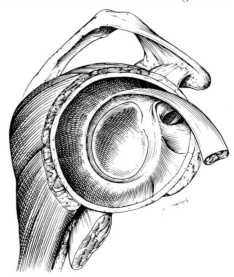

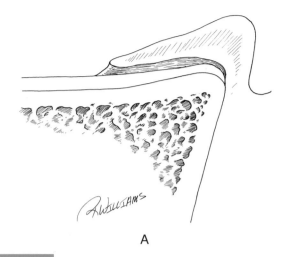

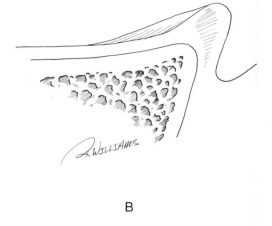

A

B

Figure 10-2

Two types of labral attachment can occur. *A.* The meniscoid-type labrum is found most frequently in the superior quadrant, but also may be found anterior or posterior. The portion of the labrum overhanging the articular surface has a leaf-like free edge resembling the meniscus of the knee. The ligaments attach at the periphery of this "meniscus" and then to the glenoid, around the corner from the articular surface. *B.* The more common situation occurs when the ligaments and capsular tissue insert directly into the labrum, which is continuous with the articular surface at the edge of the glenoid, with no free edge of labrum overhanging the articular surface.

attachment. When present, this meniscoid-type labrum is thought to be normal unless there are splits or fragmentation of the overhanging tissue, which can cause catching and joint irritation. Additionally, it is thought that in the normal shoulder there is always a smooth transition between the articular cartilage and the capsular attachment to the bone below the meniscoid labrum; unless this transition is disturbed, it is thought to be normal (Fig. 10-3).

In a series of 21 adult cadaver dissections, we reviewed the cross-sectional anatomy of the labrum in various positions around the joint. The inferior labrum had the most consistent appearance: triangular in shape, with a consistently attached central edge. The posterior labrum was similarly triangular, but occasionally had an unattached inferior surface that overlaid the glenoid cartilage. The anterior labrum was typically attached both centrally and peripherally, but did not have the triangular cross-sectional appearance. Instead it appeared as a thickened band of capsule still distinguishable from the rest of the capsule, both microscopically and macroscopi-

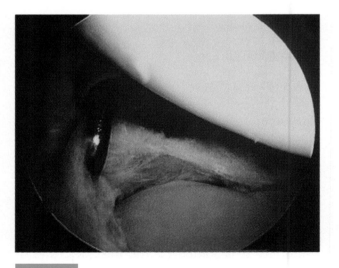

Figure 10-3

The meniscoid superior labrum is very commonly seen and should not be confused with a pathological SLAP lesion, but may be a predisposing anatomic factor in type III and IV SLAP lesions.

cally. The superior labrum was consistently attached peripherally, often around the corner from the glenoid face, but often had a free central edge of a varying degree.[1]

Biomechanical Considerations of the Labrum

The shoulder joint has more freedom of movement than any other joint in the body. Since the glenoid is a very shallow concave socket and the humeral head is much larger and hemispherical, there is little stability provided by the bony anatomy. Therefore, it is the soft tissues associated with the glenohumeral joint—specifically, the labrum, the capsular ligaments, and the muscle-tendon units—that afford the joint stability. The labrum encircling the glenoid socket increases its depth, and therefore increases the stability of the humeral head. The diameter of the glenoid surface is increased in the vertical plane to 75 percent of that of the humeral head; in the transverse direction it is approximately 57 percent. Both Reeves[2] and Perry[3] have demonstrated that the bonding strength of the fibrous labrum to the glenoid neck increases with skeletal maturity. At a younger age (less than 25 years) the bonding strength of the labrum is less than that of the capsule proper and the subscapularis tendon; therefore, dislocations tend to disrupt the labral-glenoid bond. As the tissues mature with age, the bonding strength increases, making failure at the labrum (Bankart lesion) less likely.

Two recent studies have shed more light on the contact areas of the labrum during various types of motion. Karzel et al.[4] demonstrated that when the cadaver shoulder was abducted 90 degrees and a compressive load applied, the labrum affected the distribution of the contact stresses. The posterior inferior labrum seemed to absorb most of the stress in this position, much as a meniscus does in the knee joint. Perhaps this is why the posterior labrum is uniformly strong and triangular in shape, as opposed to the anterior labrum.

Impingement of the superior labrum has been demonstrated in another cadaver study by Jobe.[5] In this study, cadaver specimens were positioned in 70 degrees of abduction and maximum external rotation, and then fixed with formalin. The fixation caused a permanent impression on both sides of the joint where the bone contacted the labrum (Fig. 10-4). On the glenoid side, the posterior superior labrum was compressed and distorted by the tuberosity and the interposed rotator cuff. With concomitant anterior instability, the posterior labral impingement appeared to worsen, perhaps giving rise to the posterior labral lesions seen in throwers along with tearing of the articular side rotator cuff.

A study of the vascularity of the labrum was performed by Burkhead et al., of Houston, Texas.[6] They showed that the vascular supply to the labrum was very rich and abundant around the entire glenoid, with the exception of the superior labrum. This may also help explain why the superior labrum is known to deteriorate with advancing age.[7] In addition, this poor superior vascularity may help explain the genesis of the SLAP lesions (injury to the superior *l*abrum from *a*nterior to *p*osterior). If a poor healing environment exists in this area, the tissues may tend not to heal after a traumatic event or repetitive microtrauma. The superior labrum and biceps anchor may then be detached, forming the pathological entity referred to as a SLAP lesion.[1,8]

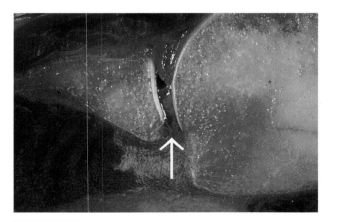

Figure 10-4
The posterior labrum and cuff can be injured by compression of these tissues between the glenoid and the greater tuberosity when the arm is in the "throwing position," as demonstrated in this cadaver specimen (*arrow*). (*Reprinted, with permission, from Ref. 5.*)

Patterns of Labral Injury

Since the labrum functions as a load-sharing structure with the glenoid, and also as a point for ligamentous attachment around the shoulder, it can be assumed that there are several potential mechanisms of injury caused by overload in these situations from a biomechanical standpoint. Therefore, compression, avulsion, shear, traction, and chronic attritional changes can occur. These injuries can occur either alone or in combinations resulting in complex patterns of labral pathology. For convenience in describing these patterns, the labrum is arbitrarily divided into six areas: (1) the superior labrum, (2) the anterior labrum above the midglenoid notch, (3) the anterior labrum below the midglenoid notch, (4) the inferior labrum, (5) the posterior inferior labrum, and (6) the posterior superior labrum. Like a meniscus tear in the knee, the tear pattern noted by the arthroscopic surgeon can be described as follows: degenerative lesion, flap tears, split non-detached tears, bucket-handle tears, and SLAP lesions.

Degenerative Lesions

A degenerative lesion appearing as a breakdown of the fibrous glenoid labrum may be representative of the continuum of degenerative joint disease. DePalma[7] suggests that, particularly in the superior labrum, this is a normal finding associated with the natural aging process of the shoulder. Acceleration of joint degeneration can occur from chronic joint abuse, particularly with repetitive compression overload. As the smooth gliding surfaces of the uninjured labrum give way to roughened irregular fibrous elements, an abrasive action may occur. This may cause injury to the adjacent humeral head articular cartilage, resulting in a kissing lesion of chondromalacia (Fig. 10-5). Alternatively, the degenerative changes in the humeral head may predispose to breakdown of the adjacent labrum, with a vicious circle resulting in progressive degeneration.

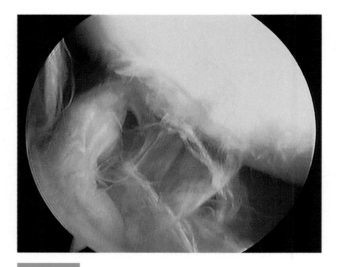

Figure 10-5
Labral damage is frequently associated with chondromalacia of the humeral head and may be a part of an ongoing degenerative process.

Flap Tears

Flap tears of the labrum are the most common pattern of acute or subacute injury noted. Most flap tears are seen in the posterior supe-

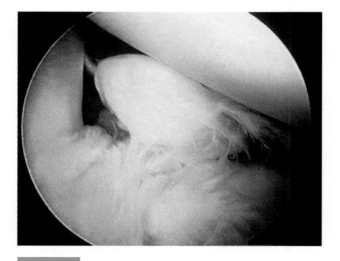

Figure 10-6
A large flap tear of the anterior labrum was causing symptoms resembling those of a loose body or subluxation of the shoulder. The diagnosis was suggested on MRI, and the lesion successfully treated by arthroscopic resection.

rior segment of the labrum, but they may be found in any location. A flap tear, like its counterpart in the meniscus, usually has a fairly broad base with a free edge corresponding to a radial tear (Fig. 10-6). The etiology of the flap lesion is not certain, but it seems often to be associated with chronic shear stress on the shoulder, such as with throwing. Perhaps the impingement of the posterior superior labrum by the greater tuberosity noted by Jobe[5] causes the typical posterior labral flap tears and fraying seen in throwers.

Vertical Split Labral Tears (Including Bucket-Handle Lesions)

The most dramatic, albeit the least common, type of anterior or posterior labral lesions is a vertical split labral tear. This may be a complete vertical disruption of labral fibers, creating a displaceable fragment, or an incomplete rent (Fig. 10-7). In order for this lesion to occur, a meniscoid-type labrum must be present overlying the glenoid surface. Since this occurs most frequently superiorly, a SLAP lesion (described below) is a common result. Otherwise, anterior and posterior vertical splits may be seen; a vertical labral tear is seldom found in the inferior labrum.

The etiology of these tears is thought to be compression injury to the joint surface, causing pinching of the labral tissue between the articular surfaces of the humeral head and the bony glenoid. This may occur from a fall on the outstretched arm or perhaps from an episode of hyperotation causing compression of the anterior or posterior labrum. The symptom complex resulting from this lesion may be that of pseudo-instability[9] with locking and catching and, sometimes, quite dramatic popping. If the fragment is not displaced, then joint irritation with painful activities is present. Seldom does pain occur at rest.

On clinical examination the findings are remarkably few. If a displaceable fragment is present then it may be trapped with a rotation compression test of the shoulder. This maneuver can be best performed in the supine position with the arm held in 90 degrees of abduction while applying a joint compression load to the shoulder. This maneuver, like McMurray's test in the knee, tends to accentuate pain and snapping in the shoulder when the arm is taken through a range of motion while maintaining the compression. Instability problems with the shoulder should be specifically sought during this exam, using apprehension, suppression, anterior and posterior translation tests (drawer testing), and the sulcus sign of inferior instability (see Chap. 12). A bucket-handle tear of the anterior or posterior labrum may be associated with clinical instability, but this is not a common finding.

Radiological imaging of the shoulder with a vertical labral tear is best accomplished using either a CT arthrogram or an MRI scan with gadolinium-enhanced image[10,11] (Fig. 10-8). The images are frequently mistaken for those of anterior instability; the pattern of capsular insertion into the labrum should be carefully evaluated.

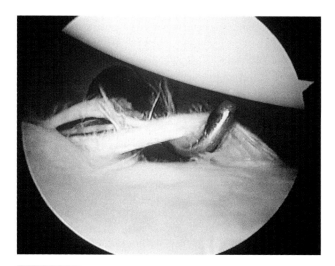

Figure 10-7
A bucket-handle tear of the anterior superior labrum is quite rare, but can cause considerable symptoms without true instability.

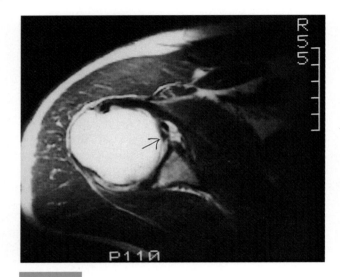

Figure 10-8
An MRI scan, particularly with intra-articular gadolinium enhancement, is often valuable in demonstrating labral pathology.

Treatment of Vertical Labral Tears

Treatment of vertical labral tears is very straightforward when they are not associated with instability. The anterior lesion is best visualized via the posterior portal. If the labral fragment is quite small, it can easily be removed using a 4.5-mm motorized shaver through the anterior superior portal. Larger fragments can be treated with resection similar to that for meniscal surgery. A small arthroscopic basket punch inserted through the anterior operating cannula can resect first the inferior attachment. The proximal attachment can then be grasped with a clamp and usually, by rotating it while maintaining a firm grasp, will avulse cleanly. The shaver is then used to complete the debridement and smooth the edges. Posterior lesions can be removed in a similar fashion while visualizing through the anterior portal and operating through the posterior portal.

A diagnostic dilemma arises when the vertical tear is not complete. The surgeon must decide whether removal of the central fragment will cause an instability problem. It has been my experience that this seldom happens if the labrum is of the meniscoid type, since the torn portion is redundant and not the true capsular attachment. Careful probing of the ligament's attachment while visualizing from the ipsilateral portal is the best assurance of capsular integrity. Video-recorded documentation in this situation is advised for future reference. Altchek et al. recently reviewed a group of 40 athletes followed a minimum of 2 years after labral debridement.[12] Forty percent of their group had instability on examination at surgery; 72 percent reported relief during the first postoperative year. At 2 years, 72 percent had symptoms.

Andrews described a lesion of the shoulder in high-level throwing athletes[13] that occurs in the anterior and superior labrum with associated avulsion and fraying of the labral tissues. This lesion was noted in 73 elite throwing athletes. Sometimes it involved a portion of the biceps tendon as well. The postulated mechanism of injury in these patients was traction to the anterior superior labrum by the long head of the biceps tendon during the deceleration phase of throwing. Some of these patients had partial rotator cuff tears in addition to their labral injuries. The lesion was treated by arthroscopic debridement of the loose fragments of the labrum, cuff, and biceps tendon, followed by a vigorous rotator cuff and throwing rehabilitation program. Andrews reported that 88 percent of these patients returned to a high level of throwing for at least one additional season following their rehabilitation.

SLAP Lesions of the Shoulder

An interesting pattern of injuries encompassing the superior aspect of the glenoid labrum and biceps tendon anchor was noted during the course of diagnostic shoulder arthroscopy. Since the superior labrum (defined as the segment between the 10 o'clock and 2 o'clock positions on the glenoid) is replete with anatomical variations, it requires extensive study and documentation to determine which elements of the anatomy were normal variants and which were truly pathological. Four distinct but related situations emerge that have been classified as SLAP lesions.

Definition of a SLAP Lesion[1,8]

A SLAP lesion is defined as an injury of the superior *l*abrum from *a*nterior to *p*osterior (in relation to the biceps tendon anchor).

Classification of SLAP Lesions

Type I lesion: Fraying and degeneration of the superior labrum with normal biceps tendon anchor (Fig. 10-9).

Type II lesion: Possible fraying of the superior labrum with pathologic detachment of the labrum and biceps anchor from the superior glenoid (Fig. 10-10).

Type III lesion: Vertical tear through a meniscoid-like superior labrum producing a bucket-

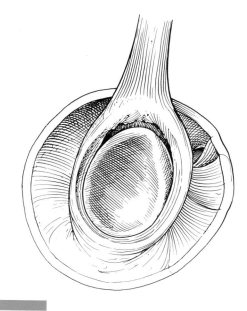

Figure 10-10
In a type II SLAP lesion the superior labrum and the biceps tendon anchor have been torn away from the superior glenoid attachment.

handle lesion which may displace into the glenohumeral joint. The biceps anchor remains intact (Fig. 10-11).

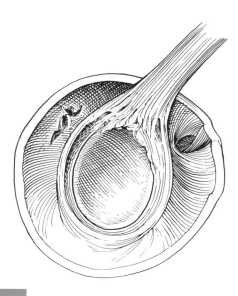

Figure 10-9
A type I SLAP lesion has fraying of the superior labrum with solid biceps tendon attachment.

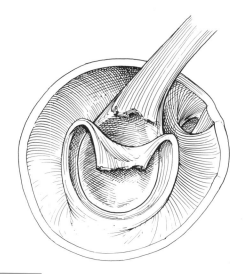

Figure 10-11
A type III SLAP lesion includes a vertical tear through the superior labrum, causing a bucket-handle fragment that can displace into the joint. The biceps anchor remains well attached.

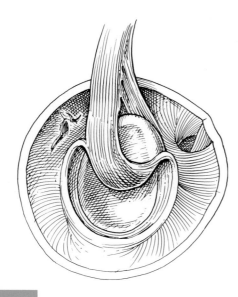

Figure 10-12
In a type IV SLAP lesion a bucket-handle tear of the superior labrum extends into the biceps tendon. This may also be associated with instability of the remaining biceps anchor and may be classified asa complex type II and IV lesion.

Type IV lesion: A tear of the superior meniscoid-like labrum which extends into the biceps tendon. The biceps anchor and remainder of the superior labrum are well attached (Fig. 10-12).

Complex lesion: A combination of two or more of the other SLAP lesions. Usually this consists of a type II and a type IV lesion.

The type I SLAP lesion is usually the most benign (Fig. 10-13). This may be seen as a component of an early degenerative glenohumeral joint disease in a middle-aged or older individual. When the superior labrum is degenerative in the younger individual, it may be considered the primary pathology and may contribute to the symptom complex. Treatment of a type I lesion is simply to shave the degenerative tissue to remove any source of joint irritation and possible catching. The shaving is best performed through the standard anterior superior and posterior superior arthroscopic portals. Care must be taken to avoid damage to the remaining superior labrum and the biceps anchor.

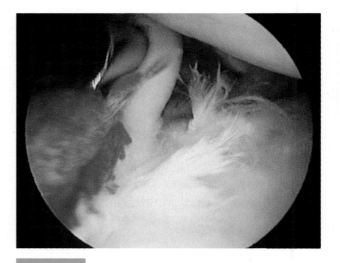

Figure 10-13
The type I SLAP lesion may be seen as part of the degenerative process of aging and is not always secondary to acute trauma.

The type II lesion is, in my opinion, the most-often-overdiagnosed type of SLAP lesion. Since the superior labrum may have a meniscoid-like appearance with a free inner edge, it may give the illusion of being pathologically loose (see Fig. 10-3). In an acute traumatic situation there is little doubt about the diagnosis, since the hemorrhagic labral tissue is easily recognized (Fig. 10-14). In a chronic situation, on the other hand, the natural healing tendency of the avulsed tissues may conceal the pathological etiology. As with Bankart lesions of the anterior labrum, the denuded bone below the avulsed labrum may appear smooth and may be covered with fibrous tissue. The articular cartilage of the superior glenoid in the normal shoulder extends to the labrum attachment. In a SLAP lesion there is a space between the articular cartilage margin and the attachment of the labrum and biceps anchor. Additionally, when traction applied to the biceps tendon causes the superior labral mechanism to arch away from the underlying bone more than 3 to 4 mm, the integrity of the labral and biceps anchor attachment should be questioned (Fig. 10-15). Often this disruption is noted in conjunction with an anterior dislocation of the shoulder. According to Rodosky et al.,[14] the disruption of the supe-

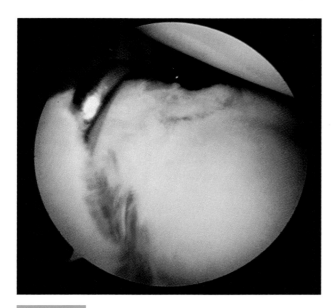

Figure 10-14
An acute type II SLAP lesion resembles an acute Bankart lesion of the anterior shoulder, with hemorrhage below the detached labrum.

rior biceps and labral attachment mechanism (type II SLAP lesion) leads to increased stress in the anterior inferior capsular and labral attachments, which may contribute to the anterior instability pattern.

Radiological diagnosis of a SLAP lesion has been difficult. Arthrogram, ultrasound, and CT scans cannot reliably demonstrate a superior labral tear. On occasion the MRI scan—especially with gadolinium enhancement—demonstrates a pathological cleft below the labrum (Fig. 10-16). Unfortunately, false-positive readings are common; the surgeon should not rely on the MRI reading alone as the reason for surgery.

Treatment of a type II lesion is similar to that for reattachment of the anterior labrum and capsule in instability surgery. Initially we believed that simply debriding the interposed fibrous membrane and decorticating the superior glenoid neck would incite a fibrovascular healing response adequate to restore the integrity of the anchor. It is now thought that this simple mechanism is not adequate and that attempts should be made to fixate the labral tissues in a juxtaposed position to the bone to ensure solid bonding.

Several authors have reported their cases of SLAP lesion repair. Savoie and Field[15] repaired 20 patients with type II and IV injuries

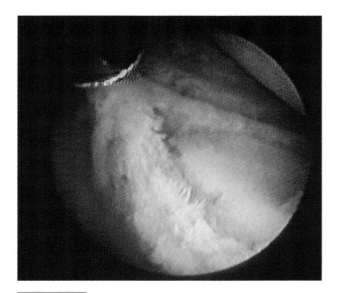

Figure 10-15
In a type II SLAP lesion the labrum arches away from the superior glenoid when traction is applied or the biceps muscle is stimulated to contract.

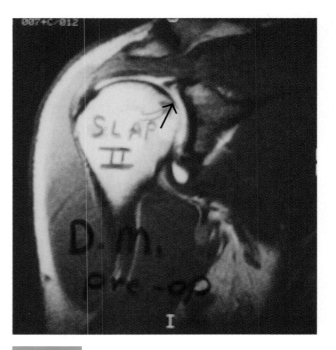

Figure 10-16
The MRI scan with intra-articular gadolinium enhancement may reveal a type II SLAP lesion (*arrow*).

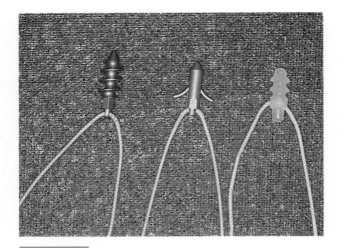

Figure 10-17
The three anchors we prefer for refixation of the type II SLAP lesion are (left to right) the Revo screw, the G2 Mitek Anchor, and the BioTak absorbable anchor (see text).

and found that all 10 lesions had healed solidly. Good and excellent results were reported in 80 percent of patients at 24 months, with failures caused by additional unrelated pathology.

At SCOI, we initially attempted to fixate the type II SLAP lesions with an absorbable polylactide BioTak. The procedure was difficult because of the acute angle of insertion, and the tack often fractured. Our present technique is much easier and uses an implantable bone anchor with strong nonabsorbable braided suture. The three anchors we prefer are the absorbable BioTak suture anchor (Concept, Inc., Largo, Florida), the 4-mm Revo titanium suture anchor screw (Concept, Inc., Largo, Florida), and the titanium G2 suture anchor (Mitek, Inc., Norwood, Massachusetts) (Fig. 10-17). (At the time of this writing, the BioTak suture anchor is experimental.)

using a trans-glenoid suture fixation technique and absorbable monofilament suture. At an average of 21 months, all patients were rated as good or excellent. In a study from Japan, 10 young athletes with type II SLAP lesions were treated by Yoneda et al. with abrasion and arthroscopic staple fixation.[16] The authors performed a second arthroscopic evaluation at 3 to 6 months for staple removal

Technique for Arthroscopic Fixation of type II SLAP Lesions (Table 10-1)

The arthroscope is kept in the standard posterior portal for viewing throughout the proce-

TABLE 10-1   Surgeon's Preference Card for Repair of Type II SLAP Lesions

1. Patient position: Lateral decubitus with bean bag
2. Standard arthroscopy set-up and instruments
3. Irrigating fluid: Synovisol
4. Arthroscopic fluid pump and cannulae
5. Shaver blades:
     4.5-mm full-radius shaver
     4.0-mm ball burr
6. Cannulae: No. 2 6-mm operating cannulae with fluid diaphragm
7. Power drill
8. Suture anchor set: Revo, Mitek G2, or BioTak
9. Arthroscopic knot-pushing device
10. 17-gauge 6-in epidural needle
11. Suture: No. 2 Ethibond
12. Dressings:
     Steri-strips
     4×4s
     ABD pads
13. Postoperative immobilization: Shoulder immobilizer—preferably with a small pillow (Ultra Sling, DonJoy, Carlsbad, California)

dure. Two anterior portals are needed to perform the repair. The anterior superior portal is developed using the transarticular rod technique. This portal is located directly anterior to the biceps tendon. This position is ideal for inserting anchors and suture needles through the anterior surface of the biceps tendon and the superior labrum. A plastic operating cannula with a flow-restricting diaphragm is useful to control fluid while still allowing instrument passage. A second anterior portal is created, using the outside-in technique, approximately 2 cm inferior to the first portal. A blunt-tipped obturator is used to insert a second plastic operating cannula at the level of the superior edge of the subscapularis tendon.

The soft-tissue shaver is inserted through the superior cannula to debride the fibrous membrane over the superior glenoid neck.

Frayed and fragmented portions of the labrum and biceps anchor are also debrided conservatively. A 4.0-mm ball-shaped burr is used to decorticate the exposed bone beneath the biceps anchor and superior labrum (Fig. 10-18). Care should be taken, when abrading, to avoid any damage to the articular cartilage. A pilot hole can be made with the burr at the exact location where the suture anchor is to be planted, directly below the biceps tendon (Fig. 10-19). This hole serves as a target to ensure perfect positioning of the drill hole and prevent skiving when drilling at an acute angle. An arthroscopic drill bit is then inserted through the anterior superior cannula and positioned in the pilot hole adjacent to the articular cartilage, just below the biceps tendon anchor point. The drill is inserted to its hub at a 45-degree angle away from the articular cartilage (Fig. 10-20). A suture anchor loaded with a no. 1 or no. 2 braided permanent suture is inserted via the superior cannula into the predrilled anchor hole below the biceps anchor and impacted or screwed into place (Fig. 10-21).

A crochet hook inserted through the midglenoid anterior portal retrieves one or both limbs of the suture out that cannula (there is less possibility for the suture to become twisted if only one limb at a time is retrieved

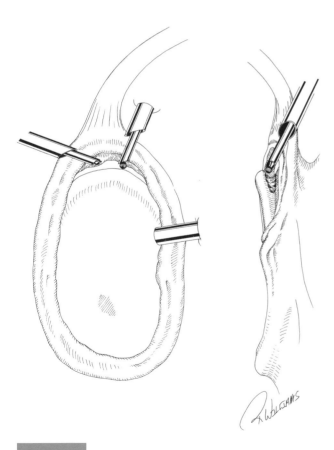

Figure 10-18
The abrasion of the superior glenoid is performed through the anterior superior portal using a high-speed ball burr.

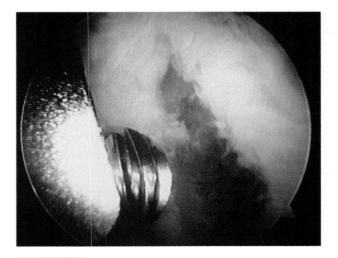

Figure 10-19
A pilot hole is created just below the articular cartilage using the 4-mm ball burr.

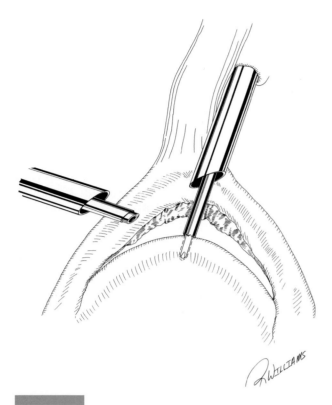

Figure 10-20
A miniature drill guide may be used to direct the drill into the superior glenoid just below the biceps tendon.

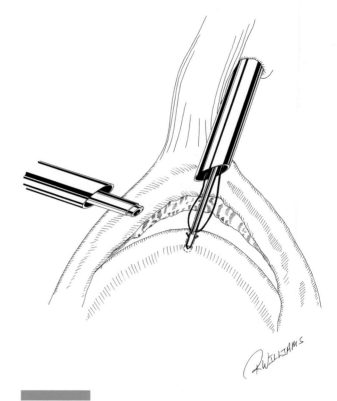

Figure 10-21
The suture anchor, preloaded with a strong, nonabsorbable braided suture, is inserted through the anterior superior cannula into the predrilled anchor hole.

out the mid-glenoid cannula (Fig. 10-22). A 6-in 17-gauge epidural needle is inserted through the anterior superior cannula and pierces the biceps and labral anchor near the anterior edge. The stylet is removed and a suture Shuttle Relay is inserted into the needle passing through the tissues and into the joint. A clamp grasps the shuttle through the lower anterior cannula, the needle is removed, and the shuttle is pulled out below (Figs. 10-23 and 10-24). One limb of the suture is threaded through the eyelet of the shuttle and carried, with the shuttle, back through the biceps and labral anchor and out the anterior superior cannula.

The epidural needle is reinserted through the anterior superior cannula, piercing the labrum and biceps anchor approximately 8 mm from the first puncture site. A second suture Shuttle Relay is passed in a similar manner and retrieved anteriorly, and the second

limb of the permanent suture is withdrawn through the biceps labral tissues and out the anterior superior cannula (Fig. 10-25). The two limbs of the suture are then tied together, using a knot-pushing device through the anterior superior cannula (Fig. 10-26). Care should be taken to ensure that the knots seat snugly on the anterior surface of the biceps tendon, so that the labrum and biceps anchor are held firmly apposed to the underlying bone (Fig. 10-27). A minimum of five single knots should be used for security before the suture tails are cut and removed. A palpating probe should test the integrity of the repair (Fig. 10-28).

If the superior labral detachment is quite large, then additional anchors may be used, either anterior or posterior to the biceps anchor. Sometimes, when an anterior superior sublabral hole is present along with the type II

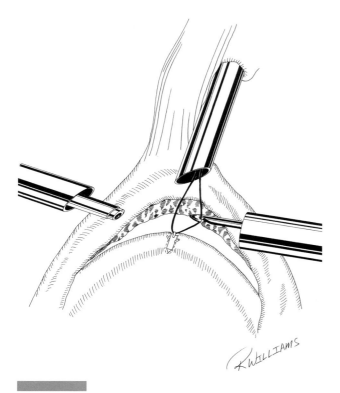

Figure 10-22
A crochet hook pulls one limb of the suture out the
anterior mid-glenoid cannula.

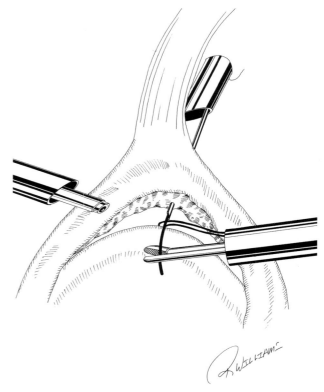

Figure 10-23
A 6-in 17-gauge epidural needle is used to insert a
Shuttle Relay through the anterior base of the biceps
tendon. The relay is pulled out the anterior midglenoid
portal.

SLAP lesion, it is best to use at least two bone
anchors for security.

The patient is treated postoperatively in an
Ultra Sling (DonJoy) and encouraged to perform gentle elbow, wrist, and hand exercises
for the first week. The therapy can progress
with protected biceps strengthening at 4 to 5
weeks. Stressful biceps activity is prohibited
for 3 to 4 months.

Treatment of Type III SLAP Lesions

Since the type III SLAP lesion occurs only
with a meniscoid-type labrum, it is adequate
to simply remove the loose segment of the
labral tissue to prevent catching and snapping
(Fig. 10-29). This debridement can be performed with standard arthroscopic basket
punches and mechanical shaving devices, using both the anterior superior and posterior
superior portals. I often prefer using an elec-

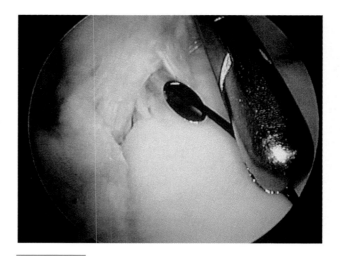

Figure 10-24
The correct location for the suture is through the
superior labrum and the base of the biceps, passing
through the detached portion of the labrum.

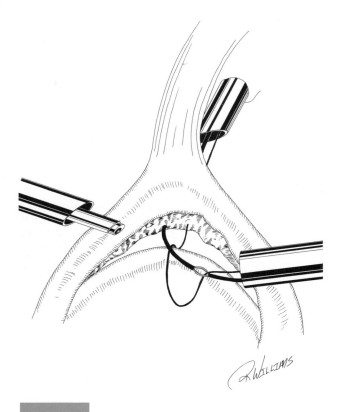

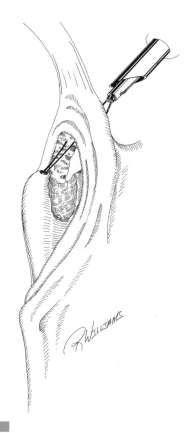

Figure 10-25
The Shuttle Relay is used to lead the suture from the anterior mid-glenoid cannula back through the biceps anchor and out the anterior superior cannula. A mattress suture is formed when both suture limbs have been passed.

Figure 10-26
A miniature knot-pusher is used through the anterior superior cannula to securely tie the mattress suture on the anterior surface of the biceps anchor.

trosurgical tool with a Subacromial Electrode tip (Concept, Inc., Largo, Florida) via an insulated operating cannula to transect the torn labrum (Fig. 10-30). By using a nonconductive surgical irrigant and the lowest possible power settings, a very clean and safe tissue debridement can be performed. Following resection of the loose tissue, a palpating probe should examine the labrum and biceps anchor to make certain that it is stable.

Treatment of Type IV SLAP Lesions

A type IV SLAP lesion presents an especially difficult problem, particularly in a young person (Fig. 10-31). If the segment of damaged

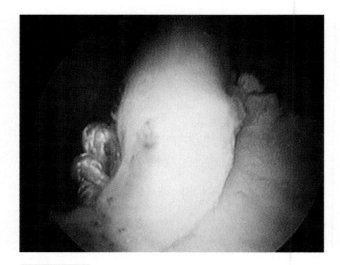

Figure 10-27
When the repair is completed, the suture knots are located away from the articular surface, on the anterior surface of the biceps tendon.

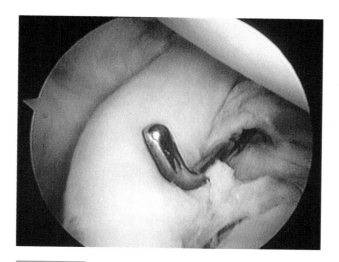

Figure 10-28
After completing the repair, the stability of the biceps anchor is tested with a palpating probe.

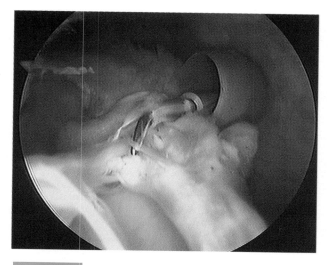

Figure 10-30
Removal of the bucket-handle portion of a type III SLAP lesion is facilitated by use of the electrosurgical tool.

biceps tendon is small, encompassing less than 10 to 15 percent of the thickness of the biceps tendon, then simply resecting the torn tissue should be adequate. When the superior labrum bucket-handle tear is associated with a tear of 30 percent or more through the biceps tendon, then consideration should be given to suture repair of the torn segment

(Fig. 10-32). In an older person with a normal rotator cuff, consideration of primary biceps tenodesis should be entertained, particularly if the remaining biceps tendon appears to be degenerative.

Repair of the type IV lesion consists of inserting multiple sutures through the labrum and biceps stump to reattach the detached segments. I prefer to use permanent sutures

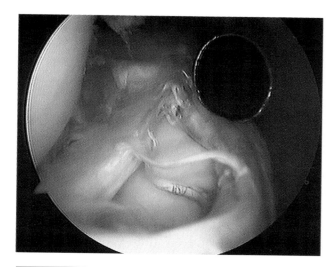

Figure 10-29
A type III SLAP lesion with a displaced bucket-handle tear of the superior labrum can cause very dramatic joint symptoms, with catching and popping in the shoulder.

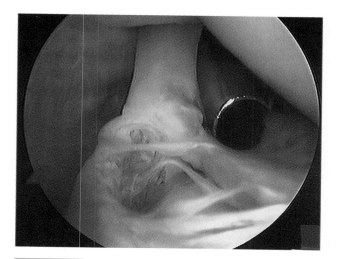

Figure 10-31
A type IV SLAP lesion with minimal biceps tendon involvement is most often treated by debridement of the torn segment.

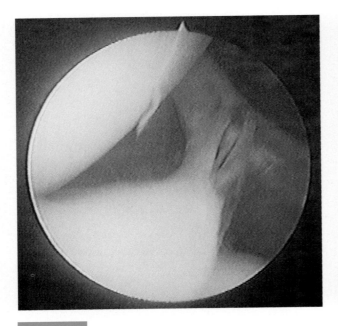

Figure 10-32
When a large segment of the biceps tendon and labrum is torn in a young patient, the surgeon may elect to perform a repair.

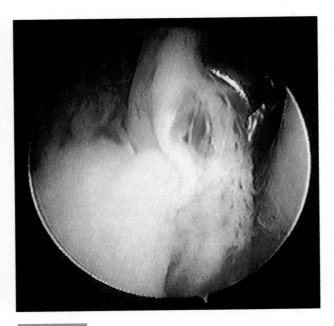

Figure 10-33
A type IV SLAP lesion is repaired using mattress sutures tied above the labrum and biceps anchor.

and a mattress technique, with the knots tied away from the articular surface above the labral rim (Fig. 10-33). To effect this repair, usually three or four mattress sutures are necessary. The first suture is placed percutaneously, using an 18-gauge epidural needle, just below the lateral acromion, through the biceps tendon, and across the split portion. A Shuttle Relay is inserted through the needle and retrieved out the anterior cannula while viewing through the standard posterior portal. The shuttle is loaded with a no. 1 or no. 2 braided permanent suture, which is carried through the tendon, across the split, and out the anterior portal. The epidural needle is removed and reinserted to puncture the biceps tendon and labrum again, 3 to 4 mm away from the first passage site. The shuttle is again inserted and retrieved with a grasping clamp out the anterior cannula. The second suture limb, previously carried out the anterior cannula by the first shuttle, is rethreaded into the eyelet of the second shuttle and withdrawn back through the biceps and labrum by withdrawing the shuttle with the opposite end. A crochet hook is inserted through the anterior

superior cannula, and both limbs of the suture are retrieved back through the anterior cannula. An arthroscopic knot-pushing device is used to tie the suture limbs together, closing the tear in the biceps and labrum. This suturing procedure is repeated, anterior and posterior to the biceps tendon, until the labral tear is adequately repaired. If the tear extends a considerable distance posteriorly, then the arthroscope is changed to the anterior portal to allow insertion of instruments through a posterior operating cannula.

Treatment of Complex SLAP Lesions

On occasion, a type IV SLAP lesion may be associated with a type II detachment of the remaining biceps stump (complex lesion). In this situation it is suggested that the torn segment of labrum and biceps be debrided. If an adequate portion of the biceps remains, it may be reattached to the superior glenoid neck using the suture anchor technique de-

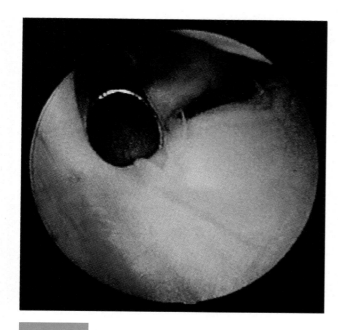

Figure 10-34
A repeat arthroscopic evaluation 4 months after repair of a type II SLAP lesion revealed excellent healing of the labrum to the glenoid neck.

scribed for the type II SLAP lesion repair. If the remaining biceps tendon appears to be fragmented or degenerative, a biceps tenodesis should be considered.

We have had opportunities to perform second arthroscopic evaluations on only two patients who have undergone this type of suture anchor repair of type II SLAP lesions. Both patients demonstrated excellent refixation of the avulsed labrum and biceps anchor, with no signs of suture irritation (Fig. 10-34). Since no long-term clinical follow-ups are currently available to document the efficacy of this method, the surgeon should use his or her best clinical judgment in each case, and should discuss with the patient the potential benefits and risks before performing this type of repair.

References

1. Snyder SJ, Rames R, Wolbert E: Labral lesions, in McGinty JB (ed): *Operative Arthroscopy.* New York, Raven Press, 1991, pp 491–499.

2. Reeves B: Experiments on the tensile strengths of the anterior capsular structures of the shoulder in man. *J Bone Joint Surg* 50B:858, 1968.

3. Perry J: Anatomy and biomechanics of the shoulder in throwing, swimming, gymnastics and tennis. *Clin Sports Med* 2:247, 1983.

4. Karzel R, Nuber G, Tautenschlager E: Contact stresses during compression loading of the glenohumeral joint: The role of the glenoid labrum. *Proc Inst Med Chicago* 42(3):64, 1989.

5. Jobe CM: Evidence linking posterior superior labral impingement and shoulder instability. Presented at the American Shoulder and Elbow Surgeons meeting, Seattle, Washington, September 1991.

6. Burkhead W: Personal communication, 11/13/92, and review of article submitted for publication: "Vascularity of the glenoid labrum."

7. DePalma AJ: *Surgery of the Shoulder,* 3d ed. Philadelphia, Lippincott, pp 212–245, 1983.

8. Snyder SJ, Karzel RP, Del Pizzo W, et al: SLAP lesions of the shoulder. *Arthroscopy* 6:274, 1990.

9. Pappas A, Goss T, Kleinman P: Symptomatic shoulder instability due to lesions of the glenoid labrum. *Am J Sports Med* 11:279, 1983.

10. Rafii M et al: CT arthrography of the capsular structures of the shoulder. *AJR* 146:361, 1986.

11. Hodler J, Kursunoglu-Brahme S, Snyder SJ, et al: The SLAP (superior labrum anterior and posterior) lesion: Standard and MR arthrography. Presented at the RSNA, 1990, paper 01246.

12. Altchek DW, Warren RF, Wickiwicz TL, Ortiz G: Arthroscopic labral debridement: A three year follow-up study. *Am J Sports Med* 20:702, 1992.

13. Andrews JR, Carson WG: The arthroscopic treatment of glenoid labral tears in the throwing athlete. *Orthop Trans* 1984:8.

11

Arthroscopic Evaluation and Treatment of the Rotator Cuff

Introduction

Over the past 10 years the arthroscope has become an important tool in the armamentarium of the shoulder surgeon. Since rotator cuff pathology is especially difficult to evaluate, both clinically and radiologically, the arthroscope has proved to be an excellent diagnostic aide. As shoulder arthroscopists have become more skillful in evaluation and surgical repair on both the glenohumeral and subacromial cuff surfaces, the treatment potential afforded by the arthroscope has also greatly increased. In this chapter I will review the current techniques used at SCOI for the clinical evaluation and surgical treatment of rotator cuff pathology, from very minor tendon irritation and impingement to severe cuff destruction. Additionally, I will highlight the salient points in our clinical and radiological preoperative evaluation. I will also discuss the *mini-open* rotator cuff repair, a technique that cannot be performed without the benefit of arthroscopic visualization.

History and Physical Examination of the Rotator Cuff

Significant pathology of the rotator cuff, requiring medical or surgical intervention, can occur at any time from the early teenage years to the eighth and ninth decades of life. The gamut of pathologies extends from minimal bursal or articular side irritation and tendinitis to the most severe rotator cuff arthropathy. Sometimes even the most obvious rotator cuff pathology can be masked by concomitant symptoms such as adhesive capsulitis, arthritis, or chronic instability. For this reason, the history and physical examination, along with imaging modalities, are important aspects of the pre-arthroscopy diagnostic phase.

History

The historical account of the patient's condition usually falls into age-related categories, although in these days of increased physical fitness and longevity there is frequently overlap.

1. *15 to 25 years.* Patients in this age group with rotator cuff problems are usually involved in active aggressive athletics or heavy labor. The common history is that of a repetitive overhead sport, such as tennis, baseball pitching, or swimming (usually freestyle). The pain occurs during the overhead portion of the activity, when the patient has mild tendinitis or bursitis. If the pain continues for several hours after cessation of the activity, a partial rotator cuff tear should be suspected. After several days of rest the patient is usually able to get back to the activity, only to have the pain recur. The concept of anterior instability contributing to rotator cuff tendinitis applies well to many of the younger patients with shoulder overuse syndrome. This situation is discussed in Chap. 12 and must always be expected in the young and middle age athletic groups.

2. *25 to 45 years.* Rotator cuff problems in this age group are frequently associated with tendinitis secondary to chronic overuse, sometimes with *true* impingement syndrome. Partial rotator cuff tears are common, but complete tears are relatively rare, in this age group. Historically, the patient usually relates chronic pain with overhead activities. There may be a notable popping in the shoulder, and symptoms frequently continue into the night. Often the patient has begun a new exercise or workout routine or has joined a team or in some way accelerated his or her sporting activities. The pain is usually described as being deep in the shoulder; the patient will point to the lateral subacromial or deltoid area. Weakness, too, may be felt by the patient during the workout program.

3. *45 to 65 years.* In this age group patients often have a true bony impingement syndrome with subsequent chronic rotator

cuff problems. Complete rotator cuff tears are common following a strenuous lifting episode or a fall, both with and without shoulder dislocation. The acute symptoms may be dramatic, with very severe pain and weakness with attempted abduction, elevation, and, sometimes, external rotation. In other cases, with chronic insidious impingement syndrome, the rotator cuff and biceps tendon may be slowly worn away by a subacromial spur. These patients report chronic pain and weakness exacerbated by lifting attempts. The pain is noticeably increased at night; the patient often requests sleeping medications and sometimes resorts to sleeping in a semi-sitting position. Crepitation may be present, and sometimes actual locking. In the most severe cases, no active shoulder elevation or external rotation is possible.

4. *65 years and above.* In the senior-citizen group, rotator cuff tears are common. Depending on the activity level of the patient and the severity of the pathology, the symptoms may be less severe than in the younger age group. Chronic aching exacerbated by activities when no arthritic changes are present on x-ray should raise suspicions of rotator cuff pathology. The most severe rotator cuff disease, called *rotator cuff arthropathy,* is usually found in this age group. The severe debilitating pain occurring with rotator cuff arthropathy is probably due to the underlying degenerative arthritis rather than the rotator cuff tear. Often, in senior citizens with limited activity, more severe rotator cuff injuries may be tolerated because of limited physical demands on the shoulder.

Physical Examination of the Shoulder

A standard comprehensive physical examination of the shoulder should be completed for all patients. Specific tests for the rotator cuff must be carefully evaluated in every shoulder workup.

Inspection may reveal atrophy of the cuff muscles, both above and below the spine of the scapula. Deltoid asymmetry may also be seen when chronic disease is present. Range of motion of the shoulder may be normal in minor disease, but there may be a "painful arc" occurring between 60 and 120 degrees of forward elevation or abduction. A locking phenomenon in this position may exist as well, if there is a bursal side or complete tear that catches beneath the acromial edge. Pain on maximum elevation may suggest an articular side rotator cuff tear impinging on the superior *glenoid* border. Passive elevation may be greater than active elevation when a complete rotator cuff tear is present. If the patient is unable to support the arm with his or her own strength, then the "drop arm" sign is present.

Palpation of the rotator cuff should include the posterior and superior aspects of the greater tuberosity, as well as the biceps groove and the lesser tuberosity. The AC joint should also be palpated, since disease there may confuse the picture. The intrinsic and extrinsic muscles of the shoulder should be tested individually. Resisted external rotation and resisted internal rotation with the elbow at the side test the infraspinatus and subscapularis muscles, respectively. Supraspinatus testing (Jobe's test) should be carefully performed (Fig. 11-1). The arm is positioned in 60 degrees of abduction and 45 degrees of forward flexion with the shoulder in internal rotation and the thumb pointing toward the ground. Pressure on the hand causes pain in the shoulder, indicating a positive test. The biceps tendon can be evaluated with Speed's test (resisted forward elevation with the arm and elbow extended and the hand in supination).

We perform the impingement no. 1 test with the patient supine on the examining table. The involved arm is compared to the opposite extremity. Full forward flexion with internal rotation and maximum elevation in the arc of the scapula (modified Neer's sign) are compared (Fig. 11-2). If pain occurs in the upper degrees of elevation, this is considered a presumptive positive test. Injection of 3 mL of lidocaine into the subacromial space should relieve the symptoms if subacromial impingement is the cause of the pain. Of course, this test may be confusing if arthritis or capsular

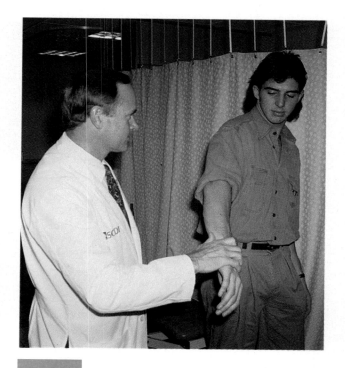

Figure 11-1
The supraspinatus resistance test is the best technique to use in examining for pain and weakness in the rotator cuff (see text).

adhesions are present, but when combined with the other aspects of the examination it is very helpful.

We perform the impingement no. 2 test, also, with the patient supine. The involved arm is positioned with the elbow in flexion and the shoulder in 90 degrees of abduction. The arm is gently moved into adduction with further elevation and internal rotation (Fig. 11-3). This maneuver causes compression of the rotator cuff structures beneath the lateral and anterior acromial arch, resulting in pain when pathology is present.

In the young throwing athlete an apprehension test should be performed. With the patient supine, the arm is placed in the provocative position of 90 degrees of abduction and external rotation. As the passive external rotation is increased, the patient may complain of posterior shoulder pain and resist further external rotation. This pain may be secondary to compression of the greater tuberosity on the posterior glenoid, with rotator cuff and su-

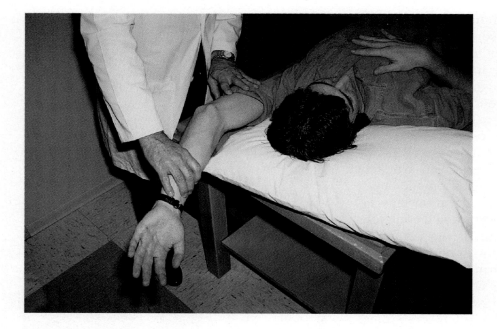

Figure 11-2
We perform the "impingement no. 1 test" with the patient supine. The arm is taken into full forward elevation and both sides are compared.

perior capsular tissue being pinched secondary to anterior subluxation. By applying a gentle reduction force with the palm of the hand over the anterior shoulder, the posterior

pain in this condition should be significantly relieved. We call this test an "apprehension suppression" test. When the hand on the front of the shoulder is removed, the posterior pain should recur if the test is truly positive (see Chap. 12). This test does not prove that the shoulder is unstable, but adds to the clinical suspicion.

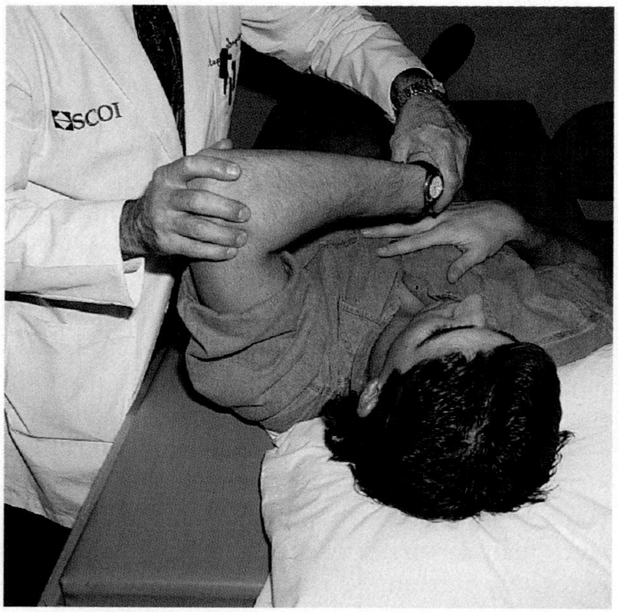

Neurological Testing

One of the most confusing clinical pictures seen in the shoulder clinic is that of suprascapular nerve dysfunction. In this clinical setting there is atrophy of the supra- and infraspinatus muscles, with marked weakness when those muscles are tested (Fig. 11-4). Pain is also present, but usually is not severe. Generally the rotator cuff is not tender to palpation. The proof of this diagnosis lies with EMG testing of the supra- and infraspinatus muscles and nerve conduction testing of the suprascapular nerve. Thoracic outlet problems also contribute to the confusion, causing muscle imbalance and secondary cuff tendonopathy. The possibility of thoracic outlet syndrome should always be remembered, and an appropriate neurological or vascular work-up ordered if suspicion arises.

Figure 11-3
The "impingement no. 2 test" is also performed with the patient supine. The shoulder is placed in forward flexion, adduction, and internal rotation, compressing the greater tuberosity against the coracoacromial arch.

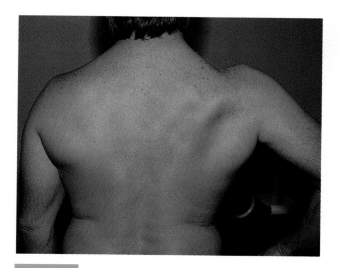

Figure 11-4
With suprascapular nerve dysfunction the atrophy of the rotator cuff muscles is very severe, but the history and symptomatology are not consistent with rotator cuff disease.

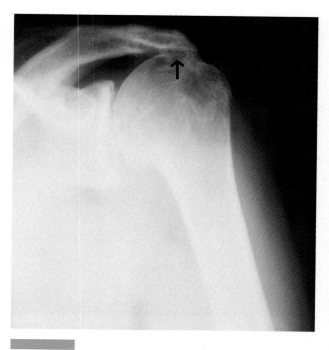

Figure 11-5
With severe rotator cuff damage, the humeral head is elevated in relation to the glenoid and there may be sculpting of the undersurface of the acromion and sclerosis of the greater tuberosity.

Imaging of the Shoulder in Impingement Syndrome and Rotator Cuff Disease

A standard x-ray series of the shoulder should be performed when evaluating for impingement or rotator cuff problems. On the AP view the greater tuberosity is evaluated for signs of sclerosis and cystic degeneration, which suggest impingement and insertional damage to the rotator cuff tendon. Additionally, the humeral/acromial space is observed; if it is narrowed significantly with proximal migration of the humerus, a massive rotator cuff tear is suspected (Fig. 11-5).

The second view is made with the humerus internally rotated and a 20-degree cephalad angulation on an AP x-ray. This view is helpful for evaluation of the AC joint. Degenerative changes in the AC joint are frequently associated with underhanging spurs. Additionally, the acromial facet of the AC joint often has an inferior osteophyte, which can be seen on this view as well (Fig. 11-6). Calcifications around the posterior aspect of the greater tuberosity of the humerus can also be noted.

The axillary lateral view is important for

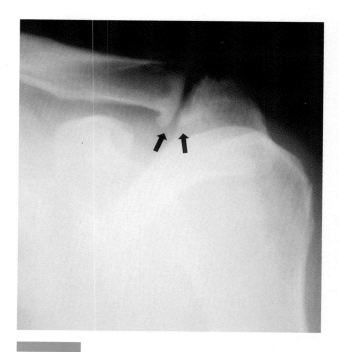

Figure 11-6
The AC joint x-ray is important in revealing potential spurs beneath the acromial and clavicular facets.

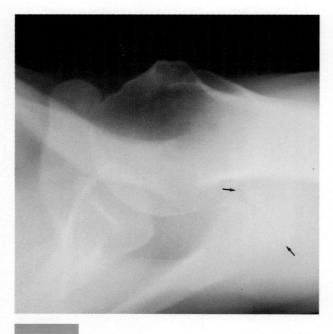

Figure 11-7
An os acromionale is difficult to see except on the axillary x-ray and MRI. It is important to recognize this entity, so as to avoid problems and confusion during arthroscopy.

evaluation of the acromial outline. If a bipartite acromion is present, it is best seen on this view. An os acromionale has been associated in the past with the impingement syndrome.[1] In our review, this has not been confirmed[2] (Fig. 11-7). It is important to recognize an os acromionale on the preoperative x-ray, so as to avoid intraoperative confusion or injury when an acromioplasty is performed.

The supraspinatus outlet or arch view is the most important of all x-ray projections for evaluating a shoulder with impingement and rotator cuff pathology (Figs. 11-8 and 11-9). An excellent outlet view is required to judge the true architecture of the coracoacromial arch. Three checkpoints will help the reviewer to determine if the x-ray is well positioned (Figs. 11-10 and 11-11):

1. The spine of the scapula should appear as a column, with both the anterior and posterior cortices well demarcated. If the spine appears widened, rotation is present.

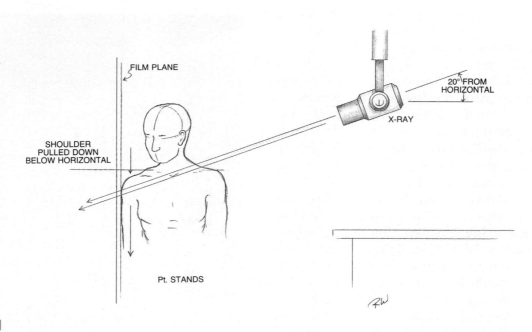

Figure 11-8
The technique for performing a consistently excellent supraspinatus outlet x-ray requires the x-ray tube to be angled 20 degrees from horizontal and directed in the plane of the scapula from posterior to anterior. The patient's shoulder is pulled inferiorly by a weight.

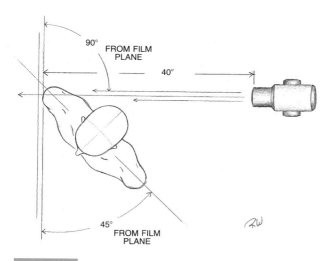

Figure 11-9
The patient stands with the involved shoulder against the film cassette at a 45-degree angle. The x-ray exposure is made from 40 inches away and perpendicular to the x-ray cassette.

2.   The film should be oriented so that a portion of the posterior acromion is visible (approximately 20 percent of the arch), as well as the larger portion of the anterior acromion (approximately 80 percent). With improper rotation only the anterior portion will be seen.

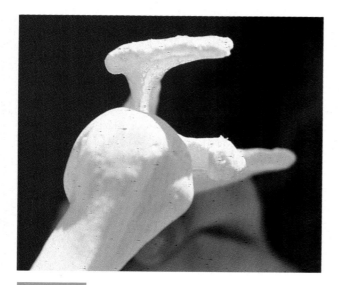

Figure 11-10
A perfectly positioned acromial outlet x-ray shows the lateral acromial outline without significant rotational distortion.

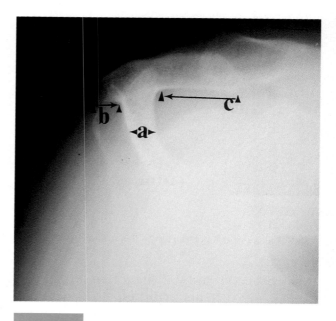

Figure 11-11
Three important checkpoints should be understood when reviewing a supraspinatus outlet x-ray: *A.* The column of the scapular spine should not be rotated (widened). *B.* The posterior lip of the acromion should be visible. *C.* The anterior inferior edge of the acromion must be clearly visible.

3.   The anterior inferior edge of the acromion should be visible so that it can be classified. If the overlying clavicle obstructs the view of the anterior inferior acromion, the x-ray is not acceptable.

This x-ray should be studied carefully to assess both the shape of the acromion, particularly in its anterior third, and its thickness. The morphological classification proposed by Bigliani and Morrison includes three acromial types based on the contour of the anterior inferior surface[3]:

Type I: Flat acromial undersurface with anterior edge extending away from the humeral head (Fig. 11-12).

Type II: Gently curved undersurface that parallels humeral head (Fig. 11-13).

Type III: Inferior-pointing anterior osteophyte, or "beak," that narrows outlet pathway of supraspinatus muscle and tendon as it exits supraspinatus fossa (Fig. 11-14).

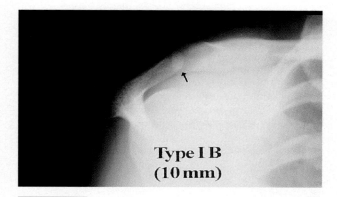

Figure 11-12
A type I acromion has a perfectly flat undersurface.

It has been shown by Bigliani that a high percentage of patients with type III acromial morphology had rotator cuff tears.

A modified acromial classification system was proposed by Snyder and Wuh.[4] This system considers the thickness of the anterior third of the acromion, measured at the intersection of the anterior and middle thirds, in addition to the morphology of the undersurface:

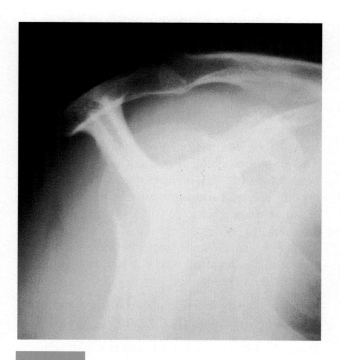

Figure 11-13
A type II acromion has a gently curved undersurface with no anterior spur.

Type A: Thin acromion—less than 8 mm thick at intersection of anterior and middle thirds.

Type B: Average acromion—between 8 and 12 mm thick

Type C: Thick acromion—more than 12 mm thick

The authors reviewed 200 outlet x-rays of patients complaining of shoulder pain, noting that in 34 percent of the female patients with type III acromions the thickness was less than 8 mm; hence the designation IIIA. The authors warned that when performing a decompression, either arthroscopic or open, on a patient with a type IIIA acromion there was a risk of inadvertent acromial fracture. We advise very careful study and classification of the acromion arch anatomy preoperatively, to minimize the risk of intraoperative iatrogenic acromial fracture (Figs. 11-15 and 11-16).

Arthrogram

The arthrogram has long been regarded by radiologists and orthopaedists as the "gold standard" imaging technique for diagnosis of rotator cuff disease. It has always been known that partial-thickness tears on the articular surface of the rotator cuff are difficult to diagnose even with double-contrast arthrograms, and that bursal surface cuff tears are not seen at all. Small full-thickness cuff tears sometimes can be missed. Because of the post-injection pain and inflammation often caused by the arthrogram contrast material, patients' acceptance of this procedure is understandably low. Since the advent of MRI and the development of dedicated coils and software for shoulder imaging, the arthrogram has been relegated to a secondary role. It is useful when a patient is claustrophobic, is physically too large to undergo an MRI scan, or has a pacemaker or other contraindication for high magnetic field exposure.

MRI Scan

In our opinion, the current "gold standard" for rotator cuff imaging is the MRI scan.[5] In order for an MRI scan to be useful and reliable, it must be of technically excellent qual-

Figure 11-14
A type III acromion has an anterior osteophyte or spur directed toward the rotator cuff below.

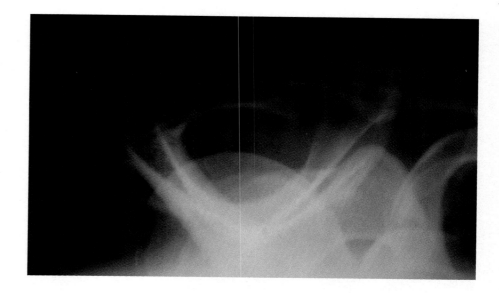

ity. Many of the original scanners used in the early MR imaging centers were of low magnetic strength (0.6 Tesla); hence, the image quality was poor (Fig. 11-17). A modern scanner, using a 1.5-Tesla magnet with dedicated shoulder coils and sophisticated software, can produce excellent-quality images that demonstrate not only the rotator cuff tendon but also the attached rotator cuff muscles. It is very important that a shoulder surgeon be proficient in evaluation of MRI scans. The report from a radiologist may misrepresent the

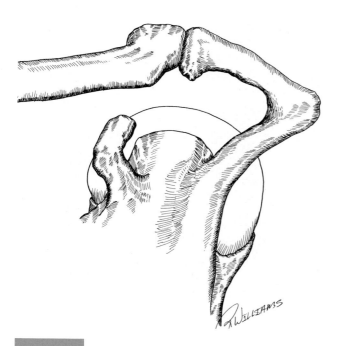

Figure 11-15
An arch classified as IIIA (Snyder and Wuh) has a definite anterior spur but a very thin acromial body. Care must be taken to avoid acromial fracture during decompression.

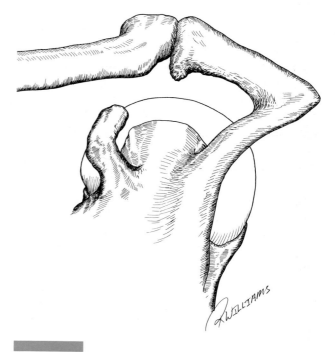

Figure 11-16
A type IIIC acromial arch (Snyder and Wuh) has, in addition to a large anterior spur, a thick acromial body, such that an aggressive acromioplasty may be performed with little fear of acromial fracture.

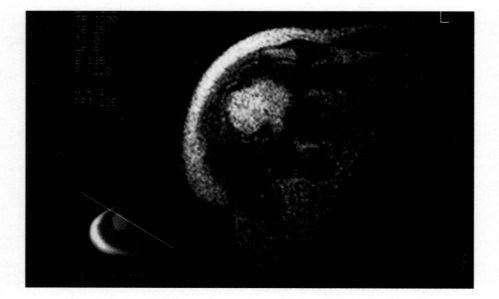

Figure 11-17
An MRI taken on a 0.6 Tesla
scanner is of marginal
quality, and interpretation of
subtle rotator cuff pathology
may be difficult.

actual condition of the rotator cuff, since his
or her interpretation may be based on dated
information or unproven radiological miscon-
ceptions. Reports of "impingement syndrome," AC joint hypertrophy, downward-
sloping acromion, or tendinitis should not be
accepted without the surgeon's personal review and confirmation with the clinical history and examination.

It is helpful to have the three standard sequences for shoulder imaging (coronal, sagittal oblique, and axial) arranged so that each
T1 weighted image is printed adjacent to the
corresponding T2 weighted image. This makes
it much easier to compare both images, looking for the presence of an abnormal high-
intensity signal in and around the rotator cuff,
which suggests inflammation or tendon disruption (Fig. 11-18). Additionally, localized atrophy of the supraspinatus, infraspinatus, or
subscapularis muscle belly—best seen on the
sagittal oblique images—strongly suggests rotator cuff damage or, possibly, neurological
deficit to that muscle (Fig. 11-19).

The MRI scan can suggest impingement of
the bony elements of the acromial arch
against the rotator cuff. It has been our experience that this is often overdiagnosed on the

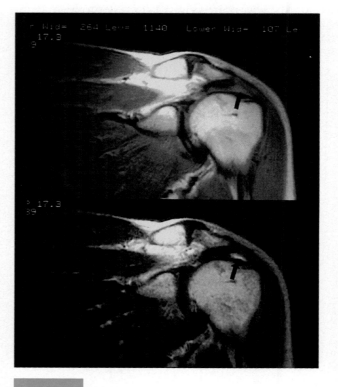

Figure 11-18
Top: This T1 weighted image reveals an intermediate
signal in the area of the supraspinatus tendon at the
attachment to the greater tuberosity. *Bottom:* The T2
weighted image proves that the signal is fluid, suggesting
a significant rotator cuff tear.

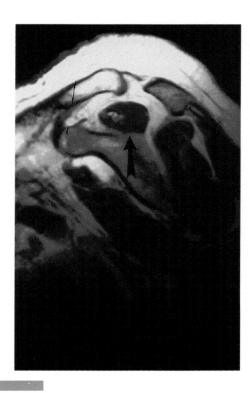

Figure 11-19
The sagittal oblique images are best suited to evaluation of the cross-sectional bulk of the rotator cuff muscles. The supraspinatus muscle is noted to be severely atrophic on this image.

radiologists' reports. We suggest that the word *impingement* be reserved for the clinical diagnosis, and that the word *impression* (of bone on the cuff) be used to describe the MRI picture.

An additional technique that has helped with the diagnosis of articular surface partial rotator cuff tears, as well as labral tears and radiopaque loose bodies, has been the gadolinium-enhanced MR arthrogram. A small amount of diluted gadolinium is injected into the glenohumeral joint and a T1 scan is performed. An articular surface partial tear is clearly outlined by the gadolinium, demonstrating the nature and size of the cuff defect[6] (Fig. 11-20).

Arthroscope-Assisted Treatment of Rotator Cuff Pathology

The techniques available to the arthroscopic shoulder surgeon to treat rotator cuff pathology include (1) cuff debridement on the articular and bursal surfaces; (2) subacromial

Figure 11-20
The partial-thickness rotator cuff tear (AIVB0C0) is easily seen with gadolinium enhancement (open arrow), as is the superior labral detachment (closed arrow). The absence of a contrast signal in the subacromial bursa confirms the "partial" nature of this lesion.

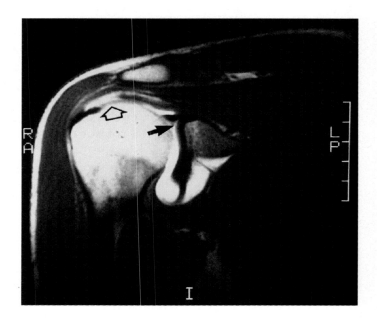

decompression, with or without partial or complete resection of the distal clavicle; (3) arthroscopic suture repair of delaminated partial cuff tears; (4) arthroscopic fixation of small rotator cuff tears to bone, using suture anchor techniques; (5) mini-open rotator cuff repair for larger lesions; and (6) arthroscopic debridement and limited decompression with no repair, for massive non-repairable tears.

Diagnostic Arthroscopic Evaluation in Rotator Cuff Injuries

As with all arthroscopic evaluations of the shoulder, a 15-point glenohumeral examination is performed and documented on videotape.[7] During this examination the rotator cuff tendon is carefully visualized from the posterior portal for the articular surface of the supraspinatus tendon located just posterior to the biceps tendon, and the infraspinatus and teres minor tendons located more posteriorly adjacent to the humeral "bare area." Visualization from the anterior portal adds further clarification, especially concerning the status of the posterior cuff. Following these observations, any cuff fragmentation should be debrided to permit classification and help decision-making.

Suture Marker Technique

For small full-thickness rotator cuff tears or significant articular surface partial rotator cuff injuries, a suture marker placed in the proximity of the lesion allows identification of the corresponding cuff area on the bursal surface. The technique for placing the marker suture should be well understood by all shoulder arthroscopists, since this is a convenient way to correlate articular and bursal side locations (Fig. 11-21). With the arthroscope viewing from the posterior portal, an 18-gauge spinal needle is inserted percutaneously through the lateral subacromial area and into the shoulder

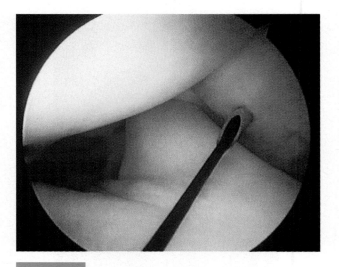

Figure 11-21
The suture marker technique is valuable for correlating the articular and bursal sides of the rotator cuff tendon, especially in the evaluation for impingement (see text).

joint, passing directly through the area of the rotator cuff damage. The correct location for the skin puncture can be determined by observing the outline of the bony landmarks on the skin. With the conventional lateral positioning for shoulder arthroscopy, the biceps tendon is located just below the anterolateral acromial margin. The supraspinatus tendon is found just posterior and lateral to the biceps tendon; thus, the location for the marker suture can be estimated before its insertion. If the articular side defect is approximately 1 to 2 cm posterior to the biceps tendon, then this area should be estimated on the skin to be approximately 2 cm posterior to the anterolateral acromial angle. By viewing the rotator cuff arthroscopically while palpating this location on the skin, one can see the indentation of the cuff surface. The spinal needle is then inserted approximately 1 cm below the acromial margin, perpendicular to the skin. Once the bone of the humeral tuberosity is felt with the needle tip, the needle is withdrawn a few millimeters, the angle changed, and the needle redirected to pass into the shoulder joint at the tendon-bone junction. If the needle is angled too proximally it will enter the bursal space and will not be seen. Therefore, the angle is changed only slightly after palpating the

Figure 11-22
A monofilament suture is inserted through a spinal needle to mark the position of a partial-thickness rotator cuff tear or, in this case, a bulging area in the supraspinatus tendon.

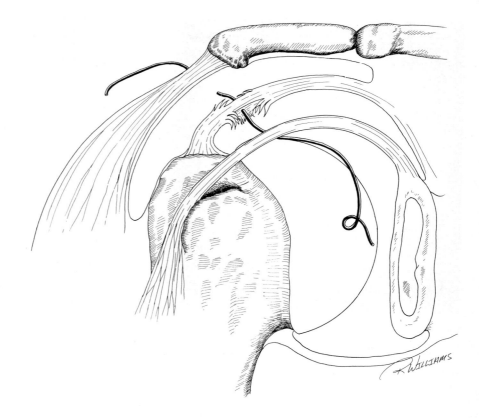

bone, which then allows the needle to enter the glenohumeral joint just adjacent to the rotator cuff attachment.

When the needle is in the proper location it is advanced to the glenoid, and the bevel is turned to face the humeral head. A no. 1 monofilament absorbable suture is inserted through the needle (Fig. 11-22). Approximately 10 cm of suture is fed into the joint before the needle is removed. This technique leaves an easily visualized marker suture crossing the subacromial space to enter the bursal surface of the rotator cuff tendon. During subsequent bursoscopy the suture marker can be identified, allowing a complete assessment of the bursal side rotator cuff tissue (Fig. 11-23).

Arthroscopic Debridement

When, during the course of glenohumeral arthroscopy, an articular surface rotator cuff

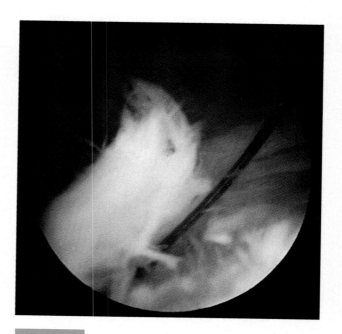

Figure 11-23
When the marker suture is located on the bursal side, it is seen to be exiting from a large flap tear in the bursal side of the supraspinatus tendon (BIV tear).

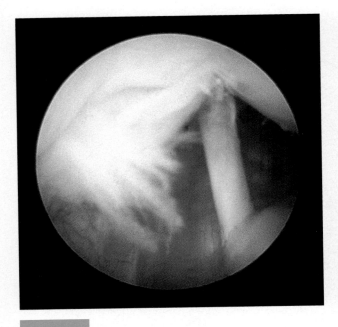

Figure 11-24
An AII partial rotator cuff tear in the supraspinatus tendon, seen from the posterior portal before debridement.

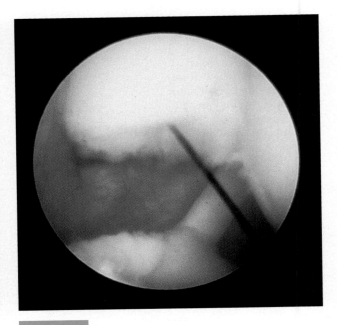

Figure 11-25
After careful debridement of the AII partial rotator cuff tear, a marker suture has been placed to help evaluate for impingement on the bursal side.

tear is noted, it is logical to proceed with careful debridement of the frayed and ragged edges (Fig. 11-24). Not only does the debridement seem to offer an element of pain relief; it

is also necessary for precise classification of the rotator cuff lesion, and as an aid in subsequent surgical planning. A 4.5-mm full-radius shaver is inserted through the anterior supe-

Figure 11-26
A second-look arthroscopic evaluation 4 months after shaving of an AIII rotator cuff tear demonstrates excellent healing and re-synovialization of the supraspinatus tendon.

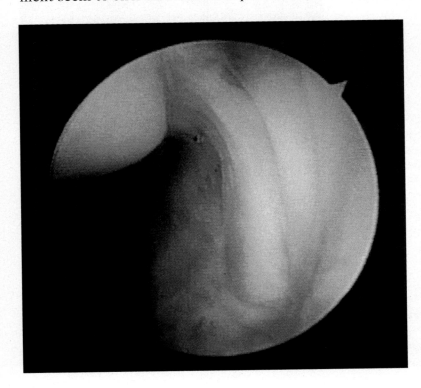

rior cannula and used to remove just the ragged edges of the rotator cuff tear (Fig. 11-25). This treatment alone is often all that is needed to promote subsequent healing when impingement is not present (Fig. 11-26).

Probing and Palpating the Rotator Cuff Tendon

To assess the thickness and quality of the remaining rotator cuff tissue, it is helpful to palpate the cuff from both the articular and bursal surfaces. Using an operating cannula with a rubber diaphragm in the anterior portal, a palpating probe can be inserted into the joint to allow manipulation and further assessment of the remaining rotator cuff tissue on the articular side. Palpation on the bursal surface is performed by first developing a lateral subacromial portal about 3 to 4 cm distal from the edge of the acromion on a line beginning at the posterior edge of the AC joint. A blunt obturator is inserted into the bursa while viewing the articular side of the rotator cuff from the posterior portal. The obturator is used to palpate the rotator cuff on the bursal surface. If a full-thickness tear is present, the palpating obturator will enter the glenohumeral joint through the defect in the cuff, thus confirming the diagnosis (Fig. 11-27). If a significant partial tear of the rotator cuff is present, then the surgeon, by viewing the indentation of the palpating probe, can better assess the thickness of the remaining tendon material.

"Bursoscopy," or Endoscopic Evaluation of the Bursal Side of the Rotator Cuff

The arm position is changed to the bursoscopy position, which requires 15 degrees of abduction and approximately 15 lb of weight for an average-sized patient. The arthroscope

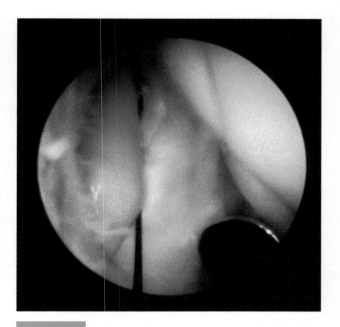

Figure 11-27
An orange blunt-tipped obturator has been inserted into the bursa to palpate the superior surface of the rotator cuff. A small full-thickness tear has been demonstrated as the probe passes into the glenohumeral joint next to the marker suture.

is inserted into the bursa using a cannula with a blunt-tipped obturator from the posterior portal. A transarticular guide rod is passed through the posterior cannula to locate the anterior skin portal. A second cannula connected to gravity drainage tubing is passed into the bursa anteriorly over the guide rod. When both cannulae are correctly positioned in the bursa, the posterior cannula should pass well anterior to the midpoint of the acromion (Fig. 11-28). The anterior cannula should be positioned only 2 or 3 cm into the anterior soft tissues, since the bursal cavity is located below the anterior third of the acromion and the anterior deltoid. The visualization of the bursa should include a systematic evaluation, which is video-recorded prior to any debridement. For this reason it is extremely important that the surgeon understand the correct technique for entering the bursa without requiring debridement of bursal tissues except in very rare cases (see Chap. 5).

Once the bursal examination has been completed, the rotator cuff debridement is

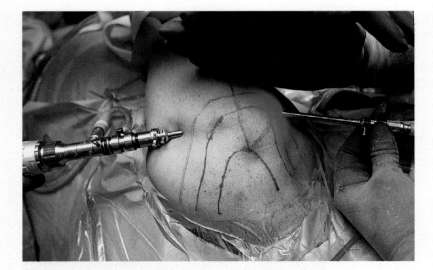

Figure 11-28
When the cannulae are properly placed in the bursa, the tip of the posterior cannula is well anterior to the midline of the subacromial space. The light of the arthroscope is seen transilluminating the fluid-filled bursa.

performed. Using a 4.5-mm full-radius shaver through the anterior cannula, the bursal surface of the cuff lesion is carefully debrided. The marker suture, if present, is located to allow precise evaluation of the bursal surface of the cuff that corresponds to an articular surface lesion. If no bursal side cuff lesion is present and the coracoacromial ligament is smooth, then the diagnosis of impingement syndrome is in doubt. If a full-thickness cuff tear is noted, the size and extent of that tear can be estimated for classification purposes.

Classification of Rotator Cuff Tears

Unless a surgeon is able to precisely evaluate and classify his or her findings in regard to rotator cuff pathology, it is difficult to record, study, and communicate with others concerning the treatment of rotator cuff lesions. Therefore, a classification system should be applied to all rotator cuff injuries, and the resulting data carefully recorded in the perma-

TABLE 11-1   Classification of Rotator Cuff Tears

	Location of Tear
A	Articular surface
B	Bursal surface
C	Complete tear, connecting A and B sides

	Severity of Tear
0	Normal cuff, with smooth coverings of synovium and bursa
I	Minimal superficial bursal or synovial *irritation* or slight capsular fraying in a small localized area; usually < 1 cm in size
II	Actual *fraying* and failure of some rotator cuff fibers in addition to synovial, bursal, or capsular injury; usually < 2 cm in size
III	More severe rotator cuff injury, including fraying and *fragmentation* of tendon fibers, often involving the whole surface of a cuff tendon (most often the supraspinatus); usually < 3 cm in size
IV	Very severe partial rotator cuff tear which usually contains, in addition to fraying and fragmentation of tendon tissue, a sizable *flap* tear and often encompasses more than a single tendon

nent operative record. A simple classification system would designate the surface of involvement and the size of the tear (Table 11-1). Partial tears would be identified as "A" (articular side) or "B" (bursal surface) lesions (Figs. 11-29 and 11-30). When a complete rotator cuff tear is found, the size of the complete tear follows the designation "C" (see Table 11-2).

Decision-Making in the Treatment of Rotator Cuff Tears

Since each situation concerning injury to the rotator cuff is unique, the shoulder surgeon must carefully evaluate the desires and needs of each patient for the intended use of the shoulder after surgery. The medical condition of the patient and the classification and quality of the rotator cuff tissue also influence the decision.

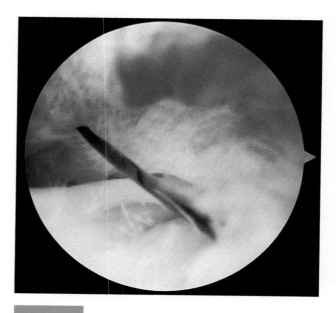

Figure 11-30

A BIII rotator cuff tear is seen with the marker suture exiting through the supraspinatus area. This tear is most likely secondary to the impingement phenomenon, since the coracoacromial ligament is frayed and there is significant surrounding bursitis.

Debridement and Subacromial Decompression

The decision to perform arthroscopic debridement and decompression is usually influenced by both preoperative and intraoperative findings. Preoperatively, the history and physical examination are important considerations. A history of pain with overhead activities, with a sense of catching or locking of the shoulder, indicates the impingement phenomenon.[8] Pain that persists for 1 h or more after the conclusion of the inciting activity usually suggests a rotator cuff tendinitis or a partial cuff tear.

The supraspinatus outlet x-ray should be carefully evaluated to determine the type of acromial contour. A type III acromion, if present, increases the probability of impingement.

If impingement signs and impingement

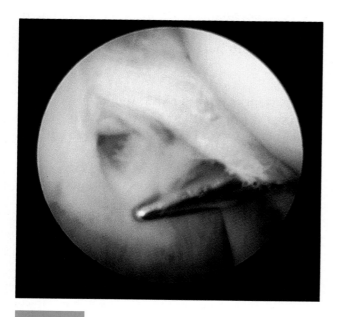

Figure 11-29

An AIII rotator cuff tear is demonstrated, with a fairly large split in the supraspinatus tendon. (See Fig. 11-20 for an MRI scan of the same patient.)

TABLE 11-2 **Classification of Complete (C) Rotator Cuff Tears**

CI	A small complete tear, such as a puncture wound.
CII	A moderate tear that still encompasses only one of the rotator cuff tendons (usually < 2 cm in size) with no retraction of the torn ends.
CIII	A large complete tear involving an entire tendon with minimal retraction of the torn edge, usually 3 to 4 cm in size.
CIV	A massive rotator cuff tear involving two or more rotator cuff tendons frequently with associated retraction and scarring of the remaining tendon ends and often an L-shaped tear. The CIV classification can also be modified with the term "irreparable," indicating that there is no possibility of direct repair.

tests are positive in the physical examination, a decompression should be considered.

Arthroscopic findings that suggest the need for subacromial decompression include (1) AIII or AIV partial rotator cuff tear; (2) BII, III, or IV partial rotator cuff tear; (3) significant fraying of the coracoacromial ligament, with subacromial spurs or ligament calcification (Fig. 11-31); (4) significant fraying of the biceps tendon, with inflammatory changes on the bursal surface of the biceps groove in the area of the rotator interval; (5) AC spurs, especially on the acromial side of the joint; and (6) any complete rotator cuff tear.

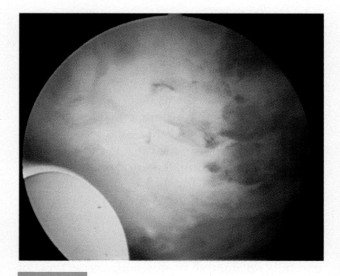

Figure 11-31
Impingement findings during bursoscopy include fraying and inflammation around the coracoacromial ligament and the undersurface of the acromion.

Technique of Arthroscopic Subacromial Decompression with Partial Inferior Clavicle Resection (Table 11-3)

The SCOI technique for arthroscopic subacromial decompression has been developed and refined over the years with valuable input from Drs. Harvard Ellman,[9] James Esch,[10] Lonnie Paulos,[11] Lanny Johnson,[12] and Tom Sampson,[13] among others. Each of these surgeons has made original contributions in arthroscopic decompression. Our technique has evolved in part from their teachings.

Patient Positioning

The patient is positioned in the lateral decubitus position and tilted approximately 30 degrees posteriorly. The body is supported by a beanbag VacuPak and the arm supported by a sterile foam STaR Sleeve (Arthrex, Inc.) in approximately 10 to 15 degrees of abduction and 0 to 10 degrees of forward flexion (Fig. 11-32).

The Procedure

Following complete glenohumeral evaluation, the arthroscope, with the pump attached, is inserted into the bursa posteriorly, and an outflow drain placed into the anterior bursal portal. The bursa is evaluated for impingement lesions. A third bursal portal is developed approximately 3 cm distal from the lateral acromial border on a line beginning at the

TABLE 11-3   Surgeon's Preference Card for Arthroscopic Subacromial Decompression (ASD)

1. *Patient position:* Lateral decubitus on beanbag
2. Standard arthroscopy set-up and instruments, with Arthrex STaR Sleeve traction apparatus
3. *Irrigating fluid:* Synovisol
4. Arthroscopic fluid pump and cannulae system
5. Electrosurgical pencil with Concept Subacromial Electrode
6. *Shaver blades:*
     4.5-mm full-radius blade
     4.0-mm acromioplasty burr
7. *Dressings:*
     Steri-strips
     4×4s
     ABD pads
8. *Immobilization:* Ultra Sling (DonJoy, Inc.)

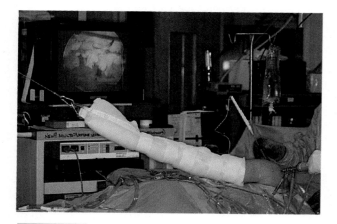

Figure 11-32
The proper position for bursoscopy and decompression includes positioning of the arm in 10 to 15 degrees of abduction and slight forward flexion with the patient in the lateral position.

Figure 11-33
The portals used for bursoscopy include the original two portals for the glenohumeral arthroscopy (anterior superior and posterior superior) as well as a mid-lateral subacromial portal in line with the posterior edge of the AC joint.

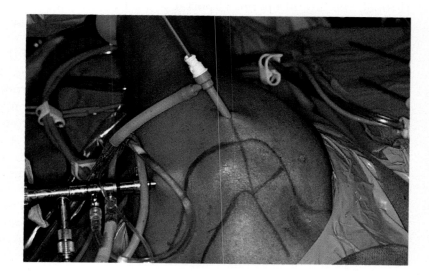

posterior edge of the AC joint and passing down the arm perpendicular to the lateral border of the acromion (Fig. 11-33). The arthroscopic shaver is inserted through an insulated operating cannula. The shaver is used to debride any tendinous or bursal elements that might obstruct the view during the decompression.

A nonconductive surgical irrigant is always used for shoulder arthroscopy, but especially for decompressions. We prefer Synovisol (2.6% glycerol), since it may be safely used for the entire procedure, regardless of whether electrosurgery is employed.[14] The electrosurgical instrument is used through the lateral portal while the arthroscope views from the posterior portal. The Subacromial Electrode tip (Linvatec, Inc.) is used with the lowest ef-

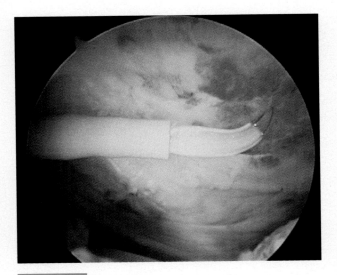

Figure 11-34
The Subacromial Electrode, from Linvatec, Inc., has an insulated, flat-bladed tip. This allows easy dissection of the coracoacromial ligament while still protecting the surrounding tissues and minimizing the power required in the electrosurgical generator.

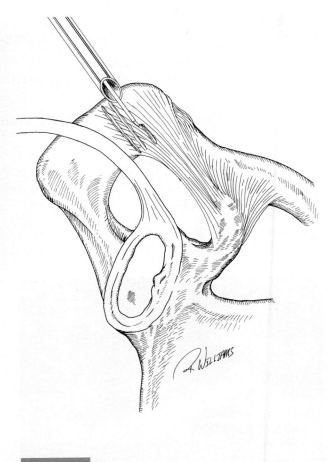

Figure 11-35
The first electrosurgical cuts begin at the AC joint and extend across to the lateral operating portal. Multiple parallel cuts are made in this fashion beneath the acromion.

fective power setting (Fig. 11-34). The coracoacromial ligament and other soft tissues beneath the acromion are removed by first creating a series of parallel cuts beginning at the posterior edge of the AC joint and extending to the lateral border of the acromion (Fig. 11-35). Additional cuts are made perpendicular to the line of the original cuts, to "checkerboard" the soft tissues for easier removal (Fig. 11-36).

A semiaggressive shaving blade inserted through the lateral operating portal is used to remove all soft tissue remnants from the undersurface of the anterior third of the acromion (Fig. 11-37). Once this has been completed, the electrosurgical instrument is reinserted and used to release the final bits of coracoacromial ligament and bursa from the anterior and lateral edges of the acromion to the position of the lateral operating portal (Fig. 11-38). This allows the surgeon to visualize the entire bony undersurface of the anterior third of the acromion and leaves no doubt about the location of the bony margins (Fig. 11-39).

The bony resection begins using a high-speed Acromionizer (Dyonics, Inc., Andover, Massachusetts) or barrel-shaped burr inserted into the bursa through an operating cannula in the lateral portal. The size of the burr is chosen on the basis of preoperative assessment of the thickness of the acromion as seen on the outlet or arch view. If the thickness of the acromion is 12 mm or more, a large acromionizer burr, such as a 5.5-mm, is used. For acromion thicknesses below 12 mm the smaller 4.0-mm acromionizer burr is recommended. The first cut of the decompression begins near the lateral operating portal and extends along the lateral acromial edge through the anterior lateral corner. The purpose of this cut is to allow the surgeon to visualize the entire anterolateral third of the edge of the acromion and to avoid accidentally

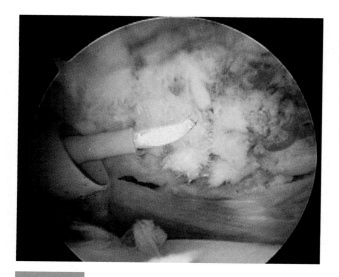

Figure 11-36
The electrosurgical tool is then used to cross-hatch the soft tissues beneath the acromion, creating small fragments that can be easily removed with the shaver.

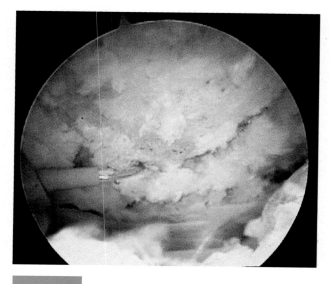

Figure 11-38
The electrosurgical tool is used one final time to outline the edges of the acromion, beginning at the AC joint anteriorly and extending around the anterolateral corner to a point adjacent to the lateral operating portal.

leaving a prominent ridge of bone along the lateral border (Fig. 11-40).

A second trough, referred to as the "orientation trough," is developed next. It begins at the lateral border of the acromion, just medial to the lateral subacromial portal, and extends across the undersurface of the acromion to

the posterior edge of the AC joint (Fig. 11-41). The proper depth of the orientation trough should be gauged from the preoperative arch x-ray view. If the thickness of the middle third of the acromion is less than 7 mm, then the

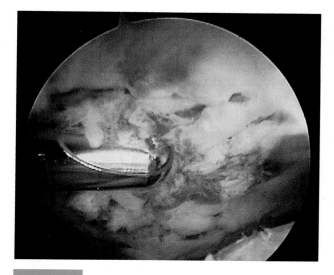

Figure 11-37
A semiaggressive soft tissue resector is used through the lateral portal to remove the soft tissue debris after it is morselized with the electrosurgical tool.

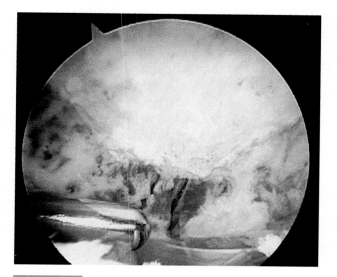

Figure 11-39
The final soft tissue debridement is completed when the undersurface of the anterior third of the acromion is completely devoid of soft tissue coverings, so that the bony anatomy can be easily recognized.

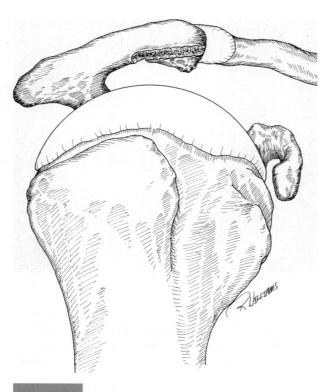

Figure 11-40
The first step in the bony decompression is to remove a
layer of bone from the lateral edge of the acromion,
beginning at the lateral operating portal and extending
to the anterolateral corner.

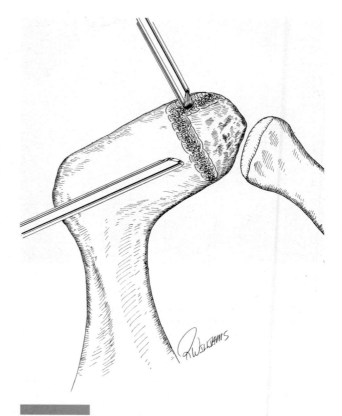

Figure 11-41
The second trough is made beginning from the lateral
operating portal and extending across the undersurface
of the acromion to the posterior edge of the AC joint.
The correct depth for this trough is determined by the
thickness of the acromion on the outlet x-ray.

orientation trough should be less than 1 mm
deep. As the measured thickness of the bone
increases, the depth of the orientation trough
should be similarly increased. With a very
thick acromion, such as a type C (greater
than 12 mm thickness), the larger-diameter
acromionizer is recommended, and a deep
trough measuring 3 to 4 mm can be cut.
During all bony abrasion, a 5.5-mm cannula
without a diaphragm is connected to a gravity drainage tubing and positioned in the anterior subacromial portal. This cannula effi-
ciently removes abraded bony debris without
over-suctioning the bursal space. In addition,
since no suction is used on the handpiece of
the acromionizer during the bony resection,
the bit seldom becomes entangled with soft
tissue.

Once the orientation trough is developed,
the arthroscope is transferred into the lateral

portal and the operating cannula switched to
the posterior portal. The shaver is first used to
remove any obstructing bursa from behind
the orientation trough (Fig. 11-42). The burr
is then used to flatten the posterior edge of
the orientation trough. The resection proceeds forward beneath the anterior third of
the acromion, removing thin layers of bone
between the area of the trough and the anterior edge. It is helpful to make the cuts by
sweeping from medial to lateral beneath the
acromion as the blade progresses from the orientation trough toward the anterior acromial
edge. By leaving a thin bony edge along the
anterior acromion the surgeon can estimate
the final amount of anterior bone removed, by
comparing the thickness of that anterior lip
with the known thickness of the acromionizer

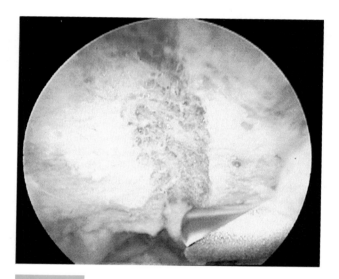

Figure 11-42
The shaver is used to remove bursa from behind the
orientation trough while viewing from the lateral portal.

blade (Fig. 11-43). The anterior spur is finally
removed beginning at the inferior edge. At the
completion of the decompression the entire
anterior third of the undersurface of the
acromion is completely flat, as is the acromial facet of the AC joint (Figs. 11-44 and
11-45).

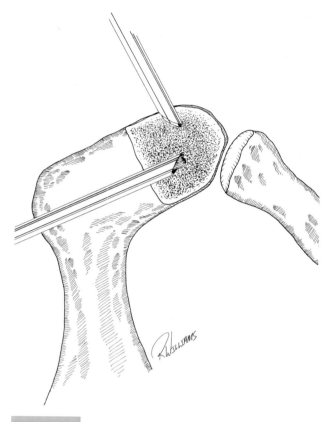

Figure 11-44
The undersurface of the anterior third of the acromion
is completely flat from the orientation trough to the
anterior and lateral edges.

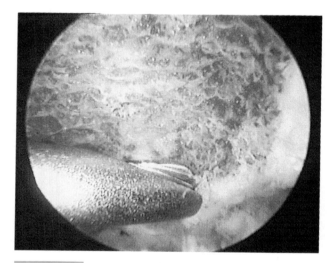

Figure 11-43
The anterior edge of the acromion is left intact until the
entire undersurface of the anterior third has been
flattened. The thickness of the remaining anterior lip is
gauged by comparing it to the known thickness of the
acromionizer blade.

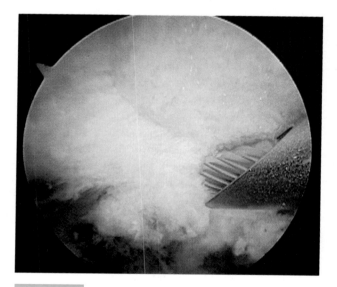

Figure 11-45
A rim of periosteum can be seen along the anterior edge
of the acromion once the decompression is completed.

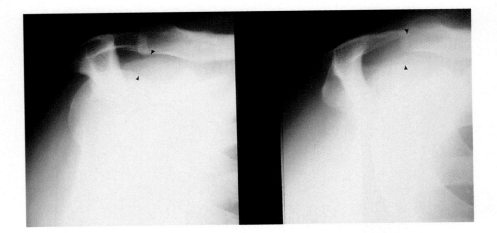

Figure 11-46
Supraspinatus outlet x-rays
taken before and after the
subacromial decompression
demonstrate a completely flat
undersurface with a wide
supraspinatus outlet beneath
the anterior acromial edge.
The deltoid attachment from
the superior aspect of the
acromion has been left intact.

The arthroscope is changed back to the posterior portal for a final visual appraisal of the adequacy of the resection, particularly around the lateral edge. If any step-off is noted, or if the surgeon wishes to contour the bone further, the acromionizer can be reinserted through the lateral portal. An arch x-ray should be taken on the first postoperative visit, to evaluate the adequacy of the decompression and the thickness of the remaining acromion (Fig. 11-46).

Mini-Mumford Resection of the Distal Clavicle (see Chap. 9)

If the preoperative x-ray demonstrates an underhanging bony spur beneath the AC joint, that spur should be removed following the subacromial decompression (Figs. 11-6 and 11-47). While viewing with the scope in the posterior portal, an electrosurgical tool in an insulated operating cannula is inserted into the lateral acromial portal to incise and morselize the capsule below the AC joint (Fig. 11-48). The shaver is used to remove the soft tissue debris prior to bony resection. An acromionizer burr is inserted into the lateral portal. With the drainage cannula inserted anteriorly, the clavicular facet of the AC joint is abraded until it is flush with the resected undersurface of the acromion (Fig. 11-49). Care must be taken to ensure that the "mini-Mumford" extends to both the anterior and posterior cortices of the clavicle. The resection is continued medially approximately 1

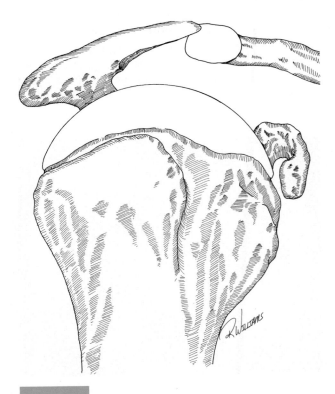

Figure 11-47
After completion of the subacromial decompression, the clavicular facet of the AC joint should be evaluated and partially resected if it appears to compromise the supraspinatus outlet.

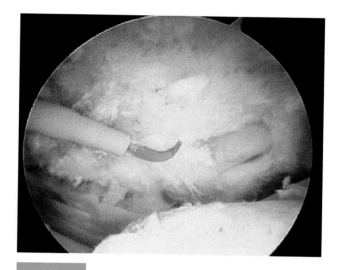

Figure 11-48
The electrosurgical tool is used via the lateral portal to open the capsule beneath the underhanging AC joint.

cm. It should be remembered that the clavicle slants in a medial and caudal direction; often it is not possible to obtain a completely flat arthroscopic appearance of the undersurface of the clavicle. If the surgeon resects too far medially the coracoclavicular ligaments may

be damaged, or the clavicle may be notched or fractured.

Arthroscopic Suture Repair of Delaminated Partial Cuff Tears

An unusual but important type of partial rotator cuff tear is the AIV lesion. In this type of tear a large flap of rotator cuff tendon, along with its overlying synovium and capsule, is delaminated on the articular surface of the rotator cuff. Visualized arthroscopically, this large flap usually has a frayed edge with some fragmented cuff tissue present (Fig. 11-50). It is my belief that this type of tear can be adequately repaired arthroscopically

The repair begins using a small full-radius shaver inserted through the anterior operating cannula to debride the frayed cuff edges (Fig. 11-51). The delaminated cuff is sutured back together using an epidural needle and a suture

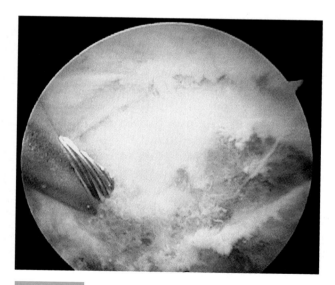

Figure 11-49
The acromionizer burr is used to flatten the underhanging clavicular tip, removing enough facet so that the distal 1 cm of clavicle is flush with the undersurface of resected acromion.

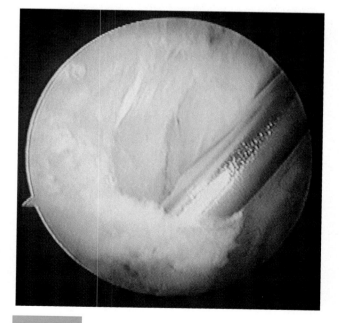

Figure 11-50
An AIV rotator cuff tear is visualized from the posterior portal after debridement of the surrounding frayed and fragmented tissue.

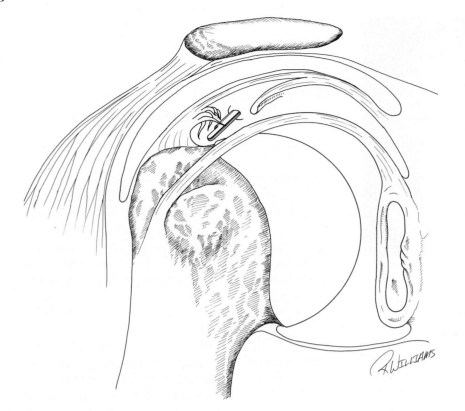

Figure 11-51
To shave and prepare an AIV tear for repair, a small full-radius motorized shaver is used through the anterior portal.

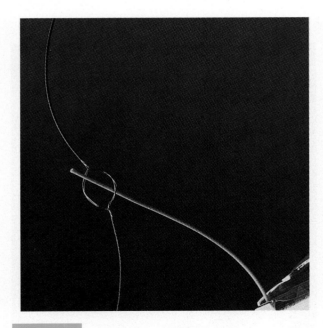

Figure 11-52
The suture Shuttle Relay (Concept, Inc.) is a 30-in suture leader composed of a central braided wire core covered with nylon coating which is open in the center, exposing a 3-mm eyelet. The shuttle is similar in size to a no. 1 monofilament suture, so it will easily pass through a hollow needle or arthroscopic suturing device.

Shuttle Relay (Concept, Inc.) (Fig. 11-52). Three cannulas are needed for the repair. A 4.5-mm arthroscopic cannula is inserted into the bursa via the lateral acromial portal, and its location within the bursal space verified by viewing with the scope. A 5.5-mm operating cannula with a diaphragm is placed into the joint through the anterosuperior portal; the arthroscope remains in the posterosuperior portal, in the 4.5-mm arthroscope cannula.

A 6-in 17-gauge epidural needle is inserted through the lateral cannula to enter the joint through the bursal side of the rotator cuff. The needle is visualized as it passes through the articular leaf of the flap tear near the free edge. With the stilette removed, a suture Shuttle Relay is passed through the needle into the joint. A grasping clamp, inserted through the anterior portal, retrieves the suture Shuttle Relay out anteriorly (Fig. 11-53). The epidural needle is removed. A nonabsorbable no. 1 or no. 2 braided suture is inserted into the eyelet of the suture Shuttle Relay and pulled down the anterior cannula, through the joint and cuff, and out the lateral

Figure 11-53
An epidural needle is passed through the lateral cannula and bursa to puncture both sides of the rotator cuff flap tear. A suture Shuttle Relay is passed through the needle and retrieved with a grasping clamp out the anterior portal.

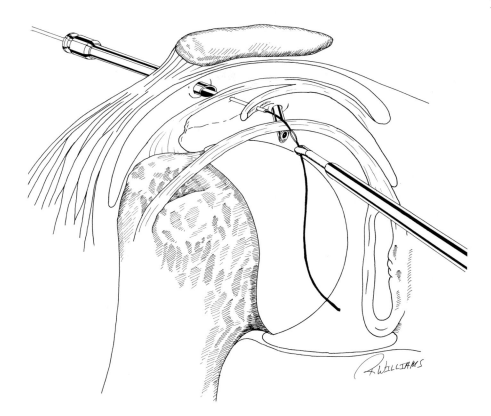

Figure 11-54
The Shuttle Relay is loaded by passing the end of a no. 2 Ethibond suture through the eyelet outside the anterior cannula. By pulling on the lateral end of the shuttle, the suture is pulled through the joint and out through the lateral cannula.

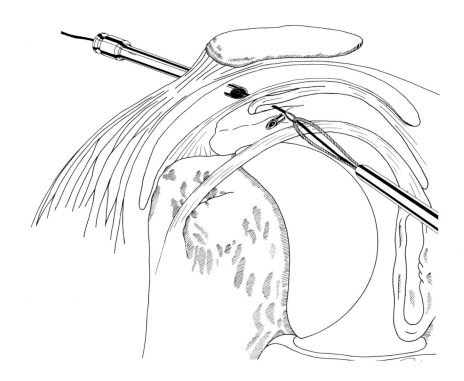

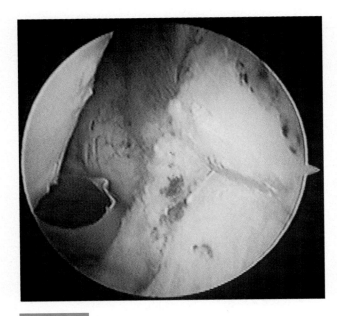

portal (Fig. 11-54). A second pass is made with the epidural needle through the same lateral bursal cannula. This time the needle pierces the rotator cuff and passes through the edge of the delaminated cuff 3 or 4 mm anterior or posterior to the first needle passage. The suture Shuttle Relay is again passed through the needle and retrieved via the anterior portal. The end of the suture limb present in the anterior portal is loaded into the eyelet of the shuttle and retrograded back out through the joint and out the lateral subacromial cannula, creating a U-shaped suture on the articular side of the cuff (Fig. 11-55). (Alternatively, the lateral limb of the suture can be loaded into the eyelet of the shuttle and brought down through the cuff and out the anterior cannula, creating a U-shaped suture on the bursal side of the cuff.) The sutures are then tied, using a knot-pushing device through the lateral subacromial cannula or the anterior cannula, thereby closing the delaminated rotator cuff (Fig. 11-56). Additional sutures are used as needed to complete the repair. A palpating probe should test the knots for security. The shoulder is protected in an Ultra Sling (DonJoy, Inc.) for 3 to 4 weeks before active exercises begin. Elbow, wrist, and hand exercises begin on the first postoperative day.

Figure 11-56
The sutures are tied down the lateral subacromial portal using an arthroscopic knot-pusher; the suture tails are then cut with a basket punch.

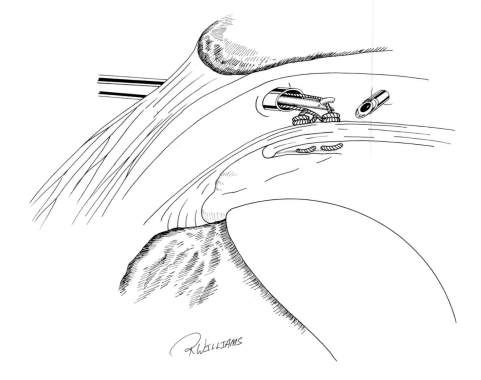

Arthroscopic Repair of Small Complete Rotator Cuff Tears

When a small non-retracted full-thickness rotator cuff tear (CI or CII) or a flap-type bursal side tear (BIV) is diagnosed arthroscopically, the surgeon may choose to perform a repair to bone using arthroscopic suture anchoring techniques. Prior to the surgery the patient must be informed that if this technique is used it will require the same amount of time for tendon healing as would an open repair. Additionally, the patient and surgeon must realize that this technique is still in the developmental stages and no long-term followups are available to aid in preoperative counseling.

The patient chosen for the arthroscopic suture anchor technique for rotator cuff repair should have good quality bone in the humeral head and the tear should not be retracted medial to the articular cartilage edge. The remaining rotator cuff tendon tissue should be of good quality.

Technique of Arthroscopic Rotator Cuff Repair (Table 11-4)

Preparing the Bone Trough

The arm is supported in the bursoscopy position, using 12 to 15 lb of distraction in approximately 15 to 20 degrees of abduction. A lateral subacromial portal is developed, and a

---

TABLE 11-4   Surgeon's Preference Card for Arthroscopic Repair of Rotator Cuff Tear

1. *Patient position:* Lateral decubitus on beanbag
2. Standard arthroscopy set-up and instruments, with Arthrex STaR Sleeve traction apparatus
3. *Irrigating fluid:* Synovisol
4. Arthroscopic fluid pump and cannulae
5. Electrosurgical pencil with Concept Subacromial Electrode
6. *Shaver blades:*
     4.5-mm full-radius blade
     4.0-mm acromioplasty burr
     4.0-mm ball burr (optional)
7. *Suture anchors:*
     Concept Revo 4-mm suture anchor screws with eyelet
8. *Suture material:*
     No. 2 Ethibond (2-colored, 2 packages)
     3-0 Vicryl (undyed, 1 package) subcutaneous
9. Suture Shuttle Relays (Concept, Inc.) no. 4
10. *Arthroscopic cannulae:*
     9-mm screw-in operating cannula with diaphragm
     5.5-mm plastic operating cannula with diaphragm
11. Power drill with appropriate drill bit for suture anchor system or hole punch from Revo System
12. *Rotator cuff suturing instrument:*
     Modified Caspari suture punch *or*
     Copper Head rotator cuff stitcher (Concept, Inc.)
13. Arthroscopic knot-pushing device (surgeon's preference)
14. *Additional instruments:*
     Large arthroscopic suction punch, crochet hook
15. *Dressings:*
     Steri-strips
     4×4s
     ABD pads
16. *Postoperative immobilization:*
     Shoulder immobilizer with small pillow spacer (Ultra Sling, DonJoy, Inc.)
     SCOI Brace (DonJoy, Inc.)

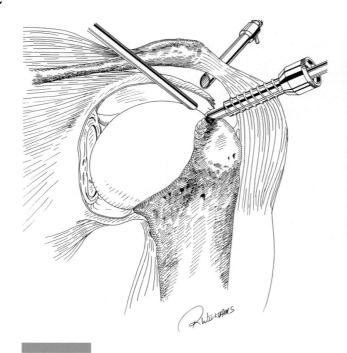

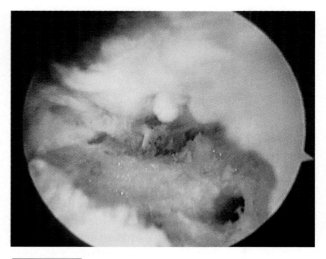

Figure 11-58
Two or three drill holes are made below the resting position of the rotator cuff in the bony trough. The holes are angled to pass beneath the articular cartilage.

Figure 11-57
A bony trough is prepared just below the resting position of the rotator cuff, adjacent to the articular cartilage of the humeral head.

subacromial decompression completed. The shaver and suction punch are used through the lateral operating cannula to debride the ragged edges of the cuff and some of the soft tissue on the greater tuberosity distal to the site of the proposed reattachment of the cuff. A 4-mm burr is used via the anterior or lateral portal to create a trough 4 to 5 mm wide adjacent to the articular cartilage of the humeral head just below the torn cuff edge (Fig. 11-57).

Creating Anchor Holes
Two or three holes are created, using the appropriate drill (or bone punch) for the chosen suture anchor either directly in the bone trough, if the bone quality is good, or at a point approximately 3 mm distal to the trough, if the bone quality is only fair (Fig. 11-58). It is necessary to create an additional small puncture for the drilling and seating of the anchors 1 cm from the lateral border of the acromion (Fig. 11-59). A spinal needle is helpful to determine the appropriate position

for the drilling or hole punching. A miniature drill guide may be used if desired, but this is not necessary if a smooth-shafted drill or punch is used. The holes should be directed proximally at a 45-degree angle to the greater tuberosity and should be placed at least 1 cm apart.

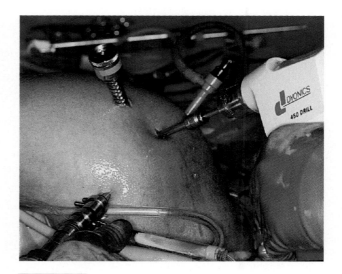

Figure 11-59
The position for the drill holes is chosen using a spinal needle as a guide. A small puncture wound serves as a portal to allow drilling, provided that a smooth drill shaft is used.

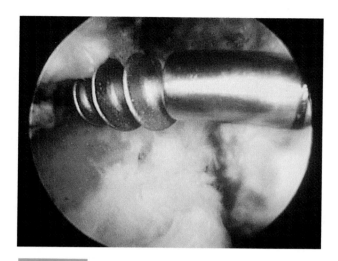

Figure 11-60
A Revo titanium suture anchor crew is inserted through the puncture site used for drilling without the need for a cannula.

Inserting Suture Anchors

A 5.5-mm operating cannula is inserted into the bursa via the anterior subacromial portal. The first suture anchor [either Mitek Super Anchor, or Concept Revo 4-mm titanium suture screw with eyelet (Fig. 11-60)] is inserted into the most anterior drill hole using appropriate arthroscopic instruments. If a Mitek anchor is used, an insertion sleeve is necessary to prevent the anchor from snagging in the soft tissue. If a Concept Revo suture anchor is chosen, it may be screwed directly through the skin stab wound and muscle without fear of entanglement in the soft tissues. The anchor is preloaded with a no. 2 braided nonabsorbable suture. Once the anchor is seated it is tested by pulling firmly on the suture. Both suture tails are pulled out the anterior cannula with a crochet hook (Fig. 11-61). One or

Figure 11-61
After the anchor is seated, the Ethibond sutures are retrieved out the anterior cannula using a crochet hook.

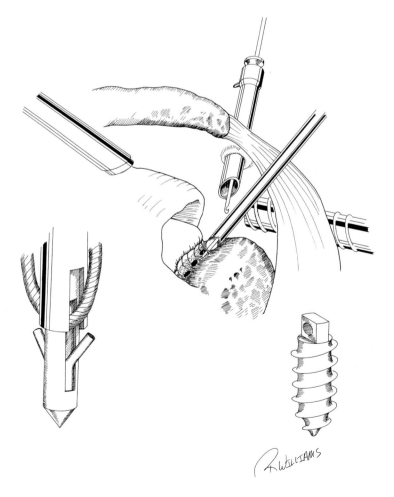

two additional anchors, preloaded with different-colored sutures, are inserted in the predrilled holes in a similar manner.

To avoid tangling of the sutures, when the second set is pulled out the anterior cannula, the first set of sutures is repositioned. This is done by first inserting a switching stick into the cannula and then removing the cannula and reinserting it over the switching stick. This maneuver separates the sutures from one another, keeping one set inside, and the other outside, the anterior cannula. If a third suture is used, both limbs are left passing through the skin puncture adjacent to the acromion so that they will not become entangled with the other two sutures anteriorly. Finally, the crochet hook is used via the lateral portal to retrieve one limb of the most posterior suture out laterally in preparation for suturing the cuff.

Passing the Cuff Suture

A *modified* Caspari-type suture punch loaded with a suture Shuttle Relay is inserted through the lateral operating cannula and used to puncture the edge of the rotator cuff tendon as far posteriorly as possible on the tear (Fig. 11-62). The punch has been modified, by the manufacturer, with a 2-mm slot

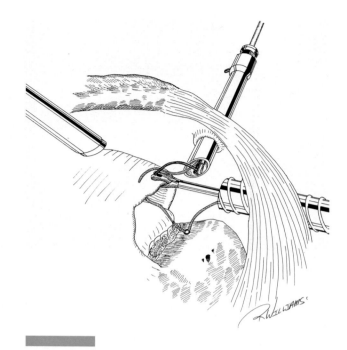

Figure 11-63
The Shuttle Relay is retrieved out the anterior portal with a grasping clamp, while the lateral end is loaded with the second limb of the Ethibond suture.

cut in the end of the loop of the upper jaw. The suture Shuttle Relay is passed through the cuff from bottom to top and into the bursa, where it is retrieved out the anterior cannula with a grasping instrument. The suture limb in the lateral cannula is threaded through the eyelet of the suture Shuttle Relay; by pulling on the anterior limb of the suture Shuttle Relay, it is carried through the cuff from bottom to top and out the anterior cannula. After pulling the second limb of the permanent suture into the lateral operating cannula, using the crochet hook, the suture Shuttle Relay is again passed, using the Caspari punch, approximately 7 to 8 mm anterior to the first puncture site, thereby placing one suture pass on either side of the anchor (Fig. 11-63). The second limb of the suture is then taken on a similar course, from lateral to anterior, by pulling on the second suture Shuttle Relay via the anterior cannula (Fig. 11-64).

The above process is repeated a second and a third time, if necessary, depending on the size of the rotator cuff tear. At the completion

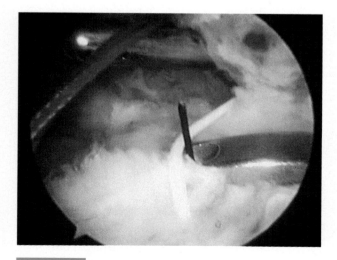

Figure 11-62
A modified Caspari punch is used to pass a Shuttle Relay through the rotator cuff, from bottom to top, to create a mattress suture.

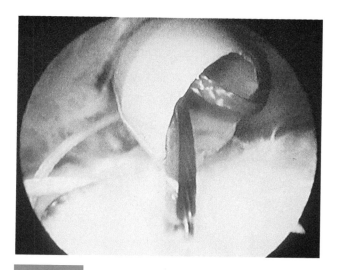

Figure 11-64
By pulling on the arm of the shuttle out the anterior portal, the second limb of the Ethibond suture is carried through the bottom and out the top of the rotator cuff, and out the anterior cannula.

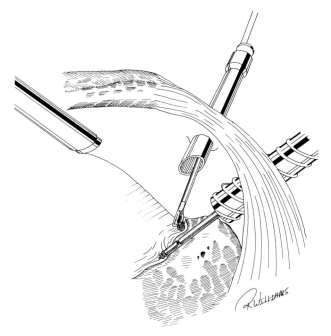

Figure 11-66
An arthroscopic punch is used to cut the suture tails after each knot is tied.

of the suturing, all but 5 lb of the weight is removed from the traction; the arm is lifted into slightly more abduction by the surgical assistant, to relax the tension on the rotator cuff. The arthroscopic knot-pusher is used down the lateral cannula to tie multiple knots securing the mattress sutures (Fig. 11-65). It is convenient to have only one of the suture pairs exiting the lateral portal at a time while tying the knots, to prevent entangling the sutures. After each suture is tied the suture ends are cut with an arthroscopic punch, and the next suture is delivered through the lateral cannula, using the crochet hook, in preparation for tying. The second and third sutures are tied in a similar manner (Fig. 11-66). Once the initial knot-tying sequence is completed, the surgeon may elect to reinforce the repair by tying one limb of each suture to one limb of an adjacent suture. This technique will create a mattress-like effect of the sutures which adds to the knots' security and distributes the suture forces over a wider area of soft tissue. The use of alternating colors for the adjacent sutures helps the surgeon identify the suture pairs, avoiding confusion when multiple strands are present in the field.

The arthroscopic incisions are closed with an inverted subcutaneous absorbable stitch. A sterile dressing is applied, and the arm is placed in an immobilizer-type splint, preferably with a small pillow (Ultra Sling, DonJoy, Inc.) (Fig. 11-67). The arm can be removed,

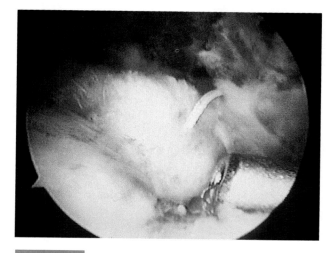

Figure 11-65
The sutures are tied using multiple stacked knots passed with a knot-pusher down the lateral cannula.

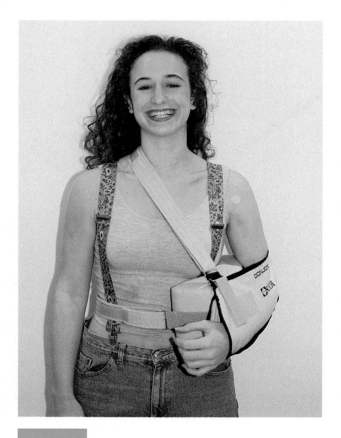

Figure 11-67
A pillow sling/immobilizer (Ultra Sling, DonJoy, Inc.) protects the arm from excessive motion while preventing an internal rotation contracture and keeping the axilla open to prevent chafing.

by opening the flap on the side of the sling, for elbow stretching and exercise (Fig. 11-68). A Polar Care icewater cooling device (Breg, Inc.) is applied beneath the dressings. The postoperative treatment is the same as for a small mini-open repair, and follows the standard rotator cuff rehabilitation program. An x-ray should be taken in the recovery room to evaluate the position of the suture anchors (Fig. 11-69).

Mini-Open Rotator Cuff Repair (Table 11-5)

The decision to perform a mini-open repair for a significant partial-thickness tear (such as an AIVBIII tear), or any complete rotator cuff

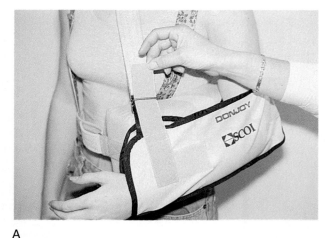

A

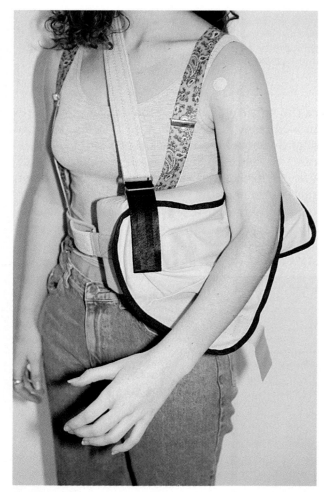

B

Figure 11-68
The Ultra Sling can be opened (*A*) by releasing the Velcro strap to allow early active elbow exercises (*B*).

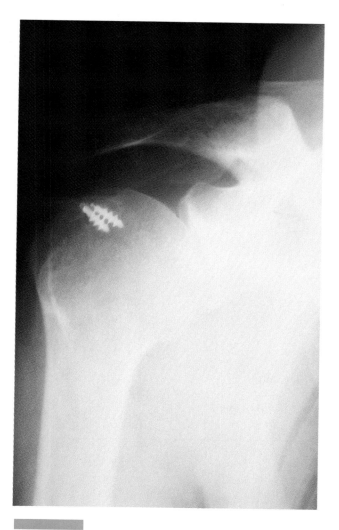

Figure 11-69
A postoperative x-ray demonstrates two Revo screws in position in the humeral head after a rotator cuff repair.

tear, is often made by the patient and the surgeon together preoperatively, on the basis of the patient's future needs for maximum strength and motion, as well as pain relief. Almost all reparable rotator cuff lesions can be managed with a mini-open repair; those that cannot probably require muscle transfers or extensive grafting procedures, which are beyond the scope of this chapter.

The Procedure

During the arthroscopic examination the severity of the tear is noted. If the free edge of the rotator cuff tendon appears to be re-

tracted significantly, a superior capsular release should be performed. Using a thin-shafted sharp-tipped elevating instrument [such as the Concept Rotator Cuff Liberator Elevator (Fig. 11-70)], the superior capsule can be released from its tethering attachment to the glenoid just above the glenoid labrum (Fig. 11-71). This release should extend to a point just anterior to the biceps tendon and posterior to the posterior superior quadrant of the glenoid. The release is performed by inserting the Liberator Elevator through the lateral subacromial portal, directly through the rotator cuff tear, and into the glenohumeral joint. With the angle of the "liberator" directed toward the superior surface of the glenoid, the sharp blade is used to puncture the capsule in multiple places (Fig. 11-72). Once this is completed, the instrument is worked around the periphery of the superior glenoid, effectively releasing the capsule with the adherent cuff from the bone. This release allows the rotator cuff to be more easily advanced laterally, since the capsule and the rotator cuff are fused in this superior area (Fig. 11-73). The Liberator Elevator can also be used to detach portions of the coracohumeral ligament from the base of the coracoid by palpating the coracoid process and stripping the ligament from the lateral aspect of its base.

The arm is then changed to the bursoscopy position, and the standard subacromial decompression is performed, along with a mini- or complete arthroscopic Mumford procedure, if needed. If a marker suture has been placed to designate the location of a significant articular surface partial tear, it is left in place to guide the surgical repair. The traction weight is reduced to 10 lb and the exposed surgical site re-prepped with povidone-iodine. New gloves and instruments are used for the open procedure, but it is not necessary to change the surgical drapes. The surgeon is positioned on the posterior side of the patient; the first assistant moves to the front of the table. When the Arthrex STaR Sleeve is used for traction, the supplemental rotation control strap is applied near the mid-forearm position to facilitate accurate rotation control.

The surgical incision is made on the previ-

TABLE 11-5   Surgeon's Preference Card for Mini-Open Rotator Cuff Tear Repair

1. *Patient position:* Lateral decubitus on beanbag
2. Standard arthroscopy set-up and instruments, with Arthrex STaR Sleeve traction apparatus
3. *Irrigating fluid:* Synovisol
4. Arthroscopic fluid pump and cannulae
5. Electrosurgical pencil with Concept Subacromial Electrode and standard electrode tip
6. *Shaver blades:*
      4.5-mm full-radius blade
      4.0-mm acromioplasty burr
7. Mini-arthrotomy tray with two Army-Navy retractors
8. High-speed 5-mm ball-shaped burr
9. Bankart punch and small mallet
10. Concept rotator cuff repair instrument system
11. *Suturing material (green & white):*
      No. 2 Ethibond with MO-7 needle (cuff)
      No. 1 Vicryl (deltoid fascia)
      2-0 undyed Vicryl (subcutaneous tissue)
      4-0 clear PDS (subcuticular)
12. *Dressings:*
      Steri-strips
      4×4s
      ABD pads
13. *Immobilization:*
      Shoulder immobilizer, with small pillow, (Ultra Sling, DonJoy, Inc.)
      SCOI postop functional shoulder brace (DonJoy, Inc.), *or*
      (for large-framed or obese patient) Quadrant shoulder brace (DonJoy, Inc.)
14. *Additional items:* Polar Care ice water dispersion pad (Breg, Inc.)

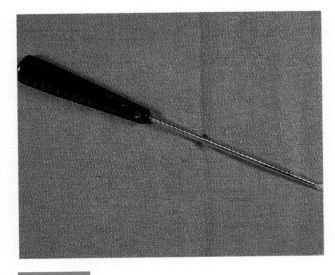

Figure 11-70
The Concept Rotator Cuff Liberator Elevator is a thin-shafted, sharp-tipped, square-bladed elevator used to release the superior capsule when a contracted rotator cuff tendon is being mobilized.

ously drawn orientation line, which extends from the posterior edge of the AC joint perpendicular to the lateral border of the acromion and on down the arm (Fig. 11-74). The incision itself is never more than approximately 5 cm in length, beginning just medial to the lateral border of the acromion and extending down the arm to the lateral subacromial operating portal.[15] If it was noted during the arthroscopic evaluation that the tear was near the rotator interval, the incision is placed 2 to 3 cm anterior to the orientation line, but it still angles toward the AC joint. Skin flaps are elevated, preserving the external deltoid fascia for later closure. The fascia is then sharply opened, but the muscle itself is bluntly separated up to the edge of the acromion. A convenient way to perform this muscle split is to insert a medium-sized periosteal elevator to carefully spread the muscle apart, beginning at the previous lateral

Figure 11-71
The Liberator Elevator is inserted through the lateral subacromial portal and used to release the superior capsule under direct vision with the arthroscope.

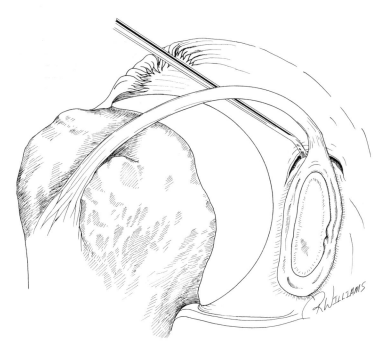

subacromial portal. Sometimes it is necessary to sharply divide a few bands of tendon tissue as the muscle split approaches the lateral border of the acromion. One must make certain that the muscle split plane intersects the lateral acromion approximately 1 to 2 cm posterior to the anterolateral corner; if the split passes too far anteriorly, it may miss the

acromion entirely and be out of position for the rotator cuff repair.

Beneath the deltoid, the submuscular layer of the subdeltoid bursa is encountered and divided. Adequate bursal tissue is removed to allow clear visualization, but it is helpful to leave a layer of bursa beneath the muscle to aid in the final closure. The bursa over the

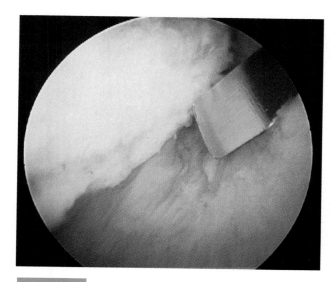

Figure 11-72
The liberator is used to puncture multiple holes in the capsule just above the superior glenoid rim.

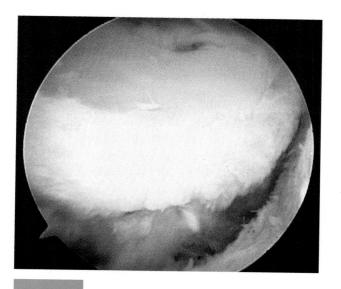

Figure 11-73
Once the release is complete, there is no further tethering of the rotator cuff by the superior capsule above the glenoid.

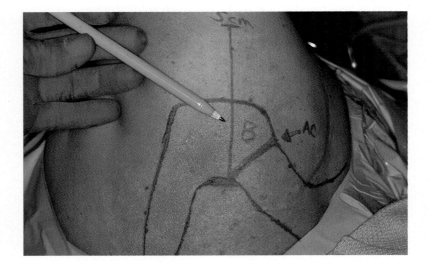

Figure 11-74
The "mini" rotator cuff incision begins just above the lateral border of the acromion and extends 5 cm down the arm.

greater tuberosity is removed in preparation for reattachment of the cuff. An electrosurgical cutter creates several parallel cuts in the bursa over the tuberosity, and a periosteal elevator covered with a surgical sponge is used to remove the bursal tissue and expose the bone. The amount of area exposed depends on the size of the rotator cuff tear and, consequently, on the number of suture tunnels that will be needed.

The free edge of the rotator cuff tendon is sharply debrided, removing only nonviable-appearing hyalinized tissue. When a significant partial tear is being repaired, it is usually necessary to excise the damaged portion of cuff tendon. If a marker suture has been used, it will guide the surgeon to the location of the partial tear. Otherwise, the area can be located by recalling its position relative to the biceps tendon. The biceps groove can be palpated and the dissection begun on the tuberosity, progressing proximally until the cuff is elevated from its bony attachment. By everting the cuff, the damaged portion of the tendon can be visualized and excised. The repair of this injury then follows that of a routine rotator cuff repair.

A 6-mm ball burr is used to create a shallow bone trough adjacent to the articular cartilage of the humeral head (Fig. 11-75). Care should be taken to protect the biceps tendon and remaining rotator cuff while burring. The free edge of the cuff tendon is secured with nonab-

sorbable no. 2 braided sutures. The use of alternating blue- and white-colored sutures facilitates identification of the correct suture pairs at the time of knot tying. If the cuff tendon quality is good, either a horizontal mattress suture or a "W" suture will give an adequate hold on the free edge of the tendon. If the tendon is frayed and of poor quality, we suggest that an SCOI stitch be used (Fig. 11-76). This suture technique is a modification of the Kessler stitch, which was designed for the repair of flexor tendons of the hand. Using the

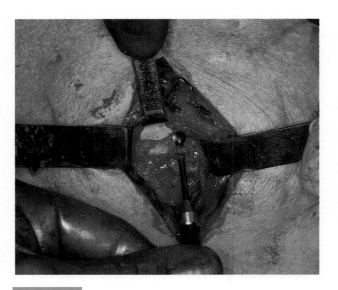

Figure 11-75
A 6-mm ball burr is used to create a trough adjacent to the articular surface of the humeral head.

Figure 11-76
The SCOI stitch is used to secure the free edge of the tendon when it is degenerative or delaminated.

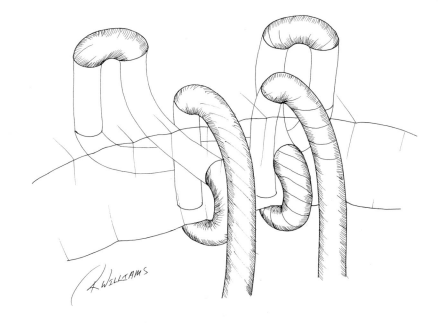

SCOI stitching technique ensures that traction forces are distributed medially into better-quality tendon, using small circular loops. Another proximal loop passes from the bursa to the articular side and back again, thereby closing intratendinous laminations. Additionally, the torn edge of the tendon is rolled by the leading loops of the stitch into the bony trough, preventing pouting of the lip.

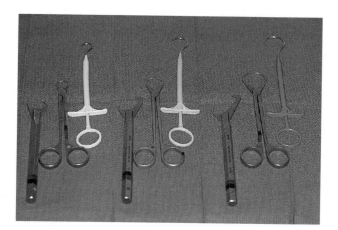

Figure 11-77
The Concept rotator cuff repair system includes nine instruments. There are three sets of three instruments each: gauge punches, circle rasps, and suture retrievers in small, medium, and large sizes.

The Concept rotator cuff suturing instruments are helpful for passing the sutures through the bony trough and out the tuberosity where they are to be tied (Fig. 11-77). These instruments consist of nine tools—three sizes each of a gauge punch, a circular rasp, and a suture retriever.

The decision as to which size of instruments to use in a particular case depends on the surgical exposure and the quality and size of the patient's bone. We prefer to use the large and medium instruments in most cases, and plan so that adjacent tuberosity holes are placed on different horizontal lines. This staggered placement is important so that a postage stamp–like stress riser effect is not created, weakening the bone.

The first instrument used in the repair is the gauge punch. The sharp end of the punch is used to create the first hole in the center of the bone trough. If the trough is located too proximally beneath an overhanging acromion, a curved "Bankart-type punch" is easier to use than the gauge punch (Fig. 11-78A and B). The punch is removed and turned 180 degrees, and the sharp end punctures a second hole in the greater tuberosity. The measuring arm of the gauge punch is used to determine the correct position to create the tuberosity hole (Fig. 11-79A and B). The blunt tip of the

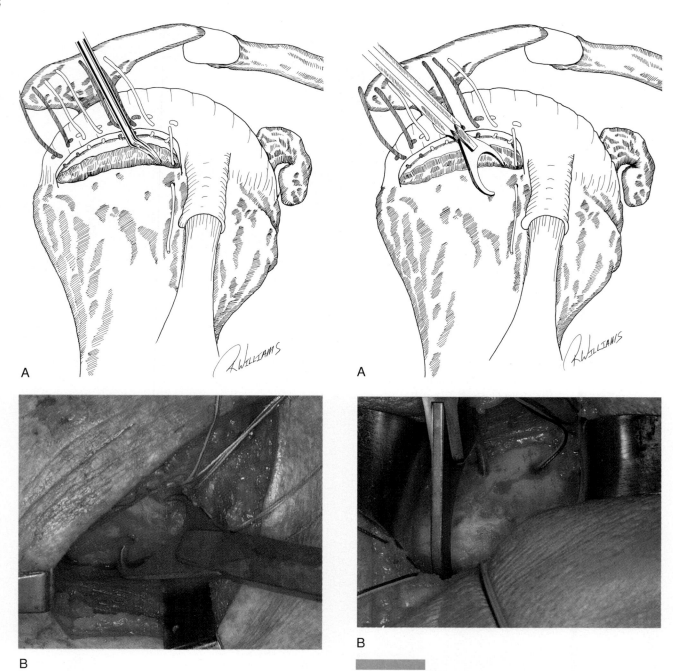

A

B

Figure 11-78

A and *B*. The first hole is made in the trough using either the punch portion of the gauge punch or a curved Bankart punch, whichever is easier.

A

B

Figure 11-79

A and *B*. The positions for the holes in the greater tuberosity are determined by measuring from the first hole, using the gauge punch.

measuring arm is held just above the original hole in the trough, and the handle of the punch is aligned toward that point as the punch is impacted into the tuberosity. Once

the cortex has been perforated, the handle of the punch is lowered so that the curve of the punch heads toward the initial hole in the bone trough. After removing the punch, the circle rasp is inserted first into the hole in the tuberosity. By applying thumb pressure on the

Figure 11-80
The first tine of the circle rasp is inserted into the punch hole in the greater tuberosity. It is worked down through the hole, using thumb pressure over the convex surface, until the second tine can be inserted into the hole in the bone trough.

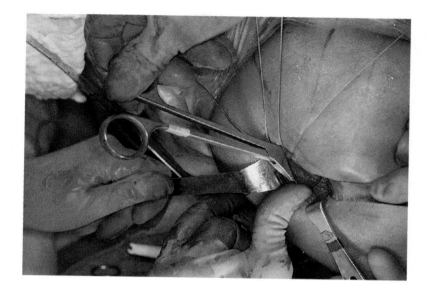

convex surface of the rasp near the tuberosity hole, the surgeon can guide it along the same path as the punch (Fig. 11-80). The second tine of the circle rasp can then be easily seated in the appropriate hole in the trough. With finger and thumb pressure exerted on the two convex surfaces of the circle rasp, the handles are gently closed with a back-and-forth rocking motion. Once the tips come together, a circular rasping motion is used to smooth the tunnel (Fig. 11-81).

The rasp is removed, and the suture retriever inserted through the tuberosity hole. It is allowed to follow the path of the circle rasp out the bone trough (Fig. 11-82). The plunger is depressed on the handle of the suture retriever, and a wire loop is exposed at the tip. One limb each of the two most central rotator cuff sutures is inserted into the wire loop. The plunger is retracted, locking the sutures inside the needle. The retriever is rolled back out the tuberosity hole, carrying the sutures with it (Fig. 11-83). The second set of holes in the trough and tuberosity are made, either anterior or posterior to the central hole. Since it is recommended that adjacent holes be at different levels on the tuberosity, the medium-sized instrument set is usually used. The second set of sutures is passed in a similar manner to the first. Additional anterior and posterior holes are made as needed. When all the sutures have been passed the arm is slightly ab-

ducted and the sutures are pulled distally, to seat the rotator cuff tendon in the trough. Continuous distal traction is applied to all but the central suture, which is the first to be

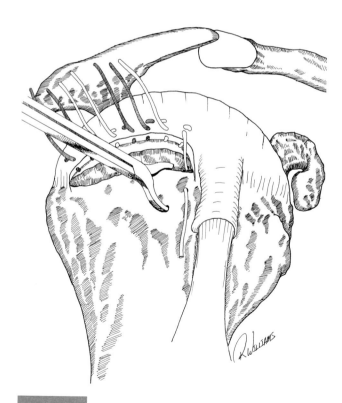

Figure 11-81
With the handles closed, the circle rasp is worked through the bony tunnel to smooth the path for the suture.

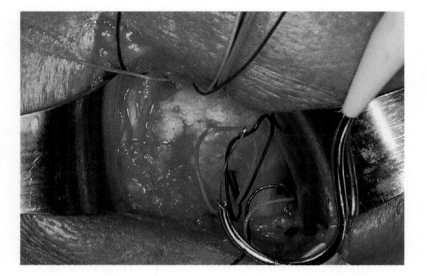

Figure 11-82
The suture retriever is inserted in the tuberosity hole and its tip passed out the bony trough where the sutures are inserted into the wire loop in the tip of the retriever.

tied. The remaining sutures are then tied (Fig. 11-84).

If the bone beneath the sutures is osteoporotic and the surgeon is concerned that the suture may cut through the bone bridge, a small pledget of Gore-Tex soft tissue patch may be inserted under the suture knot (Fig. 11-85). This pledget should measure approximately 2 mm in width and approximately 4 mm in length. Any excess material should be removed after the knot is tied over the pledget.[16]

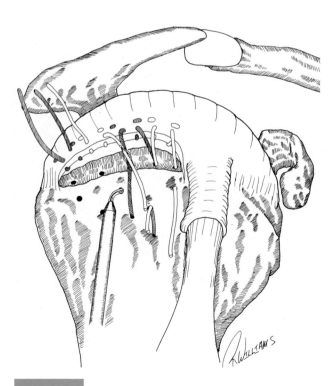

Figure 11-83
The plunger is retracted and the retriever is removed from the tuberosity hole, carrying the sutures with it.

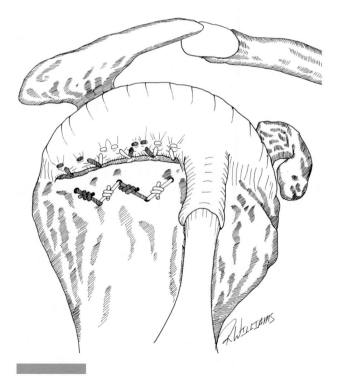

Figure 11-84
The sutures are tied over the bony bridge in the tuberosity in a staggered array so that no "postage stamp" stress riser will occur.

Figure 11-85
Sometimes, when the bone is soft, it is necessary to use a Gore-Tex soft tissue pad beneath the suture knots.

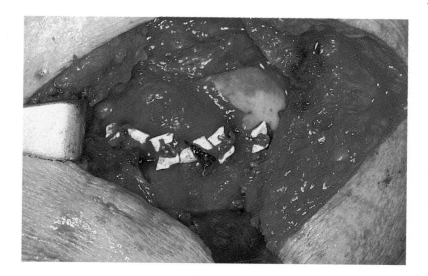

The deltoid muscle is closed in two layers using no. 1 absorbable suture. The first layer closed is the subdeltoid bursal surface, followed by the superficial deltoid fascia. Subcutaneous tissues are closed in a routine fashion, and a subcuticular skin closure performed with no. 4-0 clear monofilament absorbable suture. A Polar Care ice pack is in-corporated in the dressing, over a thin layer of sterile cotton padding (Fig. 11-86).

Postoperative Immobilization

In most cases the arm is protected for 3 to 4 weeks with a shoulder sling and a small pillow (Ultra Sling, DonJoy, Inc.) (see Fig. 11-68). The purpose of the pillow is to prevent the forearm from resting in an internal rotation position. Also, the few degrees of abduction afford a better healing posture for the rotator cuff and permit air circulation to the axilla for better hygiene (Fig. 11-87).

If the bone is soft or the rotator cuff tendon tissue is of poor quality, the arm is placed in a functional abduction brace. The brace we pre-fer, the SCOI shoulder brace, is made by DonJoy, Inc. (Carlsbad, California) (Fig. 11-88). The SCOI brace permits the patient to exercise the elbow, wrist, and hand early in the postoperative period. As soon as the patient is alert, he or she begins active elbow flexion and extension by releasing the elbow hinge lock (Fig. 11-89). Also, the exercise ball on the forearm cradle is squeezed frequently to maintain forearm muscle tone. The abduction support is set at approximately 40 degrees after surgery. In large-framed or obese patients the SCOI brace may not offer a good fit; a Quadrant brace (DonJoy, Inc.) may be needed. This brace has the same basic benefits as the SCOI, but is more adaptable to larger patients (Fig. 11-90).

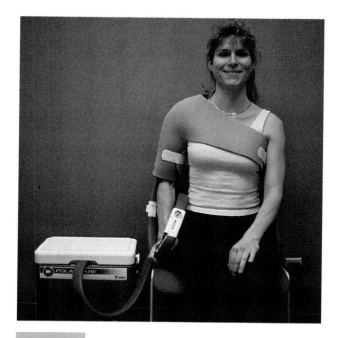

Figure 11-86
A Polar Care ice pad (Breg, Inc.) is incorporated into the postoperative dressing to aid in pain control and reduce inflammation.

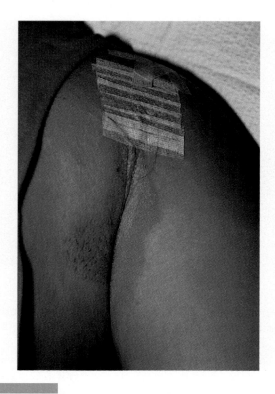

Figure 11-87
If the arm is held in adduction in the postoperative period with no air circulation to the axilla, a rash may occur and become secondarily infected.

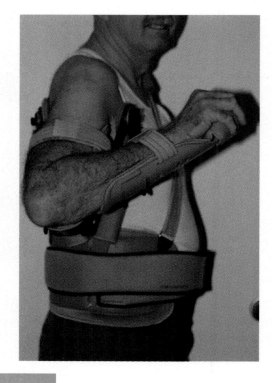

Figure 11-89
The elbow hinge is released in the postoperative period to allow the patient free motion of the elbow, wrist, and hand while still protecting the shoulder.

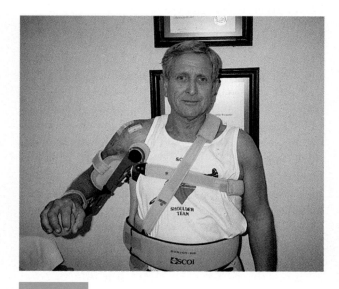

Figure 11-88
The SCOI shoulder brace can hold the arm in a comfortable position of abduction to relieve tension on the rotator cuff repair.

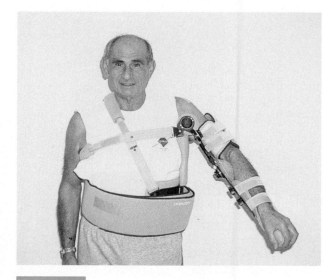

Figure 11-90
The Quadrant brace (DonJoy, Inc.) allows more universal positioning in flexion, abduction, and rotation than the SCOI brace. It also is more adaptable to larger-framed patients.

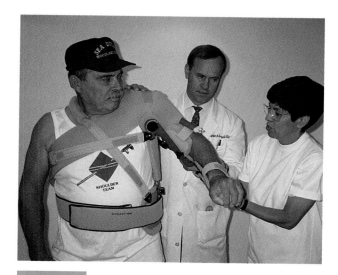

Figure 11-91
After the first week in the postoperative brace, a family member or therapist can be instructed to perform passive range-of-motion exercises of the shoulder several times during the day.

At 1 week post-surgery, the shoulder is moved passively in an abduction arc between 30 and 70 degrees. This passive mobilization requires the help of a reliable family member, friend, or therapist to support the arm while the abduction hinge locks on the front and back are released (Fig. 11-91). The arm can be elevated and lowered by the helper while the patient relaxes the shoulder musculature. The SCOI shoulder brace is worn continuously for 3 to 4 weeks, depending on the severity of the tear and the quality of the tissues being repaired. After the brace is removed, an Ultra Sling (DonJoy, Inc.) with its small abduction pillow is worn for an additional 2 to 3 weeks. Physical therapy begins around the third or fourth week. The patient, who has been instructed in the use of the STK (Shoulder Therapy Kit—Breg, Inc.) before surgery, follows the surgeon's prescribed instructions with the help of the therapist, both at home and during the therapy sessions.

References

1. Neer CS II: *Shoulder Reconstruction.* Philadelphia, Saunders, 1990, p 53.

2. Snyder SJ, Patterson MD: Acromial morphology and rotator cuff injury. (Personal communication.)

3. Bigliani LU, Morrison DS, April EW: The morphology of the acromion and its relationship to rotator cuff tears. *Orthop Trans* 10:216, 1986.

4. Snyder SJ, Wuh HCK: A modified classification of the supraspinatus outlet view based on the configuration and the anatomic thickness of the acromion. Presented at American Shoulder and Elbow Surgeons Annual Closed Meeting, Seattle, Washington, September 1991.

5. Rafii M, Firooznia H, Sherman O, et al: Rotator cuff lesions: Signal patterns at MR imaging. *Radiology* 177:817, 1990.

6. Hodler J, Kursunoglu-Brahme S, Snyder SJ, et al: Rotator cuff disease: Assessment with MR arthrography versus standard MR imaging in 36 patients with arthroscopic confirmation. *Radiology* 182:431, 1992.

7. Snyder SJ: A complete system for arthroscopy and bursoscopy of the shoulder. *Surg Rounds Orthop* July 1989, p 57.

8. Neer CS II: Anterior acromioplasty for chronic impingement syndrome in the shoulder: A preliminary report. *J Bone Joint Surg* 54A:41, 1972.

9. Ellman H: Arthroscopic subacromial decompression: Analysis of one to three year results. *Arthroscopy* 3:173, 1987.

10. Esch JC, Ozerkis LR, Helgager JA, et al: Arthroscopic subacromial decompression—results according to degree of rotator cuff tear. *Arthroscopy* 4:241, 1988.

11. Paulos LE, Harner CD, Parker RD: Arthroscopic subacromial decompression for impingement syndrome of the shoulder. *Tech Orthop* 3:33, 1988.

12. Johnson LL: *Arthroscopic Surgery Principles and Practice.* St. Louis, Mosby, 1986, pp 1301–1445.

13. Sampson T: Precision acromioplasty in arthroscopic subacromial decompression of the shoulder. *Arthroscopy* 7:301, 1991.

14. Marshall GJ, Kirchen ME, Sweeney JR, Snyder SJ: Synovisol as an irrigant for electrosurgery of joints. *Arthroscopy* 4:187, 1988.

15. Kessel L, Watson M: The painful arch syndrome. Clinical classification as a guide to management. *J Bone Joint Surg* 59B:166, 1977.

16. France EP, Paulos LE, Harner CD, et al: Biomechanical evaluation of rotator cuff fixation methods. *Am J Sports Med* 17:176, 1989.

12

Shoulder Instability

Introduction

Of all of the common shoulder pathologies that may benefit from shoulder arthroscopy, shoulder instability is certainly near, if not at, the top of the list. Today the orthopedic surgeon contends not only with the easily diagnosed instability of complete anterior dislocation, but also with the very subtle and difficult diagnostic problems of symptomatic subluxation and instability with secondary impingement commonly found in throwing athletes. Multidirectional shoulder laxity and various degrees of posterior laxity further complicate the diagnostic problem. Since each of these instability patterns requires an accurate diagnosis and subsequent surgical or nonsurgical treatment, the potential benefits of precise arthroscopic assessment, and in some cases surgical repair, are enormous.

When one considers the possible clinical consequences of an incorrect diagnosis in an instability situation, it is obvious that the surgeon should employ the best possible means to ensure that the diagnosis is correct. All traditional open surgical approaches required to repair labral or ligamentous avulsions involve some form of iatrogenic injury to the subscapularis or infraspinatus tendons. The surgical scars, with their subsequent cosmetic uncertainties, should not be overlooked. The arthroscope affords the orthopaedist the opportunity for minimally traumatic joint visualization, ensuring a more accurate and complete diagnosis, and in many cases allowing minimally invasive precise surgical repair of the injured tissues. In this chapter we will briefly review the history of the use of the arthroscope in instability surgery of the shoulder and discuss several alternatives to surgical repair. We will conclude with the techniques currently used at SCOI.

The Anatomy of Shoulder Stability

Although the pathology of shoulder instability was eloquently described by Bankart and others before 1950,[1] it was not until the arthroscope allowed in vivo study of the shoulder anatomy that surgeons could appreciate many of the complex and fascinating aspects of shoulder instability. The anterior capsular ligaments, together with the subscapularis tendon, the labrum, and to some extent the rotator cuff, give the soft tissues the support needed to ensure joint stability. The variable arrangements of the anterior capsular ligaments can be mistaken for pathological situations, and require careful study by the shoulder arthroscopist.

There are three distinct thickenings within the anterior shoulder capsule, called the anterior glenohumeral ligaments. They all originate from the anterior and inferior surface of the humeral head and insert on the anterior glenoid. These three glenohumeral ligaments are named for their relative points of origin on the humerus (Figs. 12-1 and 12-2). The *superior glenohumeral ligament* originates from the upper portion of the anterior humerus in the area of the lesser tuberosity and inserts anterior to the superior glenoid tubercle. The *middle glenohumeral ligament* takes origin from the area below superior ligament on the

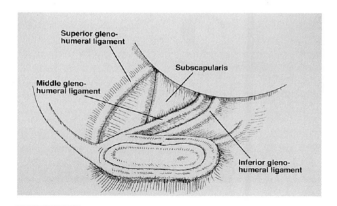

Figure 12-2
The classic arrangement of the glenohumeral ligaments includes distinct superior, middle, and inferior glenohumeral ligaments, with a recess or reflection beneath each. No capsular foramen is present.

lesser tuberosity and the anatomical humeral neck. It inserts along the anterior neck of the glenoid, 1 to 2 mm below the articular cartilage margin; or it may insert directly into the glenoid labrum in the anterior superior quadrant. The *inferior glenohumeral ligament* is composed of three distinct and recognizable structures. The superior band of the inferior glenohumeral ligament originates from an area on the humeral neck below the middle ligament. It passes across the front of the joint to insert along the anterior surface of the glenoid at the articular cartilage margin, usually combining with the anterior glenoid labrum. The insertion usually extends from the anterior inferior quadrant to an area just above the anterior epiphyseal notch. The axillary pouch is the second section of the inferior ligament. The pouch includes the ligamentous tissue below the superior band and inserts along the neck of the glenoid with the labrum from an area throughout an arc encompassing the inferior 30 to 40 percent of the glenoid margin. The third section, or posterior band, of the inferior ligament resembles the anterior superior band. Like its counterpart anteriorly, it most often enters the labrum at the articular cartilage margin near the midpoint of the glenoid.

The function of the glenohumeral ligaments

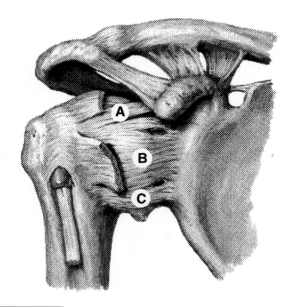

Figure 12-1
The glenohumeral ligaments are named for their respective origins on the humeral head. The superior ligament is always present; the middle ligament has variable morphology; the inferior ligament is present in most situations with a prominent superior band.

has been identified in several classic studies. Turkel, O'Brien, Rodosky,[2,3,4] and others have demonstrated that the stability provided by the ligaments is specific to the position of the arm at the time the stress is applied. The anterior superior ligament is most important with the arm near the side with little or no abduction. It provides some support for anterior inferior displacement of the humeral head, in conjunction with the coracohumeral ligament. Bosminigin demonstrated that after cutting of the anterior superior structures in the rotator interval, the humeral head tended to displace inferiorly.[5]

The middle glenohumeral ligament and the subscapularis tendon are the most important structures for guarding against anterior shoulder instability with the arm at around 90 degrees of abduction. As the arm is taken farther overhead in more abduction and external rotation forces are applied, the superior band and the inferior axillary pouch become more prominent stabilizers. Posteriorly, O'Brien et al. have demonstrated that the superior band of the inferior ligament plays an important stabilizing role.[3] In order for the humeral head to dislocate posteriorly in their cadaver model, it was necessary not only to cut the posterior capsular ligaments but to extend the release proximally as far as the anterior superior quadrant. This seems consistent with the fact that an isolated ligamentous injury is seldom enough to allow a complete dislocation, but may set the stage for a joint subluxation.

The glenoid labrum is also thought to have a certain stabilizing effect on the joint. Although the labrum is an extremely variable structure, most often it does form a complete ring around the glenoid surface. One theory concludes that the labrum serves as a vacuum seal for the humeral head, much as a rubber suction cup would against a smooth ball.[6] Additionally, the labrum is thought by some authors to serve as a buttress or wedge around the minimally concave glenoid face. This wedge effect may inhibit some excessive humeral head translation.[7] Since the anterior glenoid labrum serves as the anchor point for the anterior inferior ligamentous complex, it is also often the site of failure in shoulder dislocations. Perry[8] has shown that the bonding strength between the labrum and the anterior glenoid bone varies significantly with age. She noted that at birth the bonding strength was around 13 kg, while at 30 years of age it reached a maximum of 64 kg for male specimens; female bonding strength was 30 percent less at each age. This may explain why a Bankart lesion is so commonly seen when the first dislocation occurs in the teenage years. In later years, when the labral glenoid bond is more secure, the tissue failure allowing the anterior dislocation may occur through the capsule, the subscapularis tendon, or the rotator cuff.

The common variations in the glenohumeral ligaments were very well described by Morgan, Rames, and Snyder.[9] We described four normal variations in the ligamentous tissues, as follows: type I included the classic arrangement and was seen in 66 percent (see Fig. 12-2). In this situation, all three ligaments were present and attached in the classic pattern to the labrum. In the type II arrangement, there was confluence between the middle and inferior ligaments with an absent or poorly developed middle ligament. This was present in 7 percent (Fig. 12-3). The type III arrangement was found in 19 percent of the shoulders and included the normal-appearing superior ligament with a "cord-like" middle

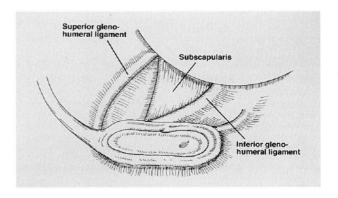

Figure 12-3
The type II arrangement includes a confluent middle and inferior glenohumeral ligament pattern in which these two ligaments present as one ligament with no recess between them. No capsular foramen is present.

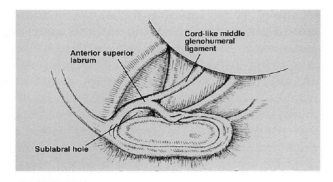

Figure 12-4
The type III pattern is that in which the middle glenohumeral ligament appears as a cord-like structure with a high-riding glenoid attachment and a large capsular foramen beneath the cord, but a normal-appearing inferior glenohumeral ligament

glenohumeral ligament and a classic inferior ligament with a well-defined superior band (Fig. 12-4). The cord-like middle ligament was described as having an appearance like that of a rounded cord with a rolled upper and lower edge. There appeared to be an opening to the subscapularis recess above and below the middle ligament. The type IV arrangement was found in 8 percent. These specimens failed to demonstrate any discernible anterior capsular ligaments (Fig. 12-5). In a follow-up study by the same authors[10] it was noted that the type III ligamentous arrangement, where the cord-like middle ligament was present,

was seldom seen in cases where the shoulder was evaluated arthroscopically for treatment of anterior instability. It was postulated that this ligamentous arrangement offered a greater element of protection against anterior instability than the other ligamentous patterns.

The anterior superior quadrant of the glenoid is known to have various other confusing anatomical variations. The "sublabral hole" has been a source of confusion to surgeons. Several anatomical studies have demonstrated this complete opening beneath the anterior superior labrum to be a non-pathological anatomical variant seen to a greater or lesser degree in approximately 9 percent of patients[9] (Fig. 12-6). Not only should this variant be appreciated by arthroscopists and not be confused with a Bankart lesion, but it should also be understood by the radiologist, who may find it confusing on MRI or CT arthrography. When a sublabral hole is present and a type III ligamentous arrangement occurs, with a cord-like middle ligament attaching to the labrum above the sublabral hole, this adds further confusion to the picture (Fig. 12-7). It appears as if the cord-like ligament had displaced the labrum, which was certainly not the case in Morgan's study.

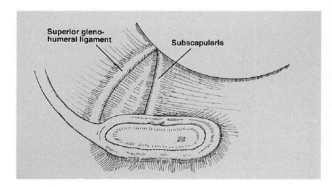

Figure 12-5
In the type IV ligament, the anterior capsule appears as a confluent sheet with no ligamentous thickenings, reflections, or recesses.

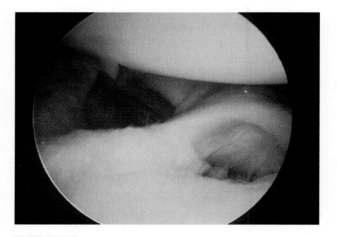

Figure 12-6
A normal sublabral hole in the anterior superior quadrant of the labrum can be mistaken for a traumatic detachment if the observer is not familiar with the superior labral anatomy.

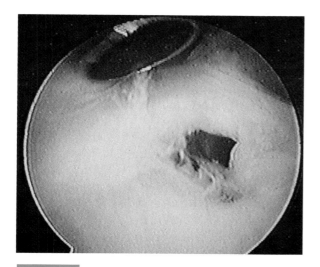

Figure 12-7
When a cord-like middle ligament attaching to the anterior superior labrum is associated with a sublabral hole, a very confusing picture will be seen, resembling a traumatic labral detachment.

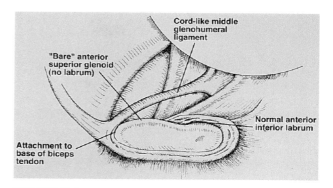

Figure 12-8
The "Buford complex" resembles a traumatic labral detachment, since no anterior superior labral tissue is seen.

A very dramatic example of a normal variant in the anterior labral structure is the so-called Buford complex.[11] The authors reviewed 200 consecutive shoulder arthroscopies and discovered this anatomic variation to be present in 1.5 percent, or 3 out of 200, of the cases studied. None of these patients had any history of shoulder instability or symptoms that could be related to the labral ligamentous anatomy.

The three anatomical elements that form the Buford complex (Figs. 12-8 and 12-9) are as follows: (1) The middle glenohumeral ligament is cord-like in structure; it blends and is continuous with the anterior superior glenoid labrum; (2) this combined ligamentous-labral structure attaches to the glenoid at a single point at the base of the biceps tendon; and (3) there is no additional anterior superior labral tissue along the anterior glenoid above the anterior epiphyseal notch. When first seen, the Buford complex appears to be a traumatic chronic avulsion of the anterior superior labrum. On further study, however, it is noted that there are no signs of fraying or ligamentous damage and the synovial and capsular tissues around the ligament labral complex appear to be undamaged. The labral struc-

tures below the epiphyseal notch anteriorly are perfectly normal. It is our feeling that the Buford complex, although bizarre in appearance, should not require surgical repair unless the biceps anchor to the glenoid has actually been disrupted or there is a transverse split near the ligament attachment to the biceps (Fig. 12-10).

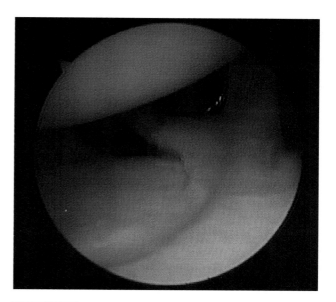

Figure 12-9
When a Buford complex is noted it should not be repaired, since this is a normal variant.

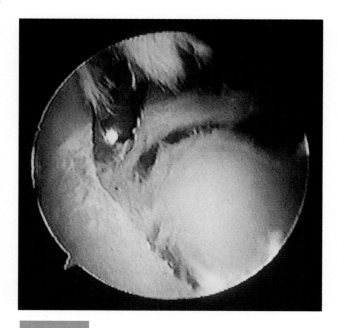

Figure 12-10
On occasion the Buford complex is associated with an actual disruption of the biceps anchor detachment; a repair may be needed.

History and Clinical Examination with Shoulder Instability

The diagnosis of shoulder instability may be obvious from a historical standpoint, as when there is a history of a classic anterior dislocation; or it may be one of the most difficult diagnoses to make, as when subtle functional subluxation is the problem. A careful review of the history will usually give important clues to the diagnosis. When a single traumatic event such as a fall or twisting of the arm—particularly in the abducted and external rotated position (throwing position)—has occurred antedating the symptoms, with or without a true dislocation, the possibility of anterior capsular damage and subsequent laxity must be considered. Following the initial event, an asymptomatic period may disguise the severity of the situation until another stress occurs in the unstable position. If the shoulder actually dislocates and requires manipulative reduction, the diagnosis is straight-

forward. When the symptoms are of slipping of the joint, or simply of pain and a "dead arm" after throwing, the diagnosis is more questionable.[12] A careful clinical examination along with a review of the x-rays, and sometimes an MRI scan, usually, but not always, solidifies the diagnosis. The pain occurring in an unstable shoulder with throwing is often felt in the posterior shoulder. The symptoms will occur with the arm in the position of risk, which is at the end of the cocking and beginning of the acceleration phase of the throw. Walsch et al.[13] and Jobe[14] have demonstrated that when there is laxity in the anterior ligamentous structures there may be posterior impingement on the rotator cuff and labrum contributing to the painful clinical picture, as well as soft tissue damage.

Physical Examination

Inspection of the shoulder may reveal hypertrophy of the musculature in the dominant arm of a thrower. Seldom is there significant atrophy present, unless previous surgery has been performed or there is neurological injury. Range of motion of the shoulder may be perfectly normal, but often the external rotation is limited either by reflex guarding or by slight capsular contraction. The classic clinical tests for instability include (1) the subacromial sulcus sign (inferior subluxation); (2) the posterior apprehension test; (3) the anterior apprehension and subsequent apprehension suppression test; and (4) anterior and posterior translation laxity.

The *subacromial sulcus test* is performed with the patient standing. With the muscles of the shoulder relaxed, the examiner places a downward stress on the patient's wrist. If there is inferior laxity of the shoulder—suggesting relaxation of the superior glenohumeral ligament, and perhaps of the coracohumeral ligament, as well as of the inferior capsule—then the shoulder will sag inferiorly in the joint and a space will be noted below the acromion (Fig. 12-11). This test should be compared to the opposite side; when congenital ligamentous laxity is present, the subacromial gap may be equally visible.

The classic *posterior instability test* is be-

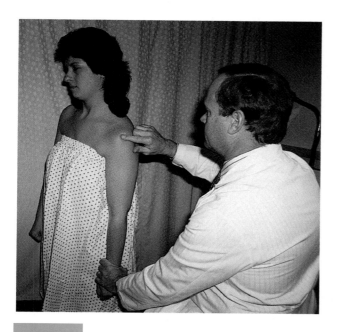

Figure 12-11
The subacromial sulcus test is used to evaluate for
inferior glenohumeral laxity (see text).

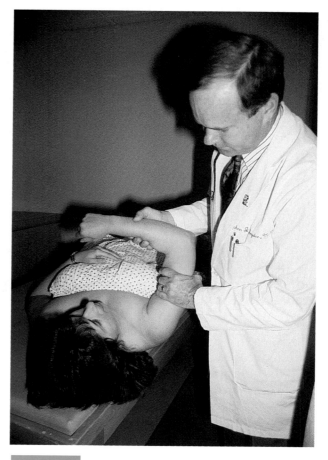

Figure 12-12
The posterior apprehension test is performed in the
supine or standing position. It is helpful in diagnosing
posterior instability (see text).

gun by having the patient position the arm in
abduction of 90 degrees. The examiner then
moves the arm into more adduction and internal rotation while applying a posterior-directed
force on the elbow. We prefer to perform this
test with the patient in the supine position. If
the patient becomes apprehensive and reports
discomfort, the test is presumably positive
(Fig. 12-12).

We prefer to perform the *anterior apprehension test* with the patient relaxed in the
supine position. The arm is placed in the 90-
degree abduction position with the forearm off
the side of the table. The arm is slowly rotated
into external rotation while the patient's reaction is observed (Fig. 12-13). If pain occurs or
a sense of apprehension is reported, the external rotation is stopped. The examiner then
tests for relief of the symptoms (*apprehension
suppression*) by placing his or her hand over
the anterior shoulder joint. By exerting gentle
posterior-directed pressure on the front of the
shoulder, the previously reported apprehension or pain should be relieved if anterior instability is the cause (Fig. 12-14). The test is
confirmed by slowly removing the hand from

the front of the shoulder without changing the
external rotation position of the arm. The
symptoms should return when the humeral
head slides back into the subluxed position.
No attempt is made to "dislocate" the shoulder, since that induces anxiety and distrust on
the part of the patient, leading to reflex guarding.

The final clinical test performed is the *anterior and posterior translation test.* With the
patient in the lateral position and his or her
head on a pillow, the arm is supported by the
examiner in 90 degrees of abduction and neutral rotation. The patient's torso should be
well toward the examiner's side of the table,
leaning slightly posteriorly. The patient must

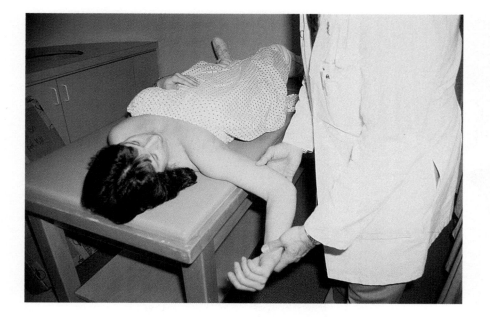

Figure 12-13
The supine abduction external rotation apprehension test helps to document anterior laxity (see text).

be encouraged to relax so that muscle guarding will not confuse the picture. The weight of the arm is allowed to compress the joint while the humeral head is translated, first anteriorly and then posteriorly, across the joint. This is the same technique used to examine for stability prior to every arthroscopic evaluation of the shoulder (Fig. 12-15).

X-Ray and MRI Evaluation in Shoulder Instability

X-Ray

The x-ray evaluation in shoulder instability is extremely important, not only to determine the presence of the problem but also to assess

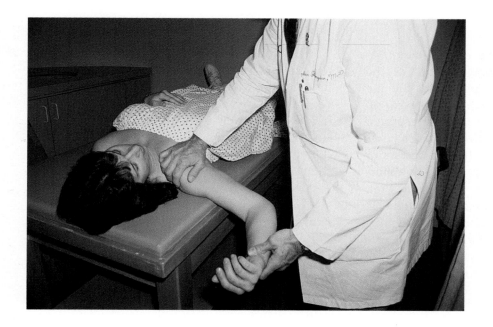

Figure 12-14
If the anterior apprehension test is positive, the symptoms should improve when a posterior force is applied to the anterior shoulder (apprehension suppression test) (see text).

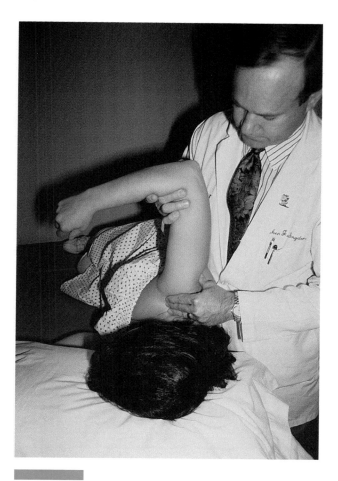

Figure 12-15
Anterior and posterior laxity are tested by translating
the humeral head with the patient in the lateral position
(see text).

the probable magnitude and chronicity of the
injury. The four standard x-ray views that we
recommend include (1) an AP view of the
glenohumeral joint, (2) an AP exposure with
20-degree cephalad angulation with internal
rotation of the arm, (3) an axillary view, and
(4) a supraspinatus outlet or lateral acromial
arch view. (See Chap. 11.)

When an acute traumatic dislocation has
previously occurred, the damage to the joint
is usually on the posterior superior aspect of
the humeral head (Hill-Sachs lesion), and
along the anterior and inferior glenoid margin
(bony Bankart lesion). These lesions can usually be seen with standard good-quality x-ray

exposures, as described above. Infrequently,
either of these bony injuries may be significant and require further study using a CT
scan.

MRI Scan

The soft tissue injuries associated with instability are best evaluated with an MRI scan. We
do not advocate performance of an MRI scan
in all cases of instability, especially if the diagnosis is evident clinically. When necessary for
planning purposes, a high-quality MRI scan
(or CT arthrogram, for that matter) will demonstrate the anterior or posterior labral and
ligamentous anatomy very well (Fig. 12-16).
In cases of more subtle instability with difficulties in diagnosis, a gadolinium-enhanced
MRI arthrogram may be warranted.[15] A Hill-
Sachs lesion is easily appreciated with this
technique, as well as the detached labral and
ligamentous tissues (Fig. 12-17).

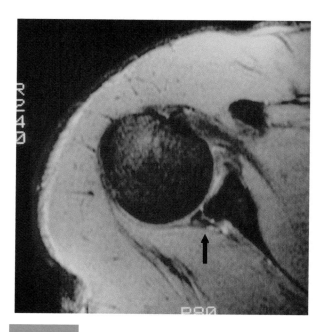

Figure 12-16
This MRI scan demonstrates a posterior labral
detachment (posterior Bankart lesion) with a normal
capsular appearance. This patient was sent for
evaluation of a suspected "anterior" instability problem.

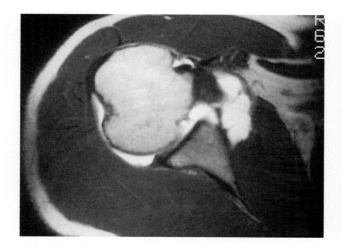

Figure 12-17
A gadolinium-enhanced MRI arthrogram readily demonstrates the damage to the anterior labrum in this case of chronic anterior subluxation.

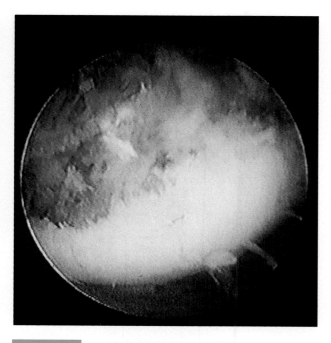

Figure 12-18
A large Hill-Sachs lesion (grade 2) is seen from the posterior portal. It should not cause problems once the anterior capsule and labrum are repaired.

Pathology of Instability—Acute and Chronic

Before the advent of arthroscopy there was no way to visualize adequately the intra-articular damage in the shoulder joint after an acute traumatic dislocation episode. Now that arthroscopy is available, several surgeons have reported their observations and have formulated certain theories that may serve as guides for future ligamentous repair options. Wheeler et al. studied a group of cadets at the United States Military Academy.[16] A similar study by Baker et al. on acute initial dislocators concluded that traumatic dislocation often inflicted very considerable damage to a shoulder joint.[17] In both studies a large percentage of patients were noted to have an acute disruption of the ligament labral attachment to the anterior glenoid (Bankart lesion). Additionally, the posterior humeral head impression fracture (Hill-Sachs lesion) was found in approximately 50 percent of the patients (Fig. 12-18). Often this fracture was not appreciated on the preoperative x-ray. Additional injuries included loose bodies within the joint, labral flaps, and biceps tendon injuries, as well as glenoid fractures. Several patients had partial-thickness rotator cuff tears as well.

Baker et al. devised a rating system to be used in assessing the damage in acute shoulder dislocations. Group 1 patients had stretching of the anterior capsular structures with possibly some hemorrhage, but no obvious tear or labral disruption. Group 2 patients had capsular tears and partial labral detachments. Group 3 patients had complete capsular labral detachment causing incompetent ligamentous tissues. It was postulated that the group 3 patients were not likely to heal spontaneously and might be considered candidates for acute repair. The other patients were thought to be more likely candidates for spontaneous healing; in these cases it was thought that surgical procedures for instability might not be necessary.

Findings in Chronic Instability

Several authors have gathered data on the intra-articular findings in chronic recurrent anterior instability of the shoulder. Johnson[18] presented his study to the American Shoulder and Elbow Surgeons meeting in Seattle, Washington, in 1991. He noted that there were partial rotator cuff tears in 13 percent of the patients. Synovitis was present in 37 percent; loose bodies were found in 19 percent; articular cartilage injury was found on the humerus in 36 percent, and on the glenoid in 15 percent; and posterior labral tears were noted in 32 percent. In our series of instability patients, we have noted similar findings.

In addition, there was a 9 percent incidence of significant damage to the superior glenoid labrum from anterior to posterior, or the so-called SLAP lesion (see Chap. 10).[19] All four types of SLAP lesion were included in the instability patients, including several cases of bucket-handle tears (type III), and bucket-handle tears that included a split into the biceps tendon (type IV). The type II SLAP lesions present a particularly difficult problem, since, as has been pointed out by Rodosky et al.,[4] when the superior labrum and biceps anchor mechanism is loose, an additional strain is placed on the anterior capsular attachment with the instability forces). For this reason, we thought it necessary to reattach all significant type II SLAP lesions to the underlying glenoid bone during instability repairs. Additionally, there were several cases of near-complete biceps tendon rupture requiring surgical debridement and, in two cases, tenodesis. Partial rotator cuff tears were not uncommon, but significant partial tears and full-thickness lesions were rare except in the older age group. Several posterior inferior flap tears of the labrum were noted; degenerative arthritis involving the humeral head and glenoid surfaces was also observed. We believe that without the arthroscopic evaluation this ancillary but important pathology would have

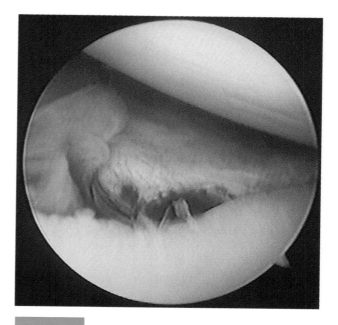

Figure 12-19
The classic Bankart lesion includes the complete detachment of the anterior labrum from the midglenoid notch to the anterior inferior corner; the capsule and ligaments are usually intact.

been missed, perhaps resulting in a less than optimal surgical outcome.

The classic pathology found with chronic anterior instability is the detached anterior labrum below the anterior epiphyseal notch extending to the inferior aspect of the glenoid (Fig. 12-19). When viewing from only a single posterior portal, it is sometimes difficult to appreciate the more subtle cases of labral detachment. The anterior superior portal affords a better view down the neck of the anterior glenoid in instability cases. With the labrum detached and displaced medially on the neck, a patulous anterior pouch with an incompetent superior band of the inferior ligament often results. Additionally, we have noted patients in whom the anterior labrum appears completely intact on the glenoid, but the ligamentous attachment to the labrum has been avulsed (Fig. 12-20). This pathological situation was appreciated only when viewing from the anterior superior portal down the neck of the glenoid.

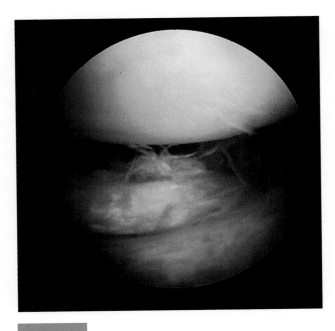

Figure 12-20
From the anterior superior portal the labrum is seen to be intact, but the ligaments are torn and deficient. This capsular lesion might have been missed had we not viewed from the anterior portal.

Wolf observed and reported on a situation in which the *humeral* attachment of the glenohumeral ligaments is disrupted. He calls this a "HAGL lesion" and suggests that it may be seen only when viewing from an anterior portal with the arthroscope rotated to look laterally toward the area of the neck of the humerus[20] (Fig. 12-21).

Neviaser has described another appearance of the labrum in chronic instability cases.[21] He noted that when the labrum is detached from the edge of the glenoid and later reattaches in a more medial location on the neck, it may create a confusing anatomical situation (Fig. 12-22). The synovium tends to fill in the space above the labrum, creating a false appearance resembling an intact labral-glenoid bond. There is always a small cleft present between the glenoid and the capsule (Fig. 12-23). He calls this pathology the ALPSA lesion (anterior labral periosteal sleeve avulsion) and suggests that the labrum must be mobilized and reduced to control the instability.

Since the detachment of the labrum may extend past the midpoint inferiorly, it is also extremely important to evaluate the posterior labrum from both the anterior and posterior portals. This again stresses the importance of the systematic 15-point glenohumeral evaluation in every arthroscopic procedure. On two occasions in our series, the preoperative diagnosis of anterior instability was changed at the time of arthroscopy on the basis of the ex-

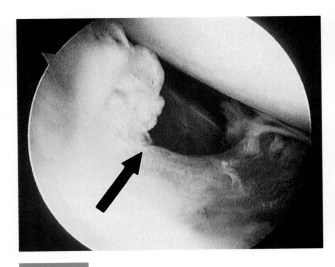

Figure 12-21
A HAGL lesion can be seen only while viewing upward from the anterior portal near the anatomical neck of the humerus (see text).

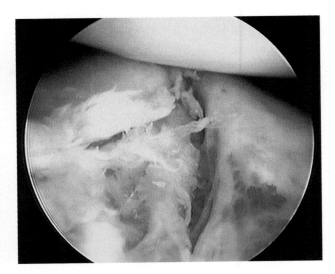

Figure 12-22
The ALPSA lesion (see text) must be understood so that a potential cause of instability is not overlooked during the arthroscopic exam. It is best visualized with the arthroscope viewing from the anterior superior portal.

Figure 12-23
The ALPSA lesion can be confusing because of the tendency for synovial scar to fill in above the displaced labrum. (*Reprinted, with permission, from Ref. 21.*)

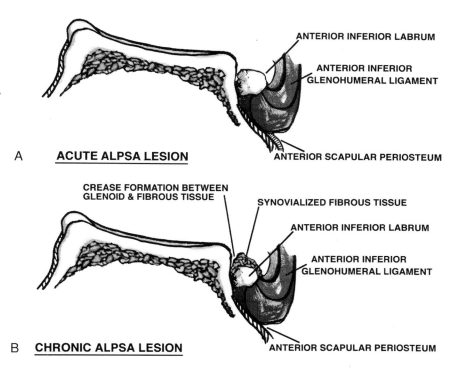

A **ACUTE ALPSA LESION**

ANTERIOR INFERIOR LABRUM

ANTERIOR INFERIOR GLENOHUMERAL LIGAMENT

ANTERIOR SCAPULAR PERIOSTEUM

CREASE FORMATION BETWEEN GLENOID & FIBROUS TISSUE

SYNOVIALIZED FIBROUS TISSUE

ANTERIOR INFERIOR LABRUM

ANTERIOR INFERIOR GLENOHUMERAL LIGAMENT

B **CHRONIC ALPSA LESION**

ANTERIOR SCAPULAR PERIOSTEUM

amination under anesthesia and the arthroscopic findings of a compete detachment of the posterior labrum with normal anterior structures (Fig. 12-24). On two additional occasions, both anterior and posterior Bankart lesions were noted at arthroscopy, directing the subsequent repair on both sides of the shoulder.

The Hill-Sachs lesion, which is present in most cases of traumatic instability, can be very minimal (grade I) with only cartilage scuffing. In more severe cases it may have a cartilage divot with a superficial bony injury (grade II), or may be quite severe and appear as a "hatchet" fracture (grade III) with a deep and fairly large defect on the humeral head. Seldom are there loose fragments around the Hill-Sachs lesion, although there may be loose chips of articular cartilage in the joint, from the more severe lesions; these are often located in the subscapularis recess.

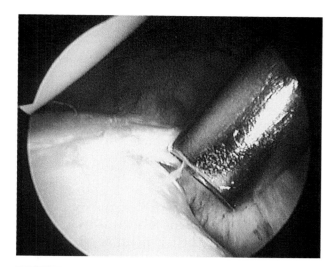

Figure 12-24
On occasion the history and physical examination can be confusing, with the arthroscopic view from the anterior portal demonstrating fraying and possibly detachment of the posterior labrum indicating posterior instability.

Arthroscopic Evaluation in Minimal Traumatic Anterior Instability ("Loose Shoulder") and Subluxation Situations

It is common knowledge now that *not* all shoulder instability is secondary to significant acute trauma. Two other types of instability exist which must be understood by the arthroscopic surgeon. The "loose shoulder" with recurrent anterior subluxation and without significant antecedent trauma, or with multidirectional laxity, is worrisome to experienced shoulder surgeons. Since these patients often have deficient collagen tissues throughout their bodies, even an excellent capsular repair may stretch out easily, allowing instability to recur. For this reason, it is important to suspect these patients from the history and clinical evaluation and confirm these suspicions with arthroscopy. The arthroscopic findings in the loose shoulder or atraumatic multidirectional instability are usually those of minimal joint damage, and often no Hill-Sachs lesion. The capsular tissues may be deficient anteriorly, inferiorly, and posteriorly, and the labrum may be attenuated or not present (Fig. 12-25). Seldom is there a significant detachment of the capsule (Bankart lesion), but often the anterior capsular ligaments are poorly defined or not visible at all. Additionally, the rotator interval area between the supraspinatus tendon and the subscapularis tendon may be very patulous. The decision to perform a surgical repair on a patient with this type of instability should be based on the surgeon's training and experience in both arthroscopic and open surgery. The patient should be carefully screened for psychosocial problems and self-destructive tendencies. If surgery is required for atraumatic laxity, most often an open capsular shift procedure is used.[22]

Findings in Overhand Thrower's Instability

When the arm is in the cocked position, as in throwing, tennis, or swimming, severe stresses are placed on the anterior capsular structures. With repetitive throwing maneuvers, particularly when the posterior rotator cuff muscles are deficient or fatigued, anterior subluxation can occur. With continued stress the anterior tissues may fail, increasing the subluxation with accompanying pain and inability to continue throwing, serving, or swimming. Glousman has classified the instability seen in throwers into three categories.[23] Group I patients have very subtle anterior instability with no visible signs of damage to their ligamentous tissues or labrum, and no Hill-Sachs lesion. Group II includes the throwers with early fraying of the labrum and a somewhat patulous capsule and a small Hill-Sachs lesion. Group III patients have significant damage to the labrum in the anterior inferior quadrant and often have a Hill-Sachs lesion. Many of these patients present with partial rotator cuff tears; some have biceps lesions as well.

Jobe has described a possible mechanism by which the classic posterior superior labral tear and partial-thickness rotator cuff tear seen in throwers may occur when subluxation is present.[14] He suggests that as the shoulder slides anteriorly, the greater tuberosity may impinge on the posterior superior labrum with the arm in the cocked and loaded position of

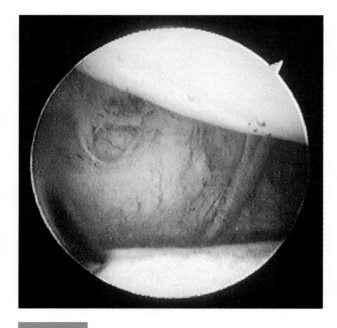

Figure 12-25
Sometimes in situations of multidirectional instability, or chronic "loose shoulder," the anterior capsular labral tissues are attenuated but no true Bankart lesion is present. (Type IV capsule.)

abduction and external rotation. Often a fold of rotator cuff tendon and posterior superior capsule is pinched between the greater tuberosity and the labrum which could damage these tissues as well. Jobe studied this hypothesis by fixing several cadaver specimens in the throwing position and sectioning the specimens. He noted that the posterior superior labrum was compressed, along with the posterior cuff, by the greater tuberosity, especially when the shoulder was rendered unstable anteriorly. We have noted this tendency as well, when viewing from the anterior portal arthroscopically, in patients with posterior shoulder lesions (Fig. 12-26). It is very important to understand that the subtle instabilities in throwers may mimic impingement syndrome. A careful history-taking and clinical examination should alert the surgeon; the arthroscopic findings, as well as the examination under anesthesia, will often confirm these suspicions and guide the subsequent care, either with physical therapy or with surgery. When surgery is needed it should address a specific pathology. Arthroscopic labral debridement is often temporarily helpful, but

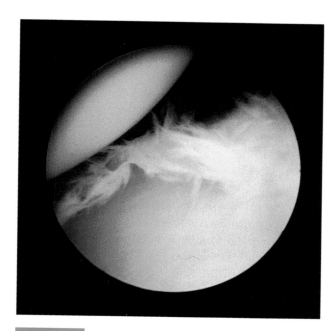

Figure 12-26

The posterior superior labral lesion seen in throwers often includes a flap tear and/or fraying of the tissues, sometimes with a posterior rotator cuff injury.

specific cuff rehabilitation or anterior or posterior capsular tightening procedures may be required in addition.[24]

Techniques for Arthroscopic Treatment of Anterior Shoulder Instability

Since the beginning of shoulder arthroscopy, surgeons have been intrigued by the prospect of being able to simplify the repair of the unstable shoulder with the use of techniques that would avoid open surgical incisions and iatrogenic injury to the otherwise uninvolved anterior structures. There are six points that we believe should be followed in the *ideal* arthroscopic surgical repair for anterior instability. Including them in the selected procedure should afford the opportunity for a safe, reproducible, and cost-effective repair by any surgeon skilled in shoulder arthroscopic techniques. The six points are:

1. Use of only absolutely safe arthroscopic portals, especially in the anterior mid-glenoid area.

2. No significant iatrogenic damage to the otherwise normal tissues (subscapularis, infraspinatus, coracoid, deltoid, or glenoid).

3. Direct repair of the avulsed labrum and ligamentous tissues on the exact edge of the glenoid rim, with the ability to adjust capsular tension when necessary.

4. Strong anchoring of the torn tissues with an implantable suture anchor (preferably long-term bio-absorbable), with no trans-glenoid drilling necessary.

5. The ability to use permanent nonabsorbable braided suture material similar to that used for open reconstructions, which is nonreactive and will eventually be incorporated into the healing tissue.

6. Relative simplicity of the instruments and the techniques for the reconstruction, so that it can be learned and perfected by any interested orthopaedist with basic shoulder arthroscopy skills.

Over the past 8 years various systems have evolved that have been used by surgeons to repair and reattach the anterior capsule tissues. The evolution of appropriate equipment for the *ideal* reconstruction has been slow. This has been due in part to the complex nature of the procedure and consequent uncertainty concerning equipment design, and in part because of the rigorous, but vitally important, requirements of the Food and Drug Administration for clinical evaluation of new implant materials.

The earliest reports of successful fixation of the anterior capsule ligaments were of surgeons using metallic staples inserted arthroscopically. Johnson popularized this technique and developed the Instrument Makar LCR (Ligament Capsule Repair) System for arthroscopic use.[25] Shortly thereafter, Wiley reported on a removable metal rivet which he used in ten patients.[26] Snyder, Gartsman, Wolf and Andrews utilized an implantable cannulated screw with a spiked washer in a similar fashion.[27] These investigators followed similar procedures for the anterior capsular fixation, which included (1) shaving and abrading the anterior glenoid neck, and (2) inserting the fixation device through the labrum and capsule and attempting to add tension to the system with proximal advancement. Unfortunately, the results of these techniques were only fair, with failure rates in the 20- to 25-percent range in the reported series.[28] There were also many reports of device-related complications, such as loosening of staples, irritation of surrounding tendons and articular surfaces, and device-related pain. Since these operations did not fulfill our six requirements for the ideal system, they were abandoned as soon as improved systems became available.

Absorbable tacks for repair of the anterior capsular structures were introduced independently for clinical trials by Warner and

Warren[29] and by Snyder in 1989. Although similar in design, the two devices were composed of different absorbable polymer; the former being polyglyconate (Acufex Microsurgical, Inc., Mansfield, MA) and the latter being homopolymer of polylactide (Concept, Inc., Largo, FL). The absorption of the polyglycolic tack took 5 to 6 weeks, while the polylactide device held for a minimum of 6 months. The investigators demonstrated that these devices could be applied in a similar fashion to the staple and screw implants, with many of the same drawbacks. It was very difficult to advance soft tissues when capsular laxity was present, and because of the size of the devices it was difficult to implant them close to the articular surface, for fear of humeral head contact. In addition, seldom could more than two tacks be used, which gave a limited number of fixation points for the repair. The angle of approach when inserting the devices was critical, and it was difficult to place the tacks in the ideal location inferiorly. If they were inserted at the wrong angle, they would easily fracture when impacted, since they were made of brittle material. The clinical trials of these devices were completed; the Acufex device is currently available on the market. Concept chose not to commercialize their product, in favor of producing a suture anchor device which is implanted completely below the bone surface (see Fig. 12-28).

Suture Repair with Transglenoid Drilling

There were four arthroscopic suturing techniques popularized by the early shoulder arthroscopy pioneers for repair of the anterior labrum and ligaments; all used transglenoid drilling techniques. The first such technique was that of Caspari.[30] He developed an ingenious instrument, called a suture punch, that allowed him to place a row of simple sutures through the avulsed anterior capsular tissues. He would then drill a single hole through the neck of the glenoid from anterior to posterior and pass all of the sutures together through this hole and out the back of the shoulder. The sutures would be divided into two bundles and then tied in a single large knot over the infraspinatus muscle fascia posteriorly.

Morgan and Bodenstab[31] used a modified Beath drill pin to spear the detached labrum and advanced it proximally. The pin was then drilled across the neck of the glenoid from anterior to posterior, carrying an absorbable suture out the back of the shoulder. A second pin was likewise used to spear another portion of the labrum and deliver a second suture out the back. These sutures were tied together in the front of the shoulder and then tied over the infraspinatus fascia posteriorly. Later, Morgan modified this technique with an interference knot tied in the suture posteriorly.[32] The knot was pulled down to the posterior cortex of the glenoid so that it was not necessary to tie it over the muscle fascia. The anterior limbs of the suture were then tied, using an arthroscopic knot-pusher, to secure the repair.

Maki,[33] in a similar technique, used a labral stitcher (Arthrex, Inc., Naples, Florida) to grasp the capsule and labrum and hold them in position while a pin was drilled across the neck of the glenoid. He popularized the use of the posterior interference knot to avoid the need for tying over the muscle and fascia. A second pin was drilled through the labrum above the first, and a second interference knot tied posteriorly. The anterior limbs were tied as in Morgan's technique. Rose et al. developed an aiming guide to help the surgeon avoid inadvertent posterior penetration near the axillary or suprascapular nerve.[34] They used a unique suturing tool, made by Acufex, to pass sutures through the labrum. They were then drilled across the joint and tied anteriorly.

All of these techniques seemed to give much better results in the hands of the investigators than the implant techniques, but they still did not fulfill our requirements for the ideal arthroscopic fixation technique. They all posed risks to the posterior neurological structures and required a low anterior portal, which threatened the musculocutaneous nerve and the cephalic vein anteriorly as well. In addition, only nonabsorbable sutures had been used, to avoid potential damage to the posterior structures. Caspari's suture punch was only able to stitch using somewhat stiff monofilament sutures.

Suture Anchor Techniques for Anterior Capsular Fixation

The development of miniature suture-holding bone anchors has allowed a completely new approach to anterior capsular ligamentous fixation. The first such anchors, made by Mitek, Inc. (Norwood, MA), utilized a small stem of titanium alloy with two lateral arcs of nitinol memory wire. An eyelet on the base of the device allowed insertion of a suture (Fig. 12-27). Another device currently being tested in an absorbable anchor. The BioTak suture anchor (Concept, Inc., Largo, Florida) is constructed of a long-lasting polylactide polymer that does not lose strength for 6 months after implantation (Fig. 12-28). The anchors are inserted into predrilled holes on the neck of the glenoid, securely fixating the suture beneath the subcortical bone. The surgeon can then use the suture to perform the labral or ligamen-

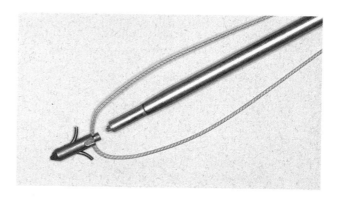

Figure 12-27
The Mitek suture anchor was the first miniature suture anchor to allow reliable fixation of sutures to bone. The eyelet in the Mitek anchor allows insertion of a no. 2 nonabsorbable braided suture.

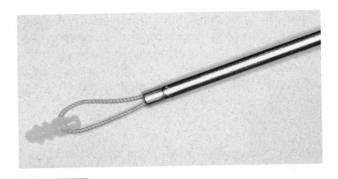

Figure 12-28
The BioTak resorbable suture anchor allows the surgeon to use any desired suture. Its holding power is maintained for 6 months, and it is radiotranslucent.

SCOI Technique for Anterior Capsular Fixation Using Suture Anchors and Permanent Braided Sutures (Table 12-1)

A new device called a suture Shuttle Relay (Concept, Inc., Largo, FL) has allowed us to fulfill two additional requirements of our ideal suturing technique and closely approximates the recommended open labral repairs of Matsen,[36] Jobe,[37] and others. The Shuttle Relay is a suture-passing device that resembles a 30-inch monofilament suture but is actually constructed of a central braided steel wire core covered with a smooth nylon coating (Fig. 12-29). In the center of the Shuttle Relay, an eyelet is formed by removing 3 mm of nylon and unwinding the wire braid. This device allows the surgeon to use the currently available stitching devices, such as the Caspari Punch or Concept suture hooks, but to pass the shuttle instead of a monofilament suture. Once the shuttle is in position the eyelet can be loaded with any nonabsorbable

tous reattachment. These anchors first became popular for open shoulder surgery, but were soon adapted to arthroscopic repairs. Wolf was instrumental in developing many of the arthroscopic techniques and has been a leader in their application. His team[35] reports using a monofilament absorbable suture through a suture hook device, allowing them to tuck the anterior capsule to eliminate laxity.

TABLE 12-1   Surgeon's Preference Card for Treatment of Anterior Shoulder Instability

1. *Patient position:* Lateral decubitus
2. Arm support: Long foam traction sleeve (STaR Sleeve, Arthrex, Inc.)
3. Traction apparatus: 2-point traction (Arthrex shoulder holder), 15 lb lateral and 5 to 7 lb distal
4. Standard arthroscopy set-up
5. *Irrigating fluid:* Synovisol or Ringer's lactate
6. Shaver blades:
   4.5-mm full-radius shaver
   4.0-mm ball burr
7. Arthroscopic fluid pump and cannulae
8. Suture anchor set: Mitek, BioAnchor, *or* other (surgeon's preference)
9. Concept Liberator Elevator
10. Crochet hook
11. Miniature arthroscopic grasper
12. 9-mm screw-in operating cannula with diaphragm (Concept)
13. Arthroscopic knot-pusher (surgeon's preference)
14. Plastic 6-mm operating cannula with diaphragm
15. Arthroscopic suture passing devices (modified Caspari Punch or Concept suture hooks)
16. Shuttle Relay (no. 3)
17. *Suturing material:* No. 2 braided permanent sutures (Ethibond or Ticron)
18. *Immobilization:* Immobilizer, preferably with a small pillow (Ultra Sling, DonJoy, Inc.)

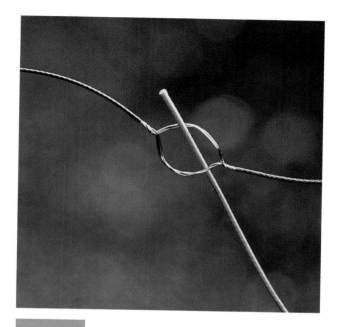

Figure 12-29
The suture Shuttle Relay is useful for passing any suture material through the joint arthroscopically. It is a 30-in suture leader the size of a no. 1 monofilament suture, constructed with a central braided wire core covered with nylon and having a 3-mm eyelet in the center.

braided suture similar to that chosen by most surgeons when doing open shoulder reconstructions, which can then be pulled back through the tissue. Mattress sutures can be created by passing the shuttle through the tissues a second time and retrieving the second limb of the original suture.

The technique that we currently employ at SCOI was modified and adapted from Wolf's original procedure, with the addition of the suture Shuttle Relay. This permits us to use a permanent nonabsorbable no. 2 braided polyester suture, sometimes in a mattress fashion, rather than a simple absorbable suture. We believe that the permanent suture affords an extra measure of security, since the monofilament absorbables lose mechanical strength by 3 weeks in the synovial joint.[38] The technique for this procedure is as follows:

1. The patient is turned to the lateral position and supported with the Vacupak beanbag. A stability examination is performed by supporting the arm with one hand at the elbow and translating the humeral head across the joint with the other hand. The weight of the arm is allowed to compress the joint so that if the head slides over the glenoid rim, a distinct jump can be felt. By rotating the arm into internal and external rotation, the ligaments will be tightened or relaxed (Fig. 12-30).

2. The arm is placed in two-point traction, as described by Gross and Fitzgibbons,[39]

Figure 12-30
The shoulder should be carefully examined for stability with the patient in the lateral position (see text).

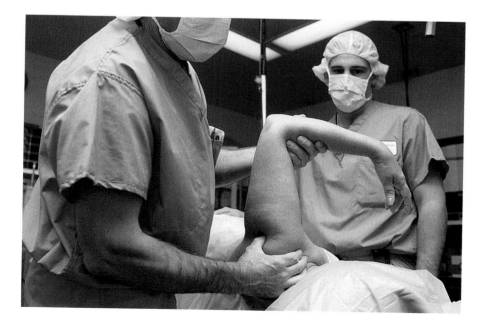

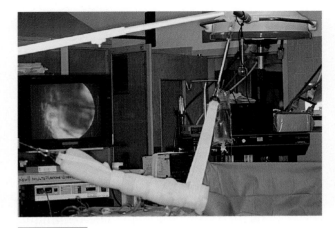

Figure 12-31
The "Gross" position is excellent for performing arthroscopic shoulder reconstruction, since the shoulder is held in internal rotation and distracted from the joint. The Arthrex shoulder holder is ideal for applying this traction.

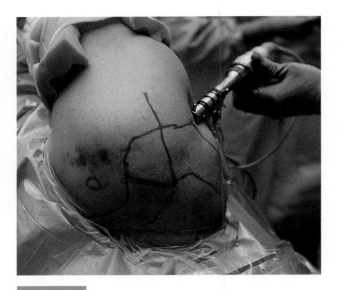

Figure 12-32
The anterior midglenoid lateral portal enters the skin 2 cm inferior to the anterior superior portal and lateral to the coracoid.

using the Arthrex shoulder holder with approximately 12 to 15 lb of traction vertically and 5 lb distally (Fig. 12-31). A sterilized foam traction apparatus (the Arthrex STaR Sleeve) is applied from the hand to the subdeltoid level.

3. A standard posterior arthroscopic portal is created, attempting to place the cannula in the upper third of the posterior glenoid at the level of the glenoid rim. The second portal is created just anterior to the biceps tendon, using an inside-out technique with a transarticular rod.

4. An anterior lateral midglenoid portal is created using an outside-in technique. While visualizing with the arthroscope from the posterior portal, a shallow stab wound is made 2 cm distal and 1 cm lateral to the original anterior superior portal; the tip of the knife blade is passed just through the skin and *not* into the muscle. This position is lateral to the tip of the coracoid process (Fig. 12-32). A blunt-tipped obturator inside a plastic operating cannula is used to tunnel through the deltoid muscle down to the capsule. The capsule is penetrated with

the blunt obturator so that it enters the joint at the upper edge of the subscapularis tendon insertion, about 2 cm lateral to the glenoid rim (Fig. 12-33). This position is much safer than the entry portal needed and advocated with most other fixation techniques, which are of-

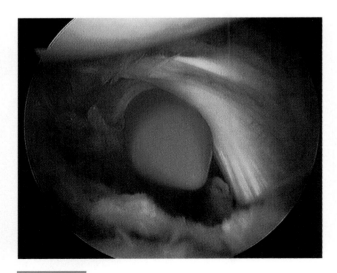

Figure 12-33
The anterior midglenoid lateral portal enters the joint near the bony attachment of the supraspinatus muscle, 2 cm lateral from the glenoid edge.

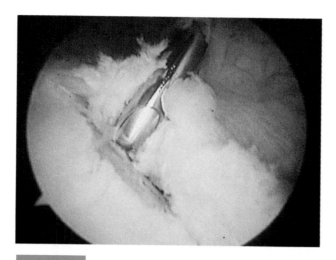

Figure 12-34
The shaver is used to debride the fibrous debris along the anterior glenoid neck.

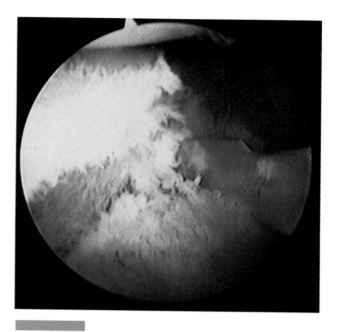

Figure 12-35
The Liberator Elevator is helpful in mobilizing the ligaments to allow advancement.

ten more medial and inferior, risking injury to the musculocutaneous nerve.

5. With the arthroscope visualizing from the anterior superior portal and a drainage cannula in the posterior portal, a shaver is inserted through the anterior lateral midglenoid operating cannula to debride the fragmented soft tissues and synovium along the glenoid neck (Fig. 12-34).

6. If the ligaments are difficult to mobilize because of scarring, a Liberator Elevator (Concept, Inc., Largo, Florida) may be used through the anterior midglenoid lateral portal (Fig. 12-35).

7. A 4-mm round burr is used through the midglenoid operating cannula to decorticate the neck of the glenoid from the edge of the articular cartilage as far medially and inferiorly as possible (Fig. 12-36). Suction to the burr is not used during this step, so as to guard against the possibility of winding-up and injuring the capsule and labral tissue. Bone chips are allowed to drain, by gravity, out the posterior cannula.

8. A suction punch is used to smooth the edge of the articular cartilage and to cre-

ate three suture anchor sites exactly at the corner of the articular surface (Fig. 12-37). The lowest anchor point should be located approximately 1 cm above the interior margin (four-thirty to five

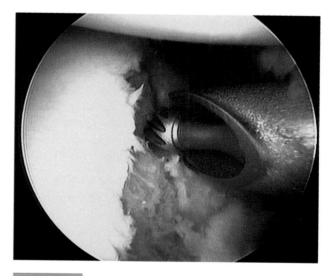

Figure 12-36
The 4-mm burr is used to decorticate the glenoid neck, allowing "friendly fibroblasts" to participate in the healing process.

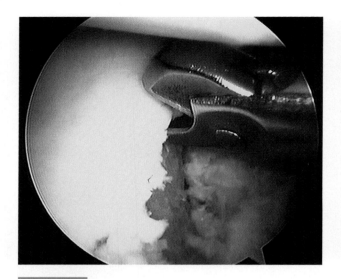

Figure 12-37
The suction punch is used to smooth the articular cartilage edge, so as to allow better visualization.

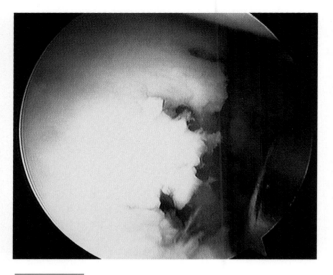

Figure 12-38
Three drill holes are made directly on the edge of the anterior glenoid at a 45-degree angle to the cartilage surface.

o'clock position), since the inferior ligaments will be pulled proximally by the suture. The other anchor sites should be more proximal, the top one being just above the midglenoid notch.

9. The appropriate drill guide and drill for the suture anchor system are used to create three anchor holes at approximately a 45-degree angle to the face of the glenoid. Since the midglenoid entry portal is lateral to the glenoid, it is quite easy to create these holes at the appropriate angle. Care should be taken not to injure the articular surface or penetrate the posterior or inferior cortex. The holes should be located exactly on the edge of the glenoid cartilage (Fig. 12-38).

10. The first anchor is loaded with a no. 2 braided polyester suture (Ethibond or Tevdek) and implanted through the anterior midglenoid cannula into the most inferior hole (Fig.12–39). Pulling on the ends of the suture will ensure that the anchor is securely seated (Fig. 12-40). The arthroscope can be placed either in the posterior or in the superior portal, or can be alternated for the remainder of

the operation, according to the preference of the surgeon. We now prefer to complete the stitching, suture passing, and knot tying visualizing from the posterior portal and working with the grasper and crochet hook via an anterior superior operating cannula.

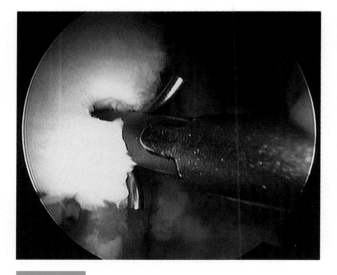

Figure 12-39
The first anchor is implanted into the most inferior drill hole and the suture ends are pulled to test for security.

Figure 12-40
See Fig. 12-39.

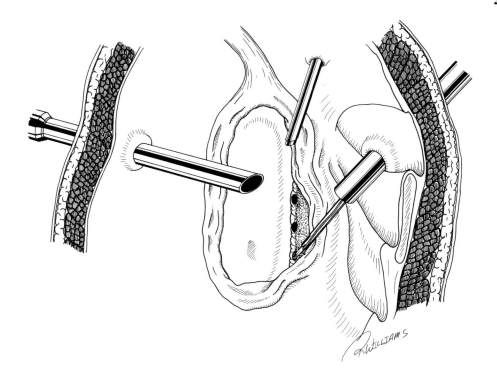

11. A crochet hook is inserted through the posterior or superior portal to snag one limb of the first suture and deliver it out the cannula (either posterior or anterior superior) that is not being used for the arthroscope (Figs. 12-41 and 12-42).

12. A suturing needle is passed through the inferior aspect of the anterior capsule and below the labrum, using either a suture hook device or a *modified* Caspari Suture Punch. The punch is modified by creating a 2-mm opening in the distal tip of the upper oval jaw. This opening allows the Shuttle Relay to be pulled out an alternative portal rather than being removed with the punch out the anterior midglenoid portal. Depending on the perceived laxity of the capsular tissues and the desired amount of reefing, a larger or smaller bite of capsule can be incorporated in the stitch (Figs. 12-43 and 12-44).

13. The suture Shuttle Relay is then passed through the suture hook or modified Caspari Punch and into the joint. An arthroscopic grasping clamp inserted

through the open cannula retrieves the lead end of the shuttle and pulls it out of the shoulder (Figs. 12-45 and 12-46).

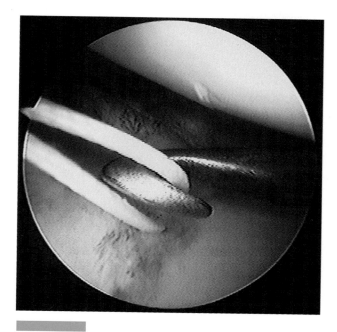

Figure 12-41
A crochet hook is used to pull one limb of the suture out an empty cannula, either superiorly or posteriorly.

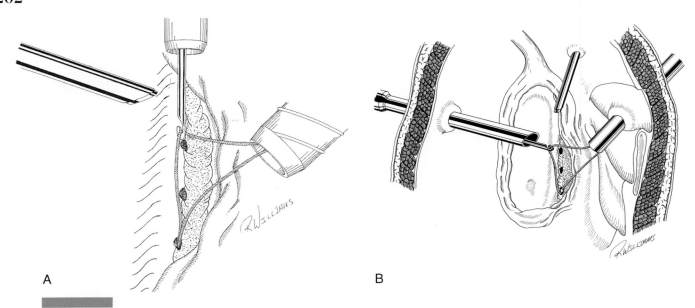

A　　　　　　　　　　　　　　B

Figure 12-42
The crochet hook is used to pull one limb of of the Ethibond suture out an alternative cannula.

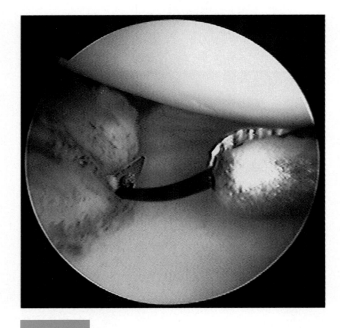

Figure 12-43
The suture hook is passed through the anterior midglenoid lateral portal through the capsular and labral tissue in the anterior inferior shoulder, gathering as much capsule as needed to eliminate laxity. The suture Shuttle Relay is passed through the needle and retrieved out an open cannula (anterior superior or posterior).

14. The first limb of the nonabsorbable suture is placed in the eyelet of the Shuttle Relay and pulled retrogradely back out the anterior midglenoid cannula and clamped (Figs. 12-47 and 12-48).

15. If a simple looped suture seems adequate, the two ends can be tied together using either a slip-knot technique reinforced with three additional knots or, preferably, a series of four stacked knots (Figs. 12-49 and 12-50).

16. If a mattress suture is desired, the second limb of the braided suture is retrieved with a crochet hook via the open portal, and a second pass of the suture hook is made approximately 3 to 4 mm proximal to the first pass, with care taken that the tip of the needle exits the joint side of the labrum near the implanted suture anchor. If too large a space remains between the tip of the needle and the anchor site, it will be difficult to advance the capsule to this area. A Shuttle Relay is then sent

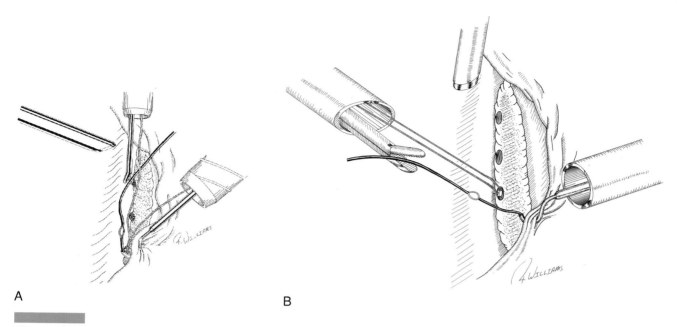

A

B

Figure 12-44
The grasping clamp catches the Shuttle Relay and leads it out the anterior superior or posterior cannula.

through the needle and retrieved out the open cannula where the second limb of the suture is located. The end of the second suture limb is placed in the eyelet of

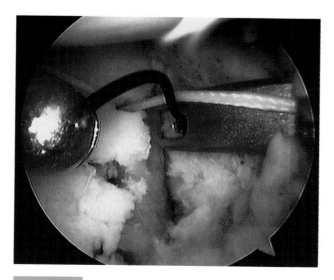

Figure 12-45
A modified Caspari Punch is also useful for passing the Shuttle Relay.

the Shuttle Relay and brought out anteriorly (Fig. 12-51).

17. It is important ensure that there are no twists in the sutures. A simple way to test this is to place one limb of the suture inside the eyelet of the knot-pushing device and run the device all the way down into the joint while visualizing it with the arthroscope. If the suture is twisted, the problem can easily be corrected at that point (Fig. 12-52).

18. The two limbs of the original suture are tied together, using an arthroscopic knot-pushing device through the anterior midglenoid cannula (Figs. 12-53 and 12-54). At least four knots should be secured before the suture ends are cut and removed.

19. The additional two remaining anchors are inserted following the same steps as used for the first suture anchor. I prefer always to visualize the anchor insertion step from the anterior superior portal,

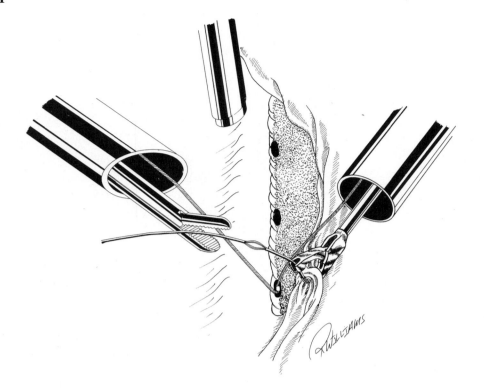

Figure 12-46
When using the modified
Caspari Punch the upper jaw
should be situated on the side
of the labrum nearest the
articular cartilage.

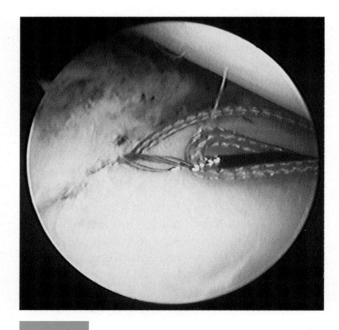

Figure 12-47
The Shuttle Relay is loaded with one limb of the
Ethibond suture and retrieved back through the labrum
and out the midglenoid cannula.

and then often change the arthroscope
to the posterior portal to visualize the
stitching and knot tying.

20. After completion of each suture, a palpating probe is used to examine the security of the knot and the placement
and security of the capsular repair (Fig.
12-55). The final inspection of the repair
site should be performed from the posterior portal, again while palpating anteriorly.

It should be remembered that with the arm
in the two-point traction system the anterior
capsular structures are relaxed, since the
shoulder is held in internal rotation. The surgeon must be careful not to involve too much
redundant capsule in the repair, since over-
tightening of the tissues can restrict external
rotation postoperatively.

Recently, a new absorbable suture anchor
has been developed. This BioTak Anchor

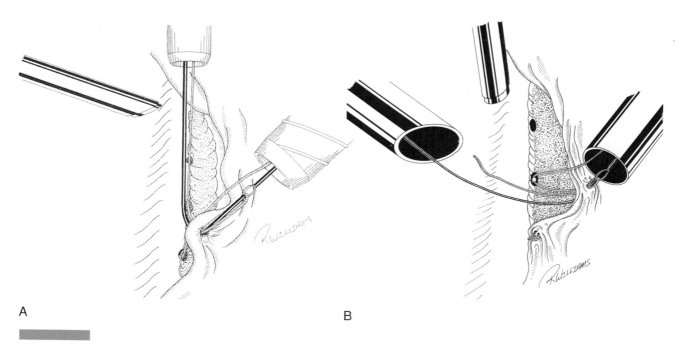

A   B

Figure 12-48
The Shuttle Relay is used to lead the Ethiband braided suture through the labrum and out the midglenoid cannula.

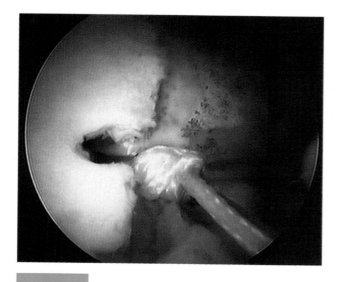

Figure 12-49
A slip knot can be used when the suture limbs slide easily through the tissues and the anchor eyelet, but the author prefers to use multiple simple stacked knots. The suture tails are cut with an arthroscopic punch.

(Concept, Inc., Largo, FL) is made of homopolymer of polylactide (see Fig. 12-28). On the basis of considerable animal and human data, it is expected that this anchor will maintain its holding strength in bone for at least 6 months. Pull-out testing of this system demonstrates that in both uniform animal and cadaveric glenoid bone, the mechanical holding strength is similar to, or better than, that of other available anchors. This new device obviously offers an additional improvement in the fixation system, allowing even closer approximation of our "ideal" six-point repair, since no metallic or other permanent implants are required. The additional steps needed to implant the absorbable suture anchor are as follows:

1. The patient set-up, soft tissue and bony debridement, and drilling are identical to those described for the Mitek anchors.

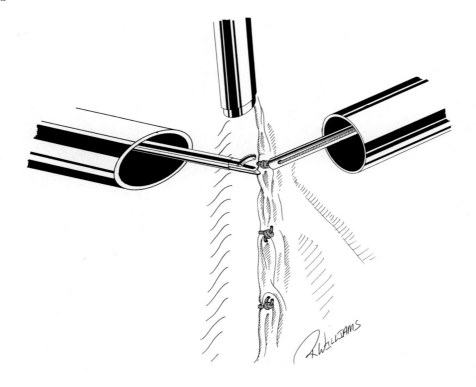

Figure 12-50
See Fig. 12-49.

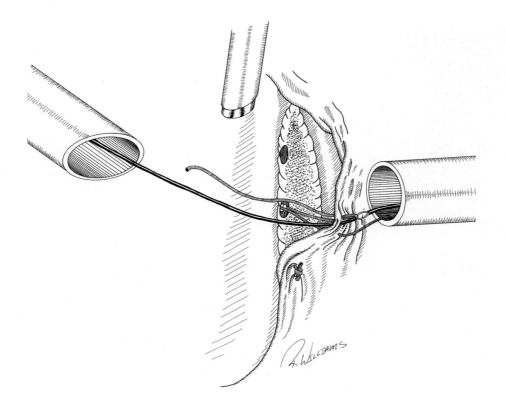

Figure 12-51
When a mattress suture is desired, the suture needle is passed a second time, along with a Shuttle Relay. The second limb of the suture is retrieved with the shuttle to complete the mattress suture.

Figure 12-52
The knot-pusher is passed down one limb of the suture before tying, to ensure visually that there are no twists present.

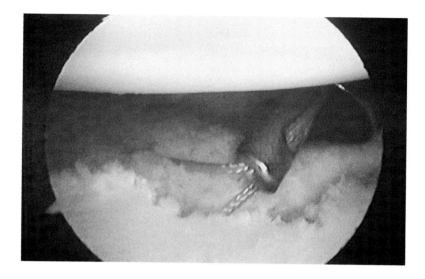

2. After the three or four anchor holes are drilled (or, in some cases, punched with a special bone punch, if the surgeon prefers) on the edge of the articular surface of the glenoid, an insertion sheath, with its centering alignment device, is passed through the midglenoid operating cannula and aligned and tapped gently to impact the device into the most inferior hole (Fig. 12-56).

3. The centering alignment device is removed while holding the insertion sheath perfectly stable in position. Care must be taken to avoid *any* change in alignment of the sheath once the alignment device is removed, as this would risk causing a fracture of the implant during seating.

4. The BioTak Anchor, preloaded with no. 2 braided nonabsorbable suture, is fixed to the anchor insertion tool and placed into the seating sheath (Fig. 12-57). The anchor is gently tapped into the lowest hole until completely seated.

5. The seating sheath is removed and the anchor is tested by pulling firmly on the

Figure 12-53
Multiple stacked knots are used when a mattress suture is desired.

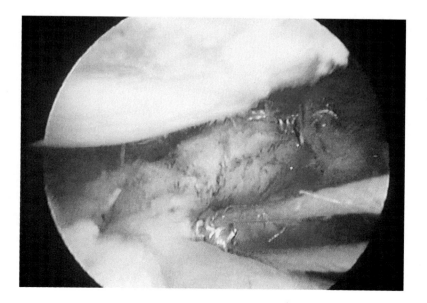

Figure 12-54
See Fig. 12-53.

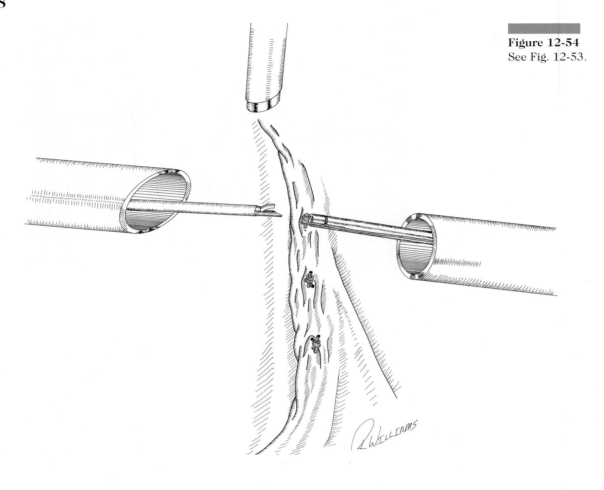

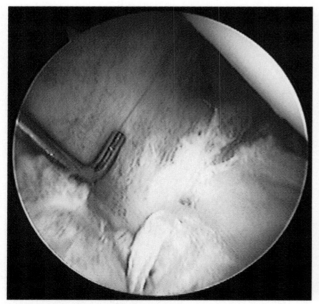

Figure 12-55
A miniature palpating probe is used to examine the security of the knot and test the capsular repair.

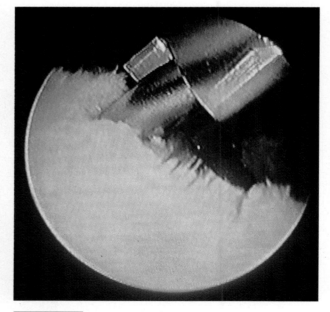

Figure 12-56
The insertion cannula for the BioTak Anchor is aligned with the drill hole using a centering alignment device.

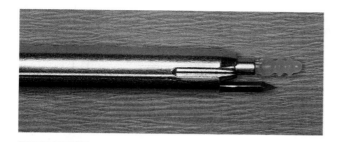

Figure 12-57
The anchor insertion tool is loaded with the BioTak Anchor holding the no. 2 braided suture and passed into the seating sheath. It is then impacted into the anterior glenoid drill holes.

sutures. If the suture anchor is not secure, or if the suture breaks, it is a simple procedure to redrill the hole, thereby removing the unwanted anchor, and replace it with another anchor.

6. The reconstruction is then continued as described above for the permanent anchor, using the suture needle and Shuttle Relay and tying the knots down through the anterior portal.

[At the time of this writing, the BioTak suture anchor is undergoing clinical testing and not yet available for general use.]

Postoperative Treatment

The arm is kept in a shoulder-immobilizing device for approximately 3 weeks postoperatively. We prefer to use an Ultra Sling (DonJoy, Inc.) a device that incorporates a pillow-spacer between the arm and the body, to prevent excessive internal rotation (Fig. 12-58). An x-ray should be taken in the recovery room to document the position of the anchors when metallic devices have been used (Fig. 12-59). The patient is encouraged to move the arm during the day for elbow, wrist, and hand exercises, and gentle external rotation to the 15- to 20-degree position during the first 3 weeks. Gentle pendulum exercises are allowed after the first postoperative visit, at approximately 10 days to 2 weeks. At 3 weeks, gentle

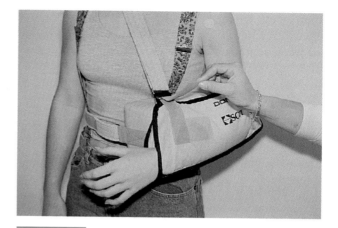

Figure 12-58
A sling immobilizer with a pillow-spacer (Ultrasling, DonJoy, Inc.) is used postoperatively to prevent an internal rotation contracture while allowing air circulation to the axilla. In addition, the arm can be removed for exercise by opening the flap and releasing the sling.

internal rotation strengthening exercises using a rubber exercise cord, such as supplied in the Shoulder Therapy Kit (STK, Breg Inc., Carlsbad, California), are encouraged. After 6 weeks, the patient begins a progressive active and active-assisted range-of-motion program using a pulley or wand. He or she continues to protect the arm from forced external rotation for an additional 3 to 4 weeks. After 10 post-

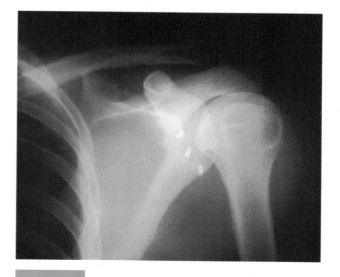

Figure 12-59
An x-ray taken in the recovery room documents the position of the fixation anchors.

operative weeks, full exercises are encouraged, except for external rotation strain in the abducted position. We recommend avoidance of severe throwing or external rotation–abduction loading stresses for approximately 5 to 6 months.

Arthroscopic Treatment of Posterior Instability

Since posterior glenohumeral instability is not commonly seen clinically, our experience with evaluation and treatment of this problem has been limited. Occasionally a posterior Bankart lesion is discovered in the preoperative workup or during arthroscopy, and the surgeon should be prepared to repair it, either arthroscopically or using standard open techniques. It is my opinion that the arthroscopic reattachment with capsular plication is a reasonable and straightforward procedure, but we have not had the opportunity to perform this procedure on a large enough series of patients to feel comfortable advocating it at this time.

Technique

When a posterior labral avulsion is present with an intact capsule and glenoid rim, the arthroscopic techniques to reattach the tissues are similar to those used for the anterior repair. A secondary operating portal is developed approximately 2 cm inferior from the original posterior superior portal. While viewing from either the anterior or the posterior superior portal, the glenoid neck is debrided and abraded. Three drill holes are made on the edge of the posterior glenoid rim along the inferior quadrant. The suture anchors, preloaded with no. 2 braided permanent suture, are inserted as for the anterior repair, and one limb of the suture is retrieved out the posterior superior cannula (Fig. 12-60). The suture Shuttle Relay is passed through the capsular and labral tissues using a modified Caspari Punch or a Concept suture hook. The shuttle is retrieved with a grasping clamp through the posterior superior portal, where the suture is

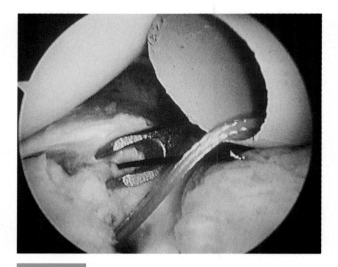

Figure 12-60

Repair of the posterior Bankart lesion is similar to an anterior repair. After the suture anchors are inserted and one limb of the suture is retrieved out the posterior superior cannula, a Shuttle Relay is passed using a modified Caspari Suture Punch or suture hook.

loaded into the eyelet. The shuttle is drawn back through the joint and capsular tissues and out the posterior inferior cannula. The sutures are tied using a knot-pusher through the posterior inferior cannula (Fig. 12-61).

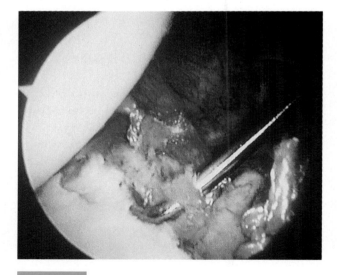

Figure 12-61

At the completion of the posterior Bankart repair the capsular tissues are slightly tucked with the sutures, and the labrum is tightly reattached exactly on the edge of the glenoid.

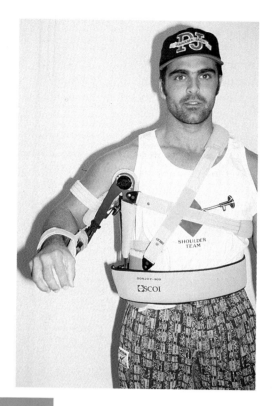

Figure 12-62
The SCOI brace can be used to hold the arm in 20 to 30 degrees of abduction and 10 to 15 degrees of external rotation by placing a firm 2-in felt pad between the two layers of the anterior pelvic support.

The suture tails are cut, and the knots and repair are tested with a palpating probe.

Postoperative Treatment

Postoperatively, the arm is held in a functional brace in approximately 25 degrees of abduction and 10 to 20 degrees of external rotation. An SCOI brace (DonJoy Inc., Carlsbad, California) can be used if a 2-in thickness of felt is placed on the anterior portion of the pelvic support of the brace, between the plastic and the foam padding (Fig. 12-62). This modification causes the arm to be comfortably held in slight external rotation. Otherwise, a Quadrant Brace (DonJoy, Inc.) allows correct positioning. The brace is used for 3 to 4 weeks. The patient begins a rehabilitation program similar to that used for the anterior reconstruction, but with protection against

posterior stress and flexion and adduction and internal rotation.

References

1. Bankart ASB: The pathology and treatment of recurrent dislocation of the shoulder joint. *Br J Surg* 26:23, 1938.

2. Turkel SJ, Panio MW, Marshall JL, et al: Stabilizing mechanisms prevention preventing anterior dislocation of the glenohumeral joint. *J Bone Joint Surg* 63A:1208, 1981.

3. O'Brien SJ, Neve S, Arnoczky SP: Anatomy and histology of the inferior glenohumeral complex of the shoulder. *Am J Sports Med* 18:449, 1990.

4. Rodosky MW, Rudert MJ, Harner CD, et al: The role of the long head of the biceps and superior glenoid labrum in anterior stability of the shoulder. Presented at the Annual Meeting of the Arthroscopy Association of North America, Orlando, Florida, 1990.

5. Bosminigin JB, Bazant FJ, Kingston CM: Factors preventing downward dislocation of the adducted shoulder joint. *J Bone Joint Surg* 41A:1182, 1959.

6. Habermeyer P, Schuller U: Die Bedeutung des Labrum glenoidale für die stabilitat des Glenohumeralgelenkes. *Unfallchirurg* 92:1989.

7. Howell SM, Galinat BJ: The glenoid-labral socket—A constrained articular surface. *Clin Orthop* 243:122, 1989.

8. Perry J: Anatomy and biomechanics of the shoulder in throwing, swimming, gymnastics and tennis. *Clin Sports Med* 2:247, 1983.

9. Morgan C, Rames RD, Snyder SJ: Anatomical variations of the glenohumeral ligaments. Presented at the Annual Meeting of the American Academy of Orthopaedic Surgeons, Anaheim, California, 1991.

10. Morgan C, Rames RD, Snyder SJ: Anatomical variations of the glenohumeral ligaments—a followup study. Presented at the Annual

Meeting of the American Academy of Orthopaedic Surgeons, Washington, DC, 1992.

11. Snyder SJ, Buford D, Wuh HCK: The Buford complex—The loose anterior superior labrum-middle glenohumeral ligament complex: A normal anatomical variant. Presented at the Annual Meeting of the American Academy of Orthopaedic Surgeons, Washington, DC, 1992.

12. Blazina ME, Saltzman JS: Recurrent anterior subluxation of the shoulder in athletes: A distinct entity. *J Bone Joint Surg* 51A:1037, 1969.

13. Walsh G, Boileau P, Noel E, Donell ST: Impingement of the deep surface of the supraspinatus tendon on the posteriosuperior glenoid rim: An arthroscopic study. *J Shoulder Elbow Surg* 1(5):238, 1992.

14. Jobe CM: Evidence linking posterior superior labral impingement and shoulder instability. Presented at the American Shoulder and Elbow Surgeons Closed Meeting, Seattle, Washington, September 1991.

15. Flannigan B, Kursunoglu-Brahme S, Snyder S, et al: MR arthrography of the shoulder: Comparison with conventional MR imaging. *AJR* 155:829, 1990.

16. Wheeler JH, Ryan JB, Arciero RB, Molinari RN: Arthroscopic versus nonoperative treatment of acute shoulder dislocations in young athletes. *Arthroscopy* 5:213, 1989.

17. Baker CL, Uribe JW, Whitman C: Arthroscopic evaluation of acute initial shoulder dislocations. *Am J Sports Med* 18:25, 1990.

18. Johnson LL: Arthroscopic acromioplasty with rotator cuff repair. Presented at the American Shoulder and Elbow Surgeons meeting, Seattle, Washington, 1991.

19. Snyder SJ, Karzel RP, Del Pizzo W, et al: SLAP lesions of the shoulder. *Arthroscopy* 6:724, 1990.

20. Wolf E: Arthroscopic management of shoulder instability. Arthroscopy Association of North America Annual Meeting, Instructional Course No. 201, Boston, Massachusetts, April 1992.

21. Neviaser T: ALPSA lesion. Presented at the Annual Meeting of the Arthroscopy Association of North America, Boston, MA, April 1992.

22. Neer CS II, Foster CR: Inferior capsular shift for involuntary inferior and multidirectional instability of the shoulder: A preliminary report. *J Bone Joint Surg* 62:897, 1980.

23. Glousman RE: Shoulder arthroscopy in the throwing athlete. *Operative Tech Orthop* 1:155, 1991.

24. Altchek DW, Warren RF, Wickiewicz TL, Ortiz G: Arthroscopic labral debridement: A three year follow up study. *Am J Sports Med* 20:702, 1992.

25. Johnson LL: *Diagnostic and Surgical Arthroscopy of the Shoulder.* St. Louis, Mosby Yearbook, 1992.

26. Wiley AM: Arthroscopy for shoulder instability and a technique for arthroscopic repair. *Arthroscopy* 4:25, 1988.

27. Snyder SJ: Anterior capsular reconstruction in the shoulder using the Dyonics cannulated screw and washer system. Presented at Arthroscopy of the Upper and Lower Extremities, Los Angeles, California, November 29–December 1, 1990.

28. Strafford BB, Snyder SJ: Arthroscopic anterior shoulder stabilization. *Orthopaedics,* 1993 (in press).

29. Warner JP, Warren RF: Arthroscopic Bankart repair using a cannulated absorbable fixation device. *Operative Tech Orthop* 1:192, 1991.

30. Caspari R: Arthroscopic reconstruction of the shoulder: The Bankart repair, in McGinty JB (ed): *Operative Techniques Arthroscopy.* New York, Raven Press, 1991, pp 507–515.

31. Morgan CD, Bodenstab AB: Arthroscopic Bankart suture repair. Techniques and early results. *Arthroscopy* 3:111, 1987.

32. Morgan CD: Arthroscopic transglenoid Bankart suture repair. *Operative Tech Orthop* 1:171, 1991.

33. Maki NJ: Arthroscopic stabilization: Suture technique. *Operative Tech Orthop* 1:180, 1991.

34. Rose DJ, Moyer RA, Marchetto P, Sidor M: Arthroscopic suture capsulorrhaphy for anterior shoulder instability. Presented at the Annual Meeting of the American Academy of Orthopaedic Surgeons, New Orleans, Louisiana, February 1990.

35. Wolf EM, Wilke RM, Richmond JC: Arthroscopic Bankart repair using suture anchors. *Operative Tech Orthop* 1:184, 1991.

36. Jobe FW, Giangarra CE, Kvitne RS, Glousman RE: Anterior capsulolabral reconstruction in athletes in overhand sports. *Am J Sports Med* 19:428, 1991.

37. Matsen FA, Rockwood C: *The Shoulder,* vol 1. Philadelphia, Saunders, 1990, pp 587–592.

38. Barber FA, Click JN: The effect of inflammatory synovial fluid on the breaking strength of new "long lasting" absorbable sutures. *Arthroscopy* 8:437, 1992.

39. Gross RM, Fitzgibbons TC: Shoulder arthroscopy: A modified approach. *Arthroscopy* 1:156, 1985.

13

Arthroscopic Evaluation and Treatment of Calcifications Around the Shoulder

Introduction

Calcifications in and around the soft tissues of the shoulder usually occur on the bursal side of the glenohumeral joint. The most common location is on the bursal surface of the supraspinatus tendon, near the attachment into the greater tuberosity. This location has been called the "critical zone" of the rotator cuff, since the blood supply to this area is poor and it corresponds to the area of maximum impingement pressure on the rotator cuff with forward elevation of the arm.[1] Additional locations for calcium deposition are the subscapularis tendon insertion into the lesser tuberosity, the musculotendinous area of the supraspinatus tendon, and the posterior attachment of the infraspinatus and teres minor tendons of the rotator cuff.

The etiology of the calcium deposition in the bursa and cuff is not known. Several possibilities exist, although none can account for all cases. Uhthoff and Sarkar believed that fluffy calcific deposits most often occurred with acute symptomatology.[2] They felt that the deposition of calcium in the rotator cuff tendon was a type of "self healing" and postulated that there was an early phase in which there was a lowering of the oxygen tension in the area secondary to inflammation. This low-oxygen milieu caused a portion of the tendon to change to fibrocartilage and encouraged chondrocyte deposition of calcium. Later, when the phagocytic cells began to engulf the calcific deposits, an inflammatory and vascular proliferation phase occurred. They postulated that the ingrowth of vascular channels caused an increase in oxygen and led to resorption. Symptoms, they believed, were intensified during the resorptive phase. Since most cases historically are spontaneous in onset, the precipitating cause of the inflammatory event is frequently unknown.

The deposits of calcium may occur as a superficial blister below the bursal covering, thereby causing little damage to the underlying rotator cuff; or they may occur within the tendinous substance, in association with more severe structural damage to the integrity of that tendon. These two forms of calcification can exist independently or together, in a combined lesion.

Incidence and History of Treatment of Calcific Tendinitis

Bosworth studied a group of 6061 adult workers with x-rays of both shoulders. He found a 2.7-percent incidence of calcium deposits in the group.[3] Most of these were located at or near the greater tuberosity and the supraspinatus tendon. Thirty-five percent of the patients with calcific deposits had previous symptomatic episodes.

Codman believed that if a calcium deposit measured more than 1.5 cm it would most likely become symptomatic.[4] He also believed that approximately 35 percent of calcifications were the cause of significant shoulder pain and disability at some time.

Historically there have been many forms of treatment advocated for calcific tendinitis, in both the acute and chronic stages. Since these lesions are known to resolve in most cases, conservative treatment when the lesion is first discovered is generally recommended. This usually consists of a sling, anti-inflammatory medication, pain medicine, and often a subacromial bursal corticosteroid injection combined with local anesthetic. Acute symptoms generally are severe for 2 to 3 days and then gradually subside. Aspiration of calcific deposits was recommended by Flint.[5] Harmon also needled almost 500 shoulders using local anesthetic and noted improvement in 79 percent of cases.[6] Barbotage, or needle lavage, was thought by Patterson and Darrach to relieve pressure within the calcific deposit, thereby relieving symptoms.[7] They treated 63 patients, 53 of whom had complete relief of symptoms.

Rowe, on the other hand, believed that needle aspiration was infrequently a good choice of treatment.[8] He believed that barbotage was

very painful and did not significantly improve the disease process. He felt that the calcium deposit would often become symptomatic again after needle aspiration. He and others believed that surgical removal of the deposit was advisable. Rowe indicates that he never experienced a recurrence of a calcific deposit after an open surgical removal.

Lichtman et al. studied 100 cases of subacromial calcium deposits and recommended surgical treatment for cases having large multi-loculated deposits with a history of chronic shoulder pain.[9]

Arthroscopic removal of calcium deposits has become quite popular in the past 5 years. Eppley et al. reported 13 shoulders with chronic calcium deposits treated by arthroscopy that were evaluated for 1 to 5 years after treatment.[10] All patients had reported marked symptomatic relief following the surgery and were glad that they had undergone the procedure.

Ellman et al. reported on 23 patients with calcific tendinitis treated arthroscopically.[11] On follow-up radiographs 14 patients had some residual calcium, while 9 had complete removal. The results were rated as good in 11 cases, as satisfactory in 10, and as unsatisfactory in only 2. The authors believed that shoulder arthroscopy was a reasonable alternative in the treatment of calcific tendinitis.

Ellman et al. reported on a multi-center study to evaluate arthroscopic treatment of calcific tendinitis.[11] Of 131 patients treated arthroscopically, the average global score (a combination of Constant functional score, activities of daily living score, and range of motion score) was 69.4 out of a possible 75. The non-operated shoulder averaged 73.7. The good results in this study had no correlation with age of the patient, size of the calcification, type of the calcification, or duration of the symptoms. Additionally, there was no benefit apparent when acromioplasty was performed (93 patients) versus no acromioplasty (37 patients). There were no significant permanent complications in this series, although one patient had a traction plexitis that resolved after 21 months. There were three cases of postoperative adhesive capsulitis, one of which required a manipulation, but all eventually resolved.

Clinical Presentation

Calcific deposits around the shoulder occur most frequently in females between 30 and 60 years old. Like many inflammatory conditions, calcific tendinitis may be characterized in three phases: acute, subacute, and chronic.

Acute calcific bursitis/tendinitis causes exquisite pain. The onset is usually spontaneous, with very rapid development of a severe clinical picture of pain; loss of motion; localized swelling, sometimes with erythema; and severe disability. There may be a trivial incidental event that seems to precede or precipitate the inflammation. Often the patient awakens with stiffness that progresses rapidly to the full syndrome in a matter of hours.

The acute pain may be so severe that any pressure of clothing or attempt to move the shoulder is vigorously resisted. The skin may be warm, and the anterior bursal contour may demonstrate a puffy appearance of swelling. Gentle palpation elicits severe tenderness within the bursa. Rotator cuff motion is inhibited by the pain; strength testing, therefore, is limited. The neurological and circulatory status of the extremity is otherwise intact. No attempt should be made to assess the full range of motion, since the pain associated with this is too severe.

Symptoms in the subacute and chronic stages of subacromial calcification depend on the size and location of the lesion as well as on the quality of the rotator cuff. Often there may be no symptoms at all in a small, flat lesion with relatively little impingement. In more prominent lesions symptoms can range from periodic catching and aching to chronic, constant pain with any abduction or elevation activity of the shoulder. In chronic subscapularis tendon calcifications, symptoms usually occur with elevation and adduction of the arm. Periodically, acute symptoms may intervene when the calcific mass ruptures or the tissues become acutely inflamed.

Diagnosis of Calcific Tendinitis/Bursitis

The standard x-ray series of the shoulder is adequate in most cases to confirm the diagnosis of calcium deposition. It is important to complete the entire four-view x-ray series in order to localize exactly and characterize the calcium. When viewing the x-ray films, several key elements should be considered. The exact localization of the calcification in relation to the impingement arch should be noted. Evaluating the arch view will reveal any anterior acromial beak or spur that may compromise the supraspinatus outlet and impinge the area of calcification (Figs. 13-1 and 13-2). The axillary view often demonstrates the location of the calcification in relation to the acromion

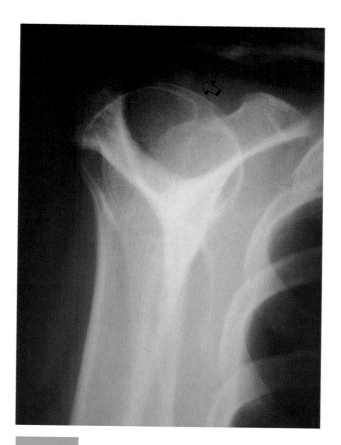

Figure 13-1

The supraspinatus outlet x-ray demonstrates the usual location of the bursal calcification beneath the anterior acromial arch.

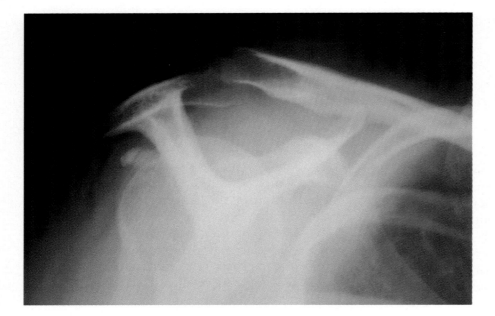

Figure 13-2
Infrequently, calcium is located in the posterior aspect of the subacromial space in the infraspinatus tendon.

as well as giving a good estimate of the anterior-to-posterior dimensions (Fig. 13-3). Finally, the biceps tunnel, or groove view, demonstrates if a subscapularis calcification crosses the biceps groove or remains medial to it in the area of the lesser tuberosity (Fig. 13-4).

The location of the calcification within the tendon proper is suggested by the proximity of the calcium to the humeral head and greater tuberosity. If the calcification extends

to the bone, the tendinous elements are likely to be involved as well.

In acute calcifications there is frequently a cloudy or puffy appearance to the calcific deposit, exhibiting rounded edges (Fig. 13-5). The more chronic calcifications may appear as either linear or stratified layers of calcium

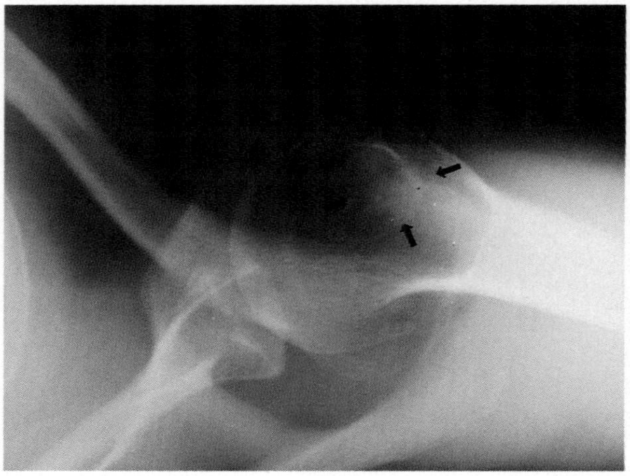

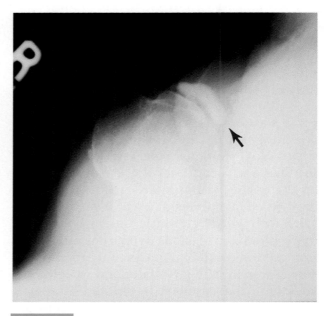

Figure 13-3
An axillary x-ray demonstrates the size of the calcification in relation to the overlying acromion.

Figure 13-4
This biceps groove x-ray demonstrates that the calcium is located over the lesser tuberosity in the subscapularis tendon.

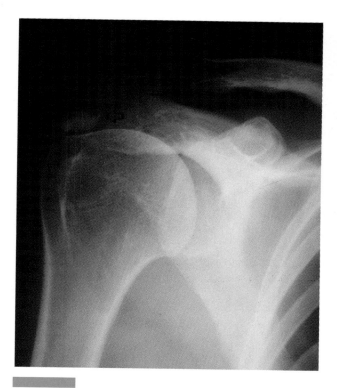

Figure 13-5
When the calcification is cloudy or puffy in appearance,
it is suspected to be relatively acute.

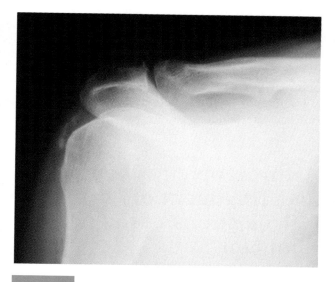

Figure 13-6
Stratified calcium is usually chronic and often very
difficult to remove entirely.

overlying the rotator cuff (Fig. 13-6). Some
chronic deposits appear as a denser material,
with the radiological appearance of bone. An
acute lesion may be less dense, with an appearance more like that of iodinated contrast
material. Often it is not possible to determine
the exact age of the calcification from the
x-ray. It seems that recurring acute symptoms
may result from an otherwise indolent-ap-
pearing chronic deposit, creating a confusing
clinical and radiological situation.

Other Imaging Modalities (MRI, Ultrasound)

The MRI scan is an excellent method for determining not only the size and location of the
calcification, but also the severity of the
tendinous involvement. Although the calcium
cannot be well differentiated from dense tendon or cortical bone by MRI techniques, an
MRI scan viewed in conjunction with an x-ray
by a knowledgeable practitioner can be ex-

tremely helpful (Fig. 13-7). Using the MRI
alone can lead to misinterpretation, since a
dense coracoacromial ligament attachment
beneath the lateral acromion may be confused
with a calcification on the superior surface of
the cuff.

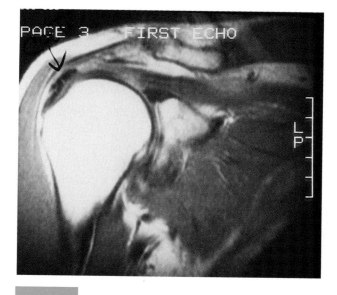

Figure 13-7
The MRI scan is helpful in determining the exact
location of the calcification in relation to the bursa and
cuff.

Ultrasound evaluation of the shoulder can also be confusing when calcium is present. Although this test may be a useful screening device in the hands of a well-trained technician, in our experience the routine use of ultrasound for evaluating calcification alone has not been satisfactory.

Arthroscopic Evaluation and Treatment of Calcifications of the Shoulder

As for all surgery of the shoulder in which the arthroscope is used, a complete systematic 15-point evaluation of the glenohumeral joint must be performed and video-recorded. Most often the glenohumeral anatomy is normal, but there may be synovitis, arthritis, biceps or cuff lesions, or significant labral problems present.

A fairly common arthroscopic finding when supraspinatus calcification is present is a unique strawberry-like vascular blotch on the articular surface in the supraspinatus tendon area (Fig. 13-8). Frequently this area serves as a marker indicating the location of the bursal side calcification. I have not seen this strawberry-like stain when the subscapularis tendon has been involved.

Suture Marker Technique

It is often difficult to locate a calcium deposit when performing the standard bursoscopy evaluation. Since there are no good identifying landmarks on the bursal side of the rotator cuff, one cannot differentiate between the surface of the supraspinatus tendon, the rotator interval, and the subscapularis. Additionally, the exact location of the tuberosity insertion of the cuff can be difficult to determine without some orientation guide. The suture marker technique has been extremely helpful in this regard. Originally, this technique was developed to aid in the correlation of an articular side rotator cuff lesion with a bursal side lesion. By inserting an absorbable monofila-

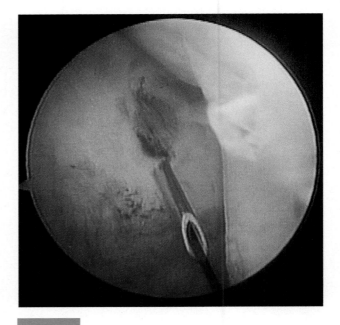

Figure 13-8
A red-colored "strawberry lesion," or vascular blotch, is seen in the supraspinatus tendon in 70 percent of cases of calcification. A suture marker passed through this area will aid location of the calcium during bursoscopy.

ment suture through a needle placed percutaneously through the lateral aspect of the subacromial space into a lesion or known location on the articular side of the cuff, a surgeon can correlate the position of the articular side lesion with the corresponding area on the bursal surface.

As I have explained above, sometimes there is a "strawberry" vascular blotch on the articular side of the cuff below the area of the bursal side calcifications. Placing a marker suture through the lesion facilitates localization of the associated calcium during bursoscopy. Additionally, after studying the x-rays and/or MRI scans, the surgeon can determine the most likely location of the calcification. When viewing the articular side of the rotator cuff arthroscopically, even if no strawberry lesion is present, a spinal needle can be inserted and a marker suture placed purely for orientation. Often the needle will pass directly through the calcium deposit; in these instances particles of calcium material can be seen passing out from around the needle or the marker suture on the articular side (Fig. 13-9).

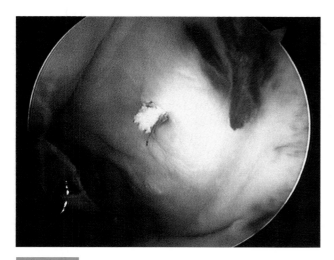

Figure 13-9
Calcium is often seen in the tip of the needle or around the marker suture that is placed for orientation.

A special orientation technique is needed when the calcification is present in the subscapularis tendon. Since the lesser tuberosity forms the lateral insertion of the subscapularis, and since this area is usually outside the anterior confines of the subacromial bursa, the suture marker technique is an extremely important aid in localization. To locate a subscapularis calcification, two marker sutures of different colors are useful (Fig. 13-10). First a spinal needle is inserted just below the anterolateral corner of the acromion, entering the glenohumeral joint anterior to the edge of the biceps tendon in the rotator interval. A violet-colored no. 1 PDS suture is inserted through the needle, which is then withdrawn, leaving the suture in place.

A second spinal needle is inserted slightly more inferiorly to enter the joint at the upper level, or even directly through the upper third of the subscapularis tendon near its insertion into the lesser tuberosity. A green-colored no. 1 Maxon suture is inserted through this needle. It is now possible to correlate these known anatomical areas with the corresponding location on the bursal side of the cuff when searching for the calcium deposit on the subscapularis tendon (Fig. 13-11).

Bursoscopy

Entry into the subacromial bursa takes place with the arm position changed to approximately 10 degrees of abduction and a few degrees of forward flexion, using approximately 15 lb for distraction. The bursa is entered via

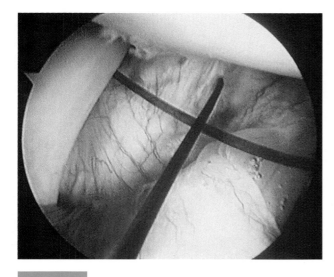

Figure 13-10
Two marker sutures are used to help locate the calcification in the subscapularis tendon. One is anterior and inferior to the biceps tendon; the second is through the upper edge of the subscapularis tendon, near the greater tuberosity.

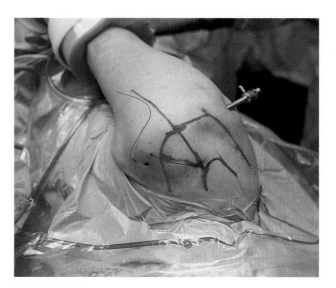

Figure 13-11
The two marker sutures are seen passing through the anterior shoulder below the anterior superior portal.

the posterior portal and distended with irrigation fluid. The anterior and lateral bursal portals are also developed. If visualization is obstructed by bursal debris, a shaver is used to remove the offending tissue. A complete bursal evaluation is then video-recorded prior to any surgical maneuvers. The marker suture or sutures are then located. The calcification frequently appears as a bulging blister on the bursal surface of the cuff (Fig. 13-12). In some cases there is a hyperemic capillary web surrounding the lesion; in others it may simply appear as an indistinct swelling of the bursa. Unless the suture marker is present to indicate the insertion of the rotator cuff, it may be difficult to differentiate between a firm calcium deposit and a bony ridge or prominence on the tuberosity inferior to the tendon-tuberosity junction.

Removal of Calcification

Two goals should be considered when removing a calcification arthroscopically: (1) Complete removal of as much calcium as possible should be a high priority, but (2) no signifi-

cant iatrogenic damage should be done to the remaining rotator cuff. Depending on the depth of the calcium deposit within the cuff tendon and the character and texture of the calcified material, the technique for removal varies. Initially, an 18-gauge spinal needle will serve to puncture the bursa around the marker suture and thereby open the calcific blister (Fig. 13-13). When the deposit is of a creamy or toothpaste-like consistency, it will flow freely from the punctured blister (Fig. 13-14). This occurs because the arthroscopic fluid pressure in the bursal space compresses the lesion. A small-diameter synovial resector blade inserted through the anterior portal can be used as a vacuum to suction up the calcium as it oozes from the blister. When the deposit seems to be empty, the tip of the shaver can be used like a rolling pin to massage the tissues with a rolling motion. Any remaining calcium will be forced toward the pinhole openings and removed by the suction (Fig. 13-15). Often this completely empties the lesion with minimal damage to the rotator cuff and the bursa.

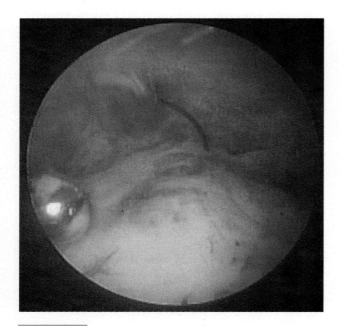

Figure 13-12
The calcific deposit frequently appears as a bulging blister on the bursal side of the rotator cuff. The marker suture passes directly through the center of the calcific nodule.

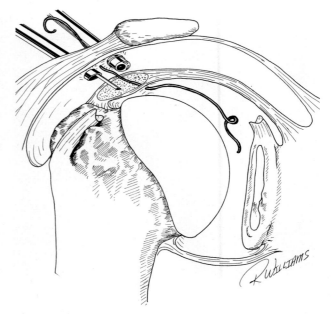

Figure 13-13
The calcific blister is opened and punctured with a spinal needle passed percutaneously lateral to the acromion.

When the calcifications are of a granular or sand-like nature, they seldom completely empty spontaneously when their bursal covering is punctured with a needle. Frequently, in this situation, the tip of the needle may locate the calcification, which presents as granular flakes in the irrigant. The outer bursal covering of the rotator cuff may then require careful removal with the synovial resector. A nonaggressive small-diameter shaver tip is recommended, to avoid inadvertent damage to the underlying cuff (Fig. 13-16). Once the bursa is removed, the calcification can be better appreciated. Often, in chronic cases, the underlying tendon has already been damaged. There may be craters and degeneration in some of the cuff fibers. The act of liberating the calcium should not cause further damage. Since the tendon damage is already present,

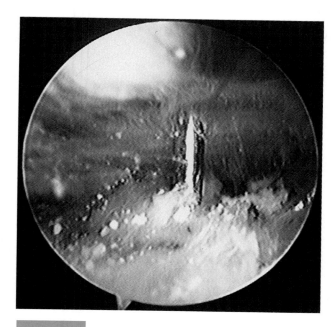

Figure 13-14
Creamy calcification can be seen flowing under pressure from the calcific blister.

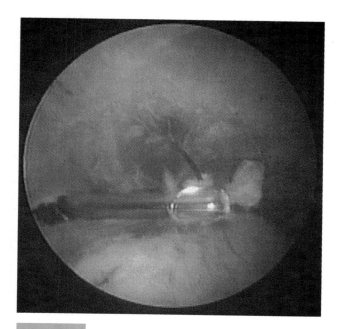

Figure 13-15
A small shaver tip can be used to roll and massage the calcium blister while the debris is suctioned from the bursal space.

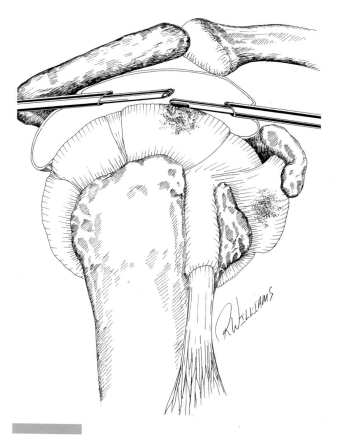

Figure 13-16
Dry calcium is removed by shaving the bursal covering to expose and liberate the underlying inspissated deposit.

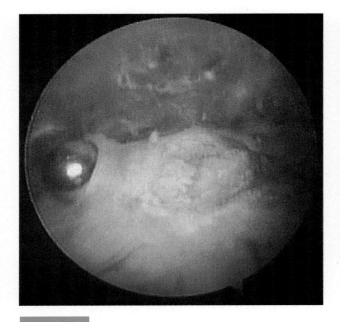

Figure 13-17
Sometimes a relatively large crater defect is present after the calcium is removed. This defect was caused by the calcium, not by the removal process.

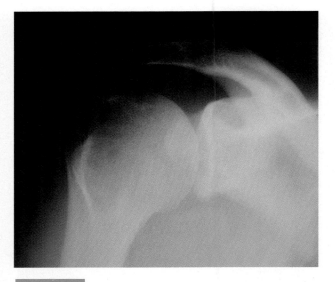

Figure 13-18
A bone-like calcium deposit is seen on the greater tuberosity. It probably should not be removed.

removal of the calcium will expose the cuff defect where calcific material was previously located (Fig. 13-17). Attempts should be made to selectively remove necrotic tendinous material with the shaver blade, but it is not possible to completely smooth the disrupted tendon. We believe that when the bursa regrows, the irregularities in the tendon surface will be covered smoothly.

Special Problem Areas

On very few occasions there may be an extremely difficult calcification located directly in the insertional fibers of the rotator cuff tendon. In this position the calcium appears on x-ray much like a tooth, with the base on the tuberosity and the point directed into the tendon. This type of calcification probably should not be removed. It is apt to be relatively chalk-like or bone-like in nature; attempts to remove it might cause more significant tendon damage (Fig. 13-18).

On rare occasions, when the calcification cannot be readily located, it is helpful to have an image intensifier in the operating room. Using this machine the calcium can be quickly located with a needle, and a marker suture inserted in the manner described above. Additionally, if there is a question about the completeness of calcium removal, a check x-ray on the operating table is helpful. Be certain that all metallic objects are removed from the bursa prior to the check x-ray, to avoid concealing any residual calcification.

Special Problems of Subscapularis Calcification

Calcific deposits in the subscapularis tendon are a special problem, since they are usually located anterior to the subacromial bursa. Using two marker sutures (as described above) as visual guides, a portion of the anterior bursal wall can be resected. Once both sutures are located, the spinal needle technique for liberating the calcium is employed (Fig. 13-19). Care should be taken, in shaving the bursa, to protect the nearby transverse humeral ligament covering the biceps tendon (Fig. 13-20). Additionally, injury to the conjoined tendon taking origin from the tip of the acromion should be avoided. Since the lesser tuberosity and its attached subscapularis tendon are directly beneath the coracoacromial

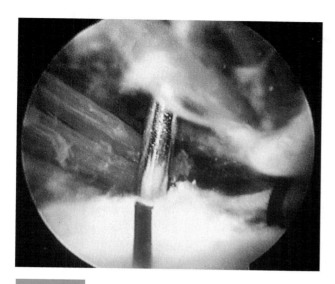

Figure 13-19
A spinal needle is also helpful to open the calcium deposit on the lesser tuberosity. Both suture markers are seen in the view (see text).

ligament, with only 1 to 2 mm of clearance, it has been our practice to remove this ligament at the time of the calcium removal from the subscapularis tendon.

To remove the coracoacromial ligament we use an electrosurgical pencil with a Subacromial Electrode (Concept, Inc.). The arthroscopic irrigant should be a nonconductive solution, such as Synovisol, which permits the surgeon to use the lowest possible power setting on the generator, thereby avoiding unnecessary injury to the overlying deltoid muscle. The tip of the electrode is used first to outline the coracoacromial ligament attachment from beneath the acromion, and then carefully to remove it. As the dissection progresses it is helpful to use a traction suture or clamp on the end of the ligament to apply tension. The traction suture can be placed using a Caspari Punch through the lateral portal, or a percutaneous epidural needle. The dissection can then proceed using the electrosurgical tool or an arthroscopic elevator such as the Concept Liberator Elevator (Fig. 13–21). When the tip of the coracoid is encountered, the entire ligament can be removed using a suction punch or large-diameter shaver. This same technique for harvesting the coracoacromial ligament may be used when performing

Figure 13-20
The bursa should be shaved only judiciously near the lesser tuberosity, with care taken to avoid injury to the biceps tendon and transverse humeral ligament.

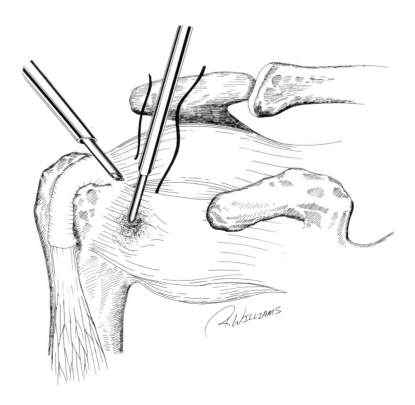

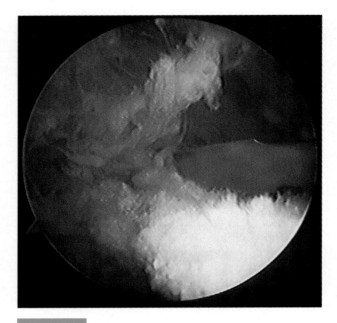

Figure 13-21
The coracoacromial ligament is totally removed in the case of subscapularis calcifications, using the Subacromial Electrode and the Concept Liberator Elevator.

an AC joint reconstruction, such as a Weaver-Dunn or Neviasser procedure.

Subacromial Decompression in Conjunction with Calcium Removal

Although the impingement phenomenon is thought to cause pain when subacromial calcifications are present in the supraspinatus tendon area, it is seldom necessary to perform a complete subacromial decompression. Unless there is a substantial anterior acromial prominence or beak compromising the area of the supraspinatus outlet, simply removing the bulk of the calcific material should provide adequate clearance for the remaining cuff and bursal tissue. On the other hand, if, after removing an inspissated calcification, a significant crater-like defect is present in the tendon, it seems logical to perform a subacromial decompression to prevent potential catching of the rough edge of the defect on the border of the acromion. In our series approximately 20 percent of the patients with arthroscopic removal of calcification required concomitant decompression.

Postoperative Treatment

The choice of postoperative treatment is governed by the severity of the initial calcification and the status of the rotator cuff tendon. In the usual situation, 1 to 2 days of rest in a sling allows local inflammation and swelling to subside before exercises are begun. Elbow, wrist, and hand exercises are begun immediately, using therapy putty. On day 3 or 4 the involved arm is passively elevated by the patient using a pulley at home. Pendulum and wand exercises are used to maintain rotation. At about 1 week progressive resistance exercises are begun, using rubber exercise tubing.

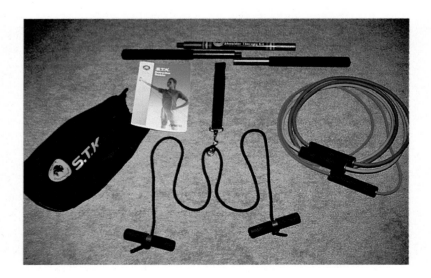

Figure 13-22
An STK (Shoulder Therapy Kit) is given to each patient preoperatively. In many cases it permits adequate home mobilization and strengthening, as an alternative to formal physical therapy.

TABLE 13-1	Surgeon's Preference Card for Calcific Tendinitis
Position:	Standard arthroscopy lateral position with overhead traction
Draping:	Shoulder arthroscopy drapes
Traction:	One-point lateral traction system
	Sterilized foam STaR Sleeve (Arthrex, Inc.) or other arm traction
Sandbags:	2-lb, 5-lb, and 10-lb
Equipment:	Standard shoulder arthroscopy equipment
	18-gauge spinal needle
	Monofilament absorbable suture (no. 1 PDS or Maxon)
	4.5-mm full-radius shaver blade Acromionizer if decompression is planned
Irrigation:	Synovisol or Ringer's lactate
Other:	Possibly x-ray, or image intensifier (fluoroscope) on standby; possible electrosurgical tools (Subacromial Electrode) for decompression

This program can progress with the help of a physical therapist; or, in the case of a motivated patient, at home or in his or her personal gym. We have found it helpful to issue an exercise kit to our patients in the preoperative period, along with physical therapy instructions. One handy kit that contains all the necessary equipment is the STK (Shoulder Therapy Kit) by (Breg, Inc., Carlsbad, California) (Fig. 13-22). The surgeon should review the exercise book included in the kit and designate the appropriate exercises to be performed during each phase of recovery. Usually the patient has returned to most normal daily living activities by 6 weeks. Return to vigorous physical activities is usually delayed for approximately 3 months.

References

1. Bateman JE: *The Neck and Shoulder.* Philadelphia, Saunders, 1978.

2. Uhthoff HK, Sarkar K: Calcifying tendinitis, in Rockwood CA, Matsen FA (eds): *The Shoulder.* Philadelphia, Saunders, 1990, pp 774–790.

3. Bosworth BM: Calcium deposits in the shoulder in subacromial bursitis: A survey of 12,122 shoulders. *JAMA* 116:2477, 1941.

4. Codman EA: *The Shoulder.* Boston, Todd Printing, 1934.

5. Flint JM: Acute traumatic subdeltoid bursitis. A new and simple treatment. *JAMA* 60:1224, 1913.

6. Harmon PH: Methods and results in the treatment of 2,580 painful shoulders with special reference to calcific tendinitis and the frozen shoulder. *Am J Surg* 95:527, 1958.

7. Patterson RL, Darrach W: Treatment of acute bursitis by needle injection. *J Bone Joint Surg* 19:993, 1937.

8. Rowe CR: *The Shoulder.* New York, Churchill Livingstone, 1988.

9. Lichtman HM et al: The surgical management of calcific tendinitis of the shoulder. *Int Orthop* 50(5), 1968.

10. Eppley RA, Snyder SJ, Brewster S: Arthroscopic removal of subacromial calcification. Presented at the Annual Meeting of the Arthroscopy Association of North America, San Diego, California, April 1991.

11. Ellman H, Bigliani LU, Flatow E, et al: Arthroscopic treatment of calcific tendinitis: The American experience. Presented at the Fifth International Conference on the Shoulder, Paris, France, July 1992.

14

Interesting and Unusual Applications for Shoulder Arthroscopy

Case No. 1: Intramuscular Cyst in the Supraspinatus Tendon

History

The patient was a 36-year-old laborer who had the spontaneous onset of pain in the right shoulder with his activities at work. Although he continued work when the initial evaluation by the company physician was negative, he developed increasing discomfort with overhead activity, weakness, and a sense of catching in his shoulder with abduction.

Physical Examination

The patient presented as a mildly obese, but otherwise very muscular, male in no acute distress. Inspection revealed no signs of significant atrophy or deformity about his shoulders. Range of motion of his shoulders was full and complete. His strength with internal and external rotation was normal, but supraspinatus strength of the dominant right shoulder

was moderately decreased in comparison to the left. The patient reported pain and became easily fatigued with supraspinatus stress testing. Neurological and circulatory status was completely intact throughout his right upper extremity. The impingement test was positive on the right (Neer's test), but the impingement II test (Hawkins' test) was negative. The biceps tension test and the liftoff test were negative.

X-Rays

X-rays were within normal limits. The arch view demonstrated a type IIB acromial arch (smooth concave curvature with no anterior spur, and average thickness measuring 10 mm). There were no other radiological abnormalities.

MRI testing was ordered because of the incomplete clinical picture. This demonstrated a large cyst within the muscular substance of the posterior aspect of the supraspinatus muscle (Figs. 14-1 and 14-2). The cyst measured approximately 2 × 2 × 4 cm and was fluid-filled.

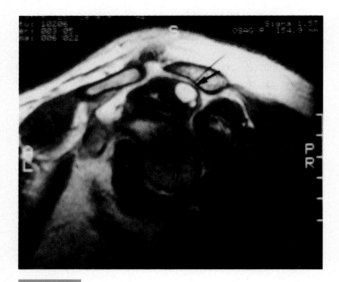

Figure 14-1
A sagittal MRI scan (T2 weighted image) showing a large fluid-filled cyst in the posterior aspect of the supraspinatus muscle.

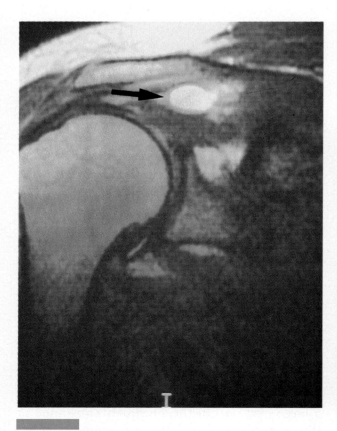

Figure 14-2
On the coronal projection of the MRI scan, the cyst is noted to be ovoid in appearance and located medial to the AC joint.

Arthroscopic Examination

The standard glenohumeral arthroscopic evaluation disclosed no signs of pathology. The bursoscopy revealed mild inflammation of the subacromial bursal tissues. The coracoacromial ligament was not frayed, and the bursal side of the rotator cuff was normal. The cyst was easily located arthroscopically by visualizing from the posterior portal while the small full-radius shaver was used to debride the bursal tissue from the superior aspect of the supraspinatus tendon in a medial direction. At the musculotendinous junction the glistening cyst wall was encountered; with gentle dissection with the tip of the shaver, the cyst was readily exposed. A pituitary rongeur was used to open the cyst and obtain a sample for pathological examination (Fig. 14-3).

The shaver was then used to debride the cyst wall in a lateral-to-medial direction. The cyst was noted to occupy approximately 25 to 30 percent of the space of the supraspinatus fossa, displacing the supraspinatus muscle anteriorly. The posterior wall of the cyst was located against the anterior edge of the suprascapular spine. The cyst wall easily peeled

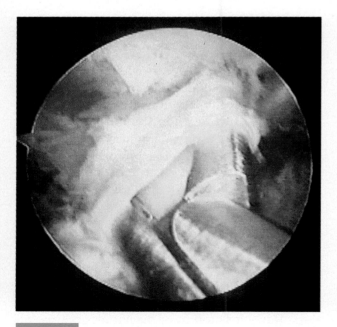

Figure 14-3
A pituitary rongeur was used to remove a segment of the cyst wall.

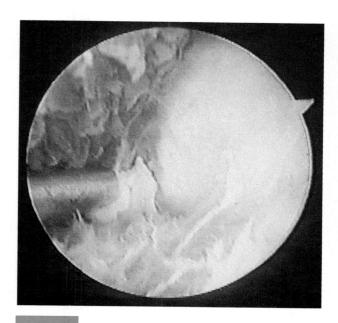

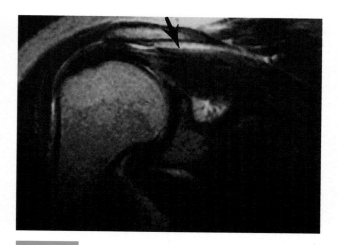

Figure 14-5
A repeat MRI scan demonstrates that the supraspinatus cyst is gone, with only minimal residual soft tissue fluid.

Figure 14-4
A shaver was used to peel off the cyst wall from the surrounding muscle. The scapular spine is on the left side of the field.

away with the shaver and seemed to have the consistency of damp wallpaper (Fig. 14-4). The entire cyst was easily removed. With the cyst gone, the muscle mass refilled the supraspinatus fossa.

Postoperative Course

The patient was treated with a sling for 1 week postoperatively. Gentle pendulum exercises and progressive active assisted range-of-motion exercises, using the pulley and exercise wand from the Shoulder Therapy Kit (STK), were begun. At 2 weeks postoperatively the patient started progressive resistance exercises using the elastic bands from the STK. Finally, at 4 weeks, he was started in physical therapy for swimming and strengthening. His range of motion had completely returned. At 8 weeks postoperatively, the patient was unable to get back to work because of a conflict, and he reported some return of his shoulder symptoms. Another MRI scan was performed (Fig. 14-5); it demonstrated that the cyst was gone and the supraspinatus muscle belly had refilled the fossa in its place.

There was some persistent effusion, but no localized fluid.

Final Outcome

The patient's job problem was resolved. He made an uneventful recovery and is back to full activities, with no further difficulties.

Discussion

This case was an interesting example of a very difficult diagnostic problem in a young, healthy, working male. The MRI was indispensable for confirming the diagnosis. The arthroscopic approach was very straightforward, allowing complete excision of this benign ganglion-type intramuscular cyst. Although the patient required 10 weeks to get back to work, he certainly had no clinical evidence of physical restrictions at the 6-week postoperative period. Several additional cases of intramuscular cysts of the infraspinatus muscle or the anterior surface of the supraspinatus muscle have been encountered, but because of fear of damage to the suprascapular nerve they have been treated with either aspiration under ultrasound or MRI control with injection (unsuccessfully), or by open resection. In this case the neural anatomy was well known, and it was believed that the cyst was not in a location that threatened the neural integrity. The local anatomy of the nerves and vessels should always be kept in mind when approaching a ganglion cyst around the shoulder, whether in an arthroscopic or in an open procedure—and especially with regard to the suprascapular and axillary nerves.

Case No. 2: Arthroscopic Excision of Osteochondroma of the Proximal Humerus

History

The patient was a 43-year-old male who had been in a motor vehicle accident, sustaining minor multiple traumatic injuries. He complained of pain in the left, non-dominant, shoulder as well as in his neck, back, and legs. His workup was unremarkable, but because of persistent shoulder problems he was sent to SCOI for an evaluation.

Physical Examination

The patient presented as a normally developed, minimally obese, muscular male with multiple tattoos on his body, in no acute distress. Inspection revealed a fullness in the posterior aspect of the left proximal humerus (Fig. 14-6). Palpation revealed a tender mass just below the posterior aspect of the greater tuberosity. There was no ecchymosis nor any skin changes in the area. The patient had full range of motion of the shoulder, but had pain with abduction at 90 degrees. His muscle testing was normal for internal rotation, but external rotation with resistance caused minor pain and weakness. Supraspinatus and biceps testing were normal. The impingement I test was negative, but the impingement II test (Hawkins' test) was positive, with pain and some restricted motion in comparison to the opposite side. Instability testing was negative.

X-Rays

X-rays as submitted by the patient's personal physician were reviewed, and were of marginal quality. New films were taken and re-

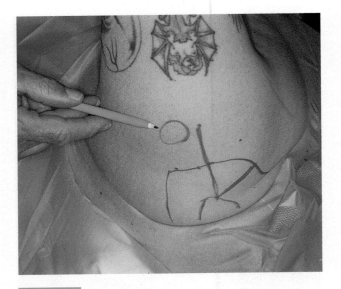

Figure 14-6
The patient had a painful bony mass located on the posterior aspect of the greater tuberosity, about 5 cm lateral to the acromion.

vealed an obvious bony deformity of the posterior aspect of the greater tuberosity of the humerus, resembling a benign osteochondroma of moderate proportions. An MRI scan revealed that the bony lesion was located just below, and posterior to, the supraspinatus and just anterior to the infraspinatus tendon attachment on the proximal humerus (Fig. 14-7). There were no signs of bony invasion or significant bone marrow disruption associated with the lesion. The rotator cuff and labral tissues appeared to be otherwise intact.

Surgical Treatment

Because of continuing complaints of localized tenderness and restricted motion, the patient was taken to surgery. Both the diagnostic arthroscopy of the glenohumeral joint and the bursoscopy examination were normal. The location of the tumor was marked using a percutaneous needle, and the synovial resector was used to remove the posterior aspect of the bursa to locate the lesion. With the arthroscope in the anterior portal and the synovial resector in the posterior portal, the periosteal and bursal coverings of the tumor were removed (Fig. 14-8). A 1/4-in curved osteotome

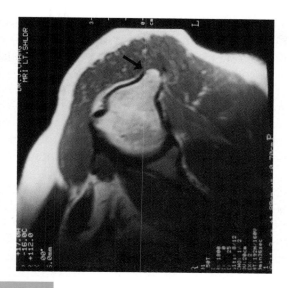

Figure 14-7
This axial view on the MRI scan demonstrates the location of the osteochondroma to be just below and posterior to the greater tuberosity, adjacent to the lowest attachment of the infraspinatus muscle.

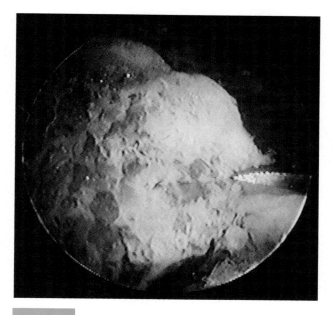

Figure 14-9
The margins of the osteochondroma were demarcated using a 1/4-in curved osteotome.

was then used to demarcate the anterior, posterior, and superior margins of the osteochondroma (Fig. 14-9). A large rongeur was used to fragment and remove the mass through the lateral portal. Care was taken to morselize the bony fragments, to avoid loosening them during removal through the deltoid muscle (Fig. 14-10).

After removal of the bulk of the lesion, a high-speed burr was used to flatten the mar-

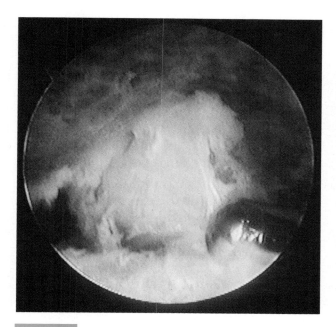

Figure 14-8
The arthroscopic shaver was used to remove the bursal covering over the osteochondroma, so as to allow better visualization.

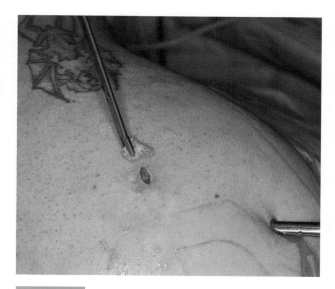

Figure 14-10
A large double-action rongeur was used to morselize and remove the bone fragments via the lateral portal.

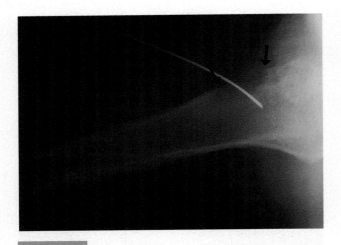

Figure 14-11
A final x-ray was taken in the operating room with a needle positioned in the center of the resected lesion.

gins of the lesion circumferentially. A final check x-ray was taken after placing a marker needle through the lateral portal into the center of the lesion. This x-ray (Fig. 14-11) demonstrated complete removal of the mass.

Postoperative Course

The patient was discharged the same day and treated with a sling. On his first postoperative visit he had no significant complaints. He started his home physical therapy program and progressed to pulley and pendulum exercises within the second week, and to progressive resistance exercises with the STK at 3 weeks. He then continued with physical therapy for 3 additional weeks, and was discharged from care with no further complaints.

The pathology report of the specimen indicated benign osteochondroma.

Discussion

The patient sustained a direct blow over a benign osteochondroma during his motor vehicle accident. The legal ramifications in regard to this patient remain to be clarified, but the surgical remedy appears to have been successful. The pointed osteochondroma served as a source of irritation to the bursa and the deltoid, and a point of contact with any pressure around the shoulder. In addition, it appeared to impinge beneath the acromion with

abduction, internal rotation, and adduction. The potential for malignant transformation of this lesion, although extremely remote, also needs to be considered.

Several technical points of this case deserve comment. The location of the lesion was fortunate, in that it did not compromise the attachment of the infraspinatus or supraspinatus tendons. Both tendon attachments could be seen at the periphery of the lesion following the resection. The axillary nerve runs within the substance of the deltoid just lateral to the location of the lesion, and care must be taken at all times to protect the nerve. For this reason, very little burring was performed, and the guard of the burr was always kept beneath the muscle, avoiding inadvertent winding-up of the soft tissues and nerve. Suction is never used on the abrader for this reason, as well. A gravity drainage cannula is inserted through a separate portal to allow removal of bone chips.

Case No. 3: Revascularization of Osteochondritis Dissecans of the Humeral Head

History

The patient was a 26-year-old female ambulance driver who had been injured in a car-versus-pedestrian accident. She had sustained a fracture of her left tibial plateau and a compression injury to her right shoulder. The tibial plateau fracture had required open reduction and internal fixation, with a fairly good result. Her right shoulder had continued to be painful and ache; she was sent to our clinic for evaluation when the diagnosis was uncertain.

Physical Examination

The patient presented as a healthy, normally muscled female, non-obese, in no acute distress. She walked with a mild limp. Range of motion of her shoulders demonstrated a 20-degree lack of forward elevation of the right

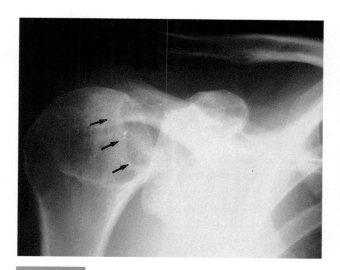

Figure 14-12
An AP x-ray demonstrates a subchondral defect with apparent bony collapse in the humeral head.

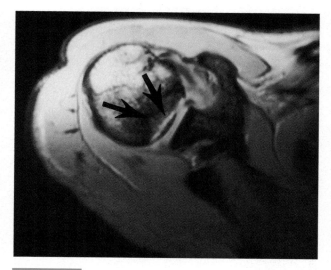

Figure 14-13
A T2 weighted MRI scan demonstrates an area of apparent bony necrosis on the medial subchondral surface of the anterior humeral head.

shoulder, with clicking and a sense of catching. External and internal rotation were normal, and abduction was normal and equal to that on the opposite side. Her strength with internal and external rotation were normal, but supraspinatus strength was moderately reduced and testing caused pain. The impingement test caused minor pain, but apprehension and instability tests were negative. The biceps tension test was negative, and her neurovascular status was completely normal.

X-Rays

The original x-rays were reviewed and were thought to be normal, but a small subchondral defect was noted on the axillary view.

Multiple additional x-rays were taken and demonstrated what appeared to be a segmental osteochondral defect in the anterior surface of the humeral head (Fig. 14-12).

On MRI scan this lesion appeared to be a segmental area of osteochondral collapse, resembling osteochondritis dissecans (Fig. 14-13).

Continued Clinical Course

Because the patient's symptoms were not severe, she elected to reduce her activities while exercising to maintain motion. After 6 months

she developed more pain and clicking in her shoulder; it was thought that the osteochondral fragment might be loose. She sought additional consultation from three orthopaedists, whose treatment suggestions ranged from benign neglect to open excision versus refixation of the lesion and bone grafting. One surgeon suggested to the patient that she would probably be a candidate for joint replacement in the near future.

Surgical Treatment

The patient elected to have diagnostic arthroscopy, followed by appropriate surgical treatment of her shoulder, when her symptoms continued to increase. Arthroscopic evaluation revealed a segmental collapse of approximately 30 percent of the subchondral bone of the anterior surface of the humeral head (Fig. 14-14). The remaining humeral head was intact with no significant arthritis, although moderate synovitis was present. There were no loose bodies within the joint. The articular cartilage over the collapsed segment was intact except at the margins, where mild fraying and a fissure were present. Because the bone fragment did not appear to be loose and the articular cartilage seemed vi-

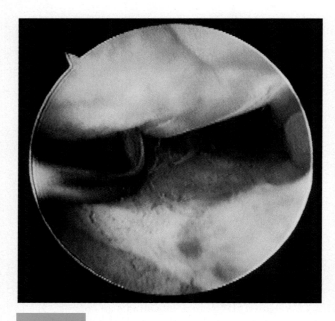

Figure 14-14
The arthroscopic evaluation of the humeral head demonstrated a segmental area of collapse on the anterior surface.

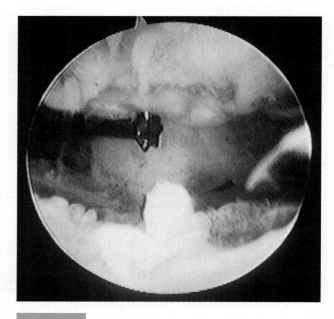

Figure 14-15
A miniature Vector (Dyonics Inc.) drill guide was used to direct a 0.62-mm K-wire into the area of the defect to create ten drill holes for vascular access.

able, it was thought best to attempt to revascularize the dead fragment. A miniature Vector guide (Dyonics, Inc., Andover, Massachusetts) was used to help visually direct a 0.62-mm K-wire through a percutaneous stab wound entering the posterior aspect of the greater tuberosity (Fig. 14-15). Ten separate drill holes were made in the osteochondral lesion, stopping just short of penetrating the articular surface. Following the drilling, the stability of the fragment was tested again with a probe.

Postoperative Treatment

The patient was discharged after one night in the hospital and treated with a simple sling. Passive motion exercises were begun on the first postoperative day, and she progressed to active assisted range-of-motion exercises, using the STK (Shoulder Therapy Kit), at 1 week. Her symptoms progressively improved, with complete resolution of her clicking and catching by 6 weeks. At 8 weeks postoperatively she returned to work as a receptionist and joined a gym to work on the strengthening of her shoulder. A repeat MRI scan was taken at 4 months, demonstrating incorporation of the previous sclerotic bone (Fig. 14-16). A final followup at 1 year postoperatively demonstrated normal motion and good strength of the shoulder. X-rays demonstrated no further subchondral collapse, although the small step-off in the subchondral bone was visible. The patient reported only minimal exertional discomfort.

Discussion

In a young, healthy, athletic patient, a segmental articular surface collapse can be devastating. The treatment for these lesions in the hip and knee has long been controversial, and the various techniques to restore circulation and reform the articular surface have been questionable at best. Coring and bone grafting procedures, particularly in the hip, have had disappointing results.

The actual diagnosis of this patient's lesion is not certain. This may have been an early

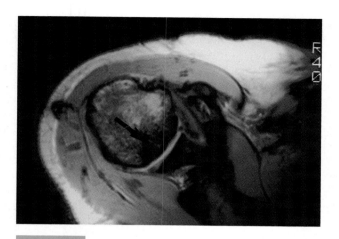

Figure 14-16
An MRI scan taken 4 months after the arthroscopically controlled drilling demonstrates apparent healing and incorporation of the osteochondral lesion, although the subchondral bone still is not perfectly smooth.

case of avascular necrosis, or an osteochondral fracture. The fact that the patient seemed to revascularize after a simple drilling procedure with a very satisfactory result was gratifying, but the step-off in the joint surface and the marginal articular cartilage damage noted at the time of arthroscopy may portend a less favorable long-term result. If the patient had no treatment, it was feared that the fragment might dislodge and lead to early degenerative changes. If the fragment had been loose at the time of surgery, to reposition it arthroscopically would have been difficult, and an open procedure might have been necessary. Thoughts of refixation of these fragments, using small cannulated screws or nonabsorbable sutures passed in a mattress fashion over a bone bridge intra-articularly and tied over the greater tuberosity externally, might be considered. A suture Shuttle Relay (see Chap. 12) would be beneficial to allow this procedure, if necessary. Additionally, if the bone fragment had been dislodged and could not be replaced, then an arthroplasty procedure removing the fragment and tapering the margins of the remaining crater might have had some benefit.

Case No. 4: Arthroscopic Removal of Loose K-Wire From the Greater Tuberosity

History
The patient was a 66-year-old female who had fallen at home 4 months previously, sustaining a comminuted three-part fracture of the right proximal humerus. The fracture had been treated by another surgeon using open reduction and internal fixation techniques employing a smooth K-wire and multiple wire loops as tension bands. The fracture was healing uneventfully, but the patient began complaining of a painful prominence in the anterior aspect of her shoulder that limited her ability to exercise and even to move her arm.

Physical Examination
The patient was an unhealthy-appearing female with obvious emphysema who appeared angry and upset but was in no acute distress. She had a well-placed anterior delto-pectoral incision on her shoulder. Her range of motion was limited by her complaints of pain, particularly of that emanating from a tender area on the anterior aspect of her shoulder near the lesser tuberosity. Palpation revealed a firm, tender mass near the lesser tuberosity that moved with humeral rotation.

X-Rays
X-rays demonstrated a healing humeral fracture with several intact wire loops employed for fracture fixation. There was a single smooth K-wire kinked posteriorly but exiting the humerus 2 cm into the soft tissue in the area of the lesser tuberosity (Fig. 14-17). It was uncertain whether the fracture was totally healed, but there were no signs of avascular necrosis or significant joint injury.

Arthroscopic Examination
The glenohumeral joint demonstrated several areas of moderately restrictive adhesions, some adherent to the articular cartilage inferi-

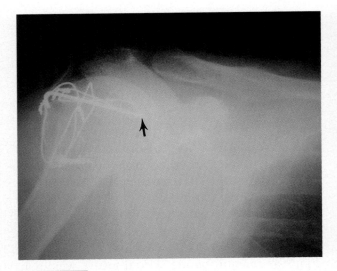

Figure 14-17
This x-ray demonstrates a healing, well-fixed fracture of the proximal humerus with a smooth K-wire protruding approximately 2 cm into the anterior soft tissues.

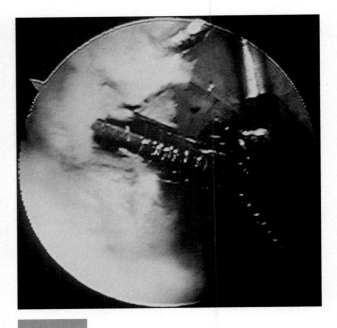

Figure 14-18
An arthroscopic view of a clamp grasping a K-wire for removal from the posterior aspect of the greater tuberosity.

orly and posteriorly, but the glenoid and articular surfaces for the most part were intact, with no fracture lines or step-offs. The rotator cuff appeared perfectly intact on the articular side. The bursoscopy demonstrated a thick bursal membrane with moderate amounts of scarring and adhesions. The knotted wire was located by shaving the bursa on the greater tuberosity. The bent pin tip was located by following the wire posteriorly. After removal of the surrounding bursal tissue the smooth K-wire was removed with a heavy arthroscopic grasping clamp via the posterior portal (Fig. 14-18).

Postoperative Course

The patient was discharged on the afternoon after surgery and treated with a sling for 1 week. Her pendulum and pulley exercises were encouraged immediately, and she progressed back to physical therapy at 2 weeks postoperatively. The tender spot on the anterior aspect of her shoulder was immediately improved; this allowed her to resume a more vigorous rehabilitation. At 4 months postoperatively her range of motion had greatly improved, and x-rays revealed that her fracture had completely healed.

Discussion

The patient had been a difficult postsurgical problem after the original surgery, because of severe lung problems from a three-pack-a-day smoking habit. Further, it was not certain preoperatively whether the rotator cuff was intact, since the patient's pain inhibited adequate testing. The location of the pin in the proximal humerus below the deltoid made it accessible to simple arthroscopic removal. One must be aware of the anatomy of the axillary nerve and the posterior rotator cuff insertion. The twisted wire knot on the greater tuberosity was easily located after shaving the bursa and could be followed back to the bent end of the offending K-wire. It was important, too, that soft tissue be removed, so that the wire could be firmly grasped with a strong clamp, ensuring that it would not be lost in the soft tissue during removal.

The postoperative course was benign and the patient had relatively little discomfort during her healing course. It was not thought advisable to remove all of the wires at this surgery, since the completeness of healing of the tuberosity fracture was still in doubt. Knowing that the rotator cuff was intact and that the articular surfaces were not damaged allowed us to encourage a much more rapid rehabilitation once the offending pin had been removed.

Case No. 5: Removal of Intra-Articular Humeral Head Bone Spur Following a Fracture

History

The patient was a 34-year-old male who had sustained a fracture of his dominant right humerus in a skiing accident. The fracture was noted on x-ray to extend into the articular surface of the humeral head, but conservative treatment had been elected by his physician. Although the fracture had healed well, the patient complained of pain and catching with overhead reaching. Often his arm became stuck in the overhead position.

Physical Examination

The patient presented as a thin, muscular, healthy-appearing male in no acute distress. His forward elevation of his right arm was limited to approximately 90 degrees, at which point the arm would lock. With traction on the arm, the arc of forward elevation increased to approximately 170 degrees without significant pain. There was crepitation and tenderness in the biceps groove; and Speed's biceps tension test was positive. Internal and external rotation strength was normal, and supraspinatus strength was normal.

X-Rays

X-rays demonstrated the residual changes of a proximal humeral fracture with an obvious step-off in the articular surface of the humeral head, best seen on the axillary view (Fig. 14-19). The step-off was located just superomedial to the greater tuberosity on the articular surface and measured approximately 6 mm.

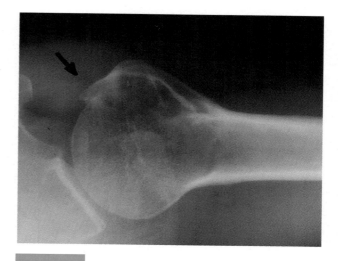

Figure 14-19
An axillary lateral x-ray demonstrates a spur on the articular surface of the anterior humeral head.

Arthroscopic Examination

The arthroscopic examination demonstrated normal glenoid articular surface. The biceps tendon had a partial tear through approximately 30 percent of its thickness, caused by fraying as it passed over the step-off of the humeral surface (Fig. 14-20). The fracture line appeared well healed but had caused a ledge-type defect by its malunion. The main

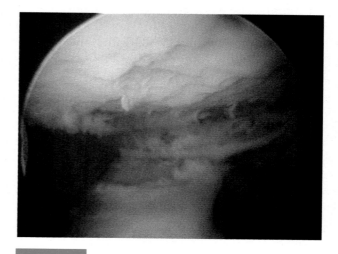

Figure 14-20
A malunion at the fracture site caused a 6-mm step-off in the humeral head, with resultant fraying of the biceps tendon.

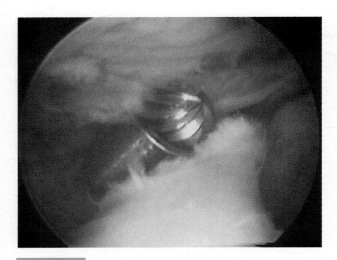

Figure 14-21
An arthroscopic burr was used to smooth the bony step-off and recreate the biceps groove.

portion of the articular surface of the humeral head was without injury. Arthroscopic treatment included flattening of the lateral portion of the humeral head to remove the step-off. A full-radius shaver was used to peel off a 5- to 6-mm width of the articular cartilage from the lateral fragment. The high-speed burr was used to fashion a new groove for the biceps tendon so that it no longer passed over the sharp fracture step-off (Fig. 14-21). The edge of the fracture step-off was also beveled so that there was a smooth transition between the remaining articular head and the greater tuberosity.

Postoperative Course

The patient was treated postoperatively with a sling and early range-of-motion exercises. He immediately noticed that there was no longer any catching as he elevated his arm and his biceps function soon returned to normal. At a 3-year follow-up evaluation the patient remained free of pain, with excellent rotator cuff and biceps tendon strength and full motion. He has returned to skiing and is an avid swimmer, and has no complaints. Follow-up x-rays demonstrate no significant interval change.

Discussion

The use of the arthroscope to evaluate glenohumeral and bursal anatomy following fractures has been very rewarding. Imaging modalities—x-ray, CT, and even MRI—can be misleading or incomplete concerning the actual status of the joint. The biceps tendon lesion found at arthroscopy would not have been suspected. Anything less than removal of the humeral head fracture step-off would probably have failed to relieve the patient's symptoms adequately. For this reason, open surgery would have been extremely difficult and probably would have required take-down of at least part of the deltoid and rotator cuff—if the lesion could have been repaired at all.

Although it was very unsettling to remove the articular cartilage from the malunited humeral head segment, it did not seem to interfere with the patient's function nor to cause him any difficulty in his medium-term follow-up. Since this case we have done six more arthroscopic fracture debridements; we have found this to be a very beneficial adjunct to improving functioning after humeral head fractures in carefully selected cases.

Case No. 6: Posterior Acromial Fracture/Spur

History

The patient was a 64-year-old female who had been injured while riding in her car on vacation. A heavy boulder had rolled down a mountain and crashed through the window of her car, striking her on the side of the neck and the shoulder. She had been knocked unconscious and later revived and taken to the emergency room by the state police. She had been evaluated for head and neck injuries and advised that she had a probable clavicle fracture which should heal in a sling. When she had not improved after approximately 8 months, she contacted her son, a physician, who ordered an x-ray and MRI scan. She was sent to our clinic because of persistent pain and weakness in her shoulder.

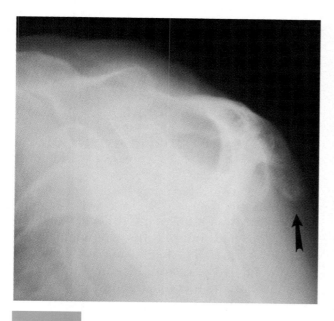

Figure 14-22
A lateral x-ray view of the acromial arch demonstrates malunion of a fracture fragment of the posterior edge of the acromion.

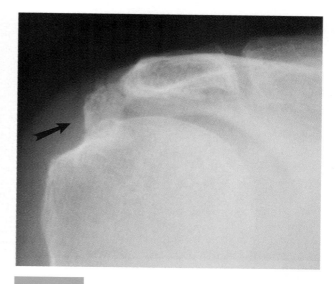

Figure 14-23
An AP x-ray demonstrates that the malunion of the acromial fracture is angled toward the humeral head.

Physical Examination

The patient presented as a healthy, non-obese female in no acute distress. She had superficial healed abrasions on the posterior aspect of her right shoulder. There was no obvious deformity of the bone to inspection. On palpation she had tenderness over the posterior aspect of her rotator cuff and acromion. Her active range of motion in forward elevation was approximately 80 degrees with severe crepitus. Abduction was limited to 60 degrees with severe pain and weakness. Internal rotation was normal, but external rotation caused pain and demonstrated severe weakness.

X-Rays

X-rays demonstrated an obvious fracture with an inferiorly tipped fragment of the posterior acromion (Figs. 14-22 and 14-23). The tip of the fracture seemed to approach the humeral head.

An MRI scan demonstrated a rotator cuff tear with retraction of the supra- and infraspinatus tendons. The *posterior* fracture fragment was contacting the humeral head at the rotator cuff.

Arthroscopic Examination

The glenohumeral arthroscopy demonstrated a moderately severe rotator cuff tear encompassing the supra- and infraspinatus tendons (CII). The biceps tendon was moderately frayed as well, but there was no glenohumeral arthritis. Bursoscopy demonstrated a moderate bursal hypertrophy and a full-thickness rotator cuff tear. There was a large bony fragment impinging on the rotator cuff from the posterior acromion. Anteriorly, there was no significant spur, and the AC joint was intact.

The surgery consisted of a "posterior subacromial decompression." With the arthroscope in the anterior subacromial portal, the bursa was resected from below the posterior acromial space, following the undersurface of the bone back to the deltoid insertion. The soft tissues were removed with the electrosurgical tool and shaver. Once the bone was outlined (Fig. 14-24), the spur was then removed so that the undersurface of the acromion was flat with no further impingement. A mini-lateral open rotator cuff repair was performed.

Postoperative Course

The patient was treated in an SCOI shoulder brace postoperatively, holding her arm in

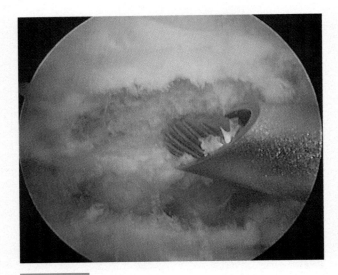

Figure 14-24
While viewing from the anterior portal, the posterior "acromioplasty" was performed with a 4.0-mm acromionizer burr.

about 30 degrees of abduction. Since no deltoid was removed, her healing progressed rapidly. At 3 weeks the brace was removed, and a sling applied. She started passive mobilization in her brace with the help of her husband at home, and started a physical therapy program in the pool at 3 weeks. By 4 months postoperatively her pain was completely gone; she had achieved forward elevation of 150 degrees with good strength and absence of night pain. Postoperative x-rays were taken, showing the bone spur to have been removed.

Discussion

The significance of the patient's acromial fracture was missed in the emergency room, probably because of the attention needed to evaluate her neurological status. The long delay between this supposedly "trivial" clavicle fracture and her final diagnosis and treatment was unfortunate, but understandable. Performing a posterior subacromial decompression while viewing from the anterior portal was actually very easy. Care must be taken posteriorly to avoid detaching any significant amount of deltoid when the fracture fragment is debrided. The goal should be to create adequate space beneath the fracture for the rotator cuff ten-

don to clear. The rotator cuff tear can then be treated in the standard fashion, with a good result expected.

Case No. 7: Arthroscopic Debridement of an Infected Bursa

History

The patient was a 68-year-old healthy retired male who had injured his dominant right shoulder in a fall. After conservative treatment had failed to restore his strength and relieve his pain, he had undergone an open rotator cuff repair and decompression by another physician. His postoperative course had been complicated by the development of a draining sinus tract on the inferior aspect of his anterior delto-pectoral incision. The sinus tract had been debrided locally, and several sutures removed. At 4 months postoperatively the patient had been sent to SCOI for a consultation, with the request for transfer of care.

Physical Examination

The patient presented as a healthy male in no acute distress. His right shoulder revealed moderate muscular atrophy. There was a small draining sinus tract around the midpoint of the otherwise well-healed delto-pectoral incision. The draining fluid was cloudy and rust-colored, but with no foul odor. The amount of drainage was minimal, requiring dressing change with a 2 × 2 pad twice daily. Active range of motion was forward flexion 40 degrees, external rotation 30 degrees, abduction 10 degrees, and internal rotation to the posterior gluteal area. Passive range of motion was limited by the patient's pain. Elbow, wrist, and hand function was normal, and the neurological status was intact.

Clinical Work-up

The patient had previously undergone a postoperative MRI scan of his shoulder, which had demonstrated intermediate signal in the area of the rotator cuff (Fig. 14-25). There was a

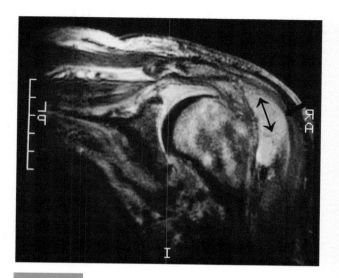

Figure 14-25
The T2 weighted MRI scan shows an area of intermediate signal in the rotator cuff tendon, with no signs of osteomyelitis. There is a huge effusion in the subacromial bursa (double arrow).

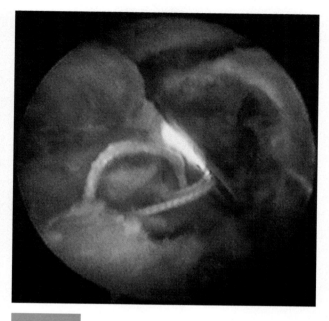

Figure 14-26
Several large fragments of heavy suture material were removed, along with necrotic bone fragments and bursal debris.

moderate amount of native joint fluid. The bursa demonstrated a large fluid collection.

X-Rays

X-rays demonstrated moderate osteopenia, but no signs of significant degenerative arthritis. There was bony irregularity around the greater tuberosity, representing the previous surgical site. An adequate subacromial decompression had been performed.

Bone scan revealed diffuse increased uptake in the right shoulder in comparison to the left, but no significant localizing focus that might suggest osteomyelitis. Multiple cultures taken using a sterile syringe into the sinus tract revealed *Staphylococcus aureus,* coagulase-positive, resistant to penicillin.

Clinical Course

The patient had a consultation with an infectious-disease specialist, who started him on oxacillin. He was taken to surgery, where an arthroscopic evaluation and surgery were performed. The glenohumeral joint was first approached from the posterior portal. The sinus tract had been sealed off with water-tight drapes to avoid contamination of the instru-

ments during the glenohumeral exam. A small amount of dilute methylene blue dye was injected through a spinal needle placed in the shoulder joint while visualizing the bursal side of the cuff. No dye was noted to leak into the bursa.

The bursa was filled with necrotic-appearing debris. Multiple large fragments of nonabsorbable braided suture were encountered and removed (Fig. 14-26). The sinus tract was located near one of the suture knots and followed out to the skin orifice, using the shaver to remove the necrotic tissue up to the skin orifice (Fig. 14-27). At that point the ostium of the sinus tract was excised. The bursa was irrigated with copious amounts of fluid, the 1-in skin incision was left open with a small wick drain.

Postoperative Course

The patient was kept in the hospital, on antibiotic treatment, for 2 days and then discharged home. He was required to return to his local emergency room twice daily for intravenous antibiotic injections. At 3 weeks he

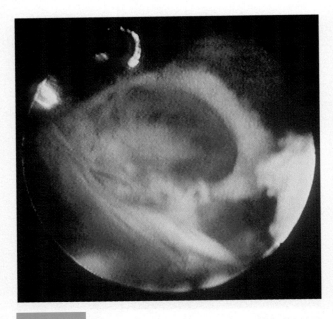

Figure 14-27
The sinus tract was followed from the area of the greater tuberosity to the ostium on the skin portal and debrided with a shaver from inside out. This photograph demonstrates the central core of the sinus tract as seen from within the bursa.

was changed to oral medication, which was continued for a total of 2 months. The surgical wound continued to drain for approximately 3 weeks postoperatively, but all cultures were negative and the patient's symptoms improved steadily. By 3 weeks he had painless forward elevation of 150 degrees and was sleeping through the night for the first time since his original surgery. The surgical wound was then closed with a skin suture and allowed to heal, without further incident.

Final Outcome

The patient was able to get back to his golf and a brisk exercise program with his upper extremities. Although he has not regained full motion, he has excellent functional use of his arm, and there have been no signs of recurrence of infection in the more than 2 years since his arthroscopic treatment.

Discussion

Infection in the shoulder is quite rare, but can be devastating. We have treated four patients with infections in the shoulder, but this was the first case involving only the bursa. This infection seemed to originate from a large retained fragment of nonabsorbable suture. It was possible, with the help of the arthroscope, to eliminate glenohumeral infection as a source of the drainage and to perform a very adequate debridement of the subacromial bursa without the need to reopen the patient's previous incision. The ostium of the draining sinus tract was excised so that the wound could continue to drain postoperatively. The final outcome was very gratifying; the patient is comfortable and is playing golf daily. The bone density was seen to have improved on his 1-year postoperative x-ray, and his rotator cuff strength is good.

15

Avoidance of Complications Associated with Arthroscopic Surgery of the Shoulder

Introduction

Like every other type of surgical procedure, shoulder arthroscopy is associated with certain potential operative risks and complications. Studying the anatomy at risk and reviewing the techniques and principles in advance of the surgery will decrease the possibilities of patient injury and complications. The surgeon who performs arthroscopic shoulder surgery should have an excellent knowledge not only of the arthroscopic anatomy but also of the surgical approaches for open procedures in and around the shoulder. This chapter will attempt to identify areas of risk and define the more common areas where complications may occur, and suggest ways to avoid them.

Potential Problems With Anesthesia

The most common types of anesthesia used for shoulder arthroscopy are general endotra-

cheal anesthesia and interscalene brachial plexus nerve block. At SCOI these two methods are used together, affording the patient a 10- to 14-h interval, following the surgery, when the block is still effective and the extremity is numb and without pain. During this extended anesthetic time, the postoperative swelling subsides and the general anesthetic agent metabolizes before the patient requires additional narcotic pain medication.

The potential problems associated with interscalene block should be reviewed with the patient by both the surgeon and the anesthesiologist. The anesthesiologist should be trained in administration of this block and should have appropriate injection needles and monitoring equipment available. The block should be performed with the patient awake and responsive. Since the local anesthetic is injected around the brachial plexus, an atraumatic flat-beveled needle may be safer than one with a standard cutting tip. The paresthesia reported by the patient should alert the doctor to the correct needle location prior to injection. Several complications can occur with improper interscalene block technique.

If the anesthesiologist inadvertently injects a bolus of marcaine intravascularly, the patient may experience a toxic reaction culminating in a grand mal seizure. The seizure can cause patient injury and require delay or postponement of the intended procedure. By carefully avoiding any superficial vein penetration and intermittently aspirating during the anesthetic injection, this complication should usually be avoided. Usually, if a seizure does occur, it is self-limited or can be controlled by administration of a general anesthetic agent.

Paralysis of the recurrent laryngeal nerve also occurs. Although phonation and cough are somewhat inhibited for the duration of the block, no long-term effects should result.

Inadvertent block of the phrenic nerve occasionally occurs. This situation is recognized postoperatively when the patient has tachypnea and inability to cough well. The involved hemidiaphragm is elevated on a chest x-ray, with no signs of pneumothorax. Phrenic nerve paralysis will resolve, with no residual effects, when the local anesthesia wears off. The blood oxygen levels should be monitored in any patient with pulmonary compromise, to avoid serious hypoxia while awaiting resolution of the block.

Infrequently there can be direct toxicity to the nerves from some anesthetic agents. One such agent, Nesacaine (chloroprocaine), has been known to cause extended paralysis for days and weeks following injection. For this reason, unless the anesthesiologist has personal knowledge and experience with an alternative anesthetic, the injection should be made with the safest effective medications, usually Marcaine (bupivacaine) and Xylocaine (lidocaine).

Frequently there is a small hematoma present at the site of the injection, caused by injury to the superficial veins. This is usually transient but can be alarming to the patient. The anesthesiologist should advise the patient that this may occur, and should use compression over the injection site for several minutes to reduce the chances of hematoma formation.

It is possible for nerve damage to occur with anesthetic injection directly into a nerve.

Although rare, this complication may cause serious permanent damage to the nerve. The anesthesiologist must be aware of this potential problem and must never continue injecting if the patient reports severe pain. The pressure used during the injection should be gentle when the needle is in the proper location; the injection should never require force. If an extended anesthesia is noted postoperatively, a neurosurgical consultation should be requested.

Complications of Endotracheal Anesthesia

For most shoulder arthroscopic procedures the patient is placed in the lateral decubitus position, and an intratracheal tube is required. The complications related to endotracheal anesthesia include those of any surgery, including vocal cord and tracheal inflammation and damage, as well as aspiration. Care must be taken during the intubation to avoid these problems. Once the tube is in place, it should be secured with tape or a tie around the patient's head. During the procedure, particularly after positioning the patient, the breath sounds should be checked carefully and frequently to ensure proper ventilation. Monitoring of the oxygen saturation and expiratory CO_2 levels insures that the patient is ventilating satisfactorily.

Patient Positioning (see Chap. 3)

Following intubation, the patient is repositioned for the surgical procedure. Care must be taken to prevent pressure concentration areas from occurring. Placement of an axillary roll between the dependent torso and operating table is particularly important. A 1-L IV bag wrapped in a towel makes an excellent axillary roll. The radial pulse of the dependent arm should be palpated, and the arm positioned on a padded arm board in 90 degrees of forward flexion. The elbow is flexed about 40 degrees, and the epicondyles are padded. The wrist and hand are slightly flexed to relax any tension on the medial nerve.

The patient's head and neck should be supported in line with the spine, preferably using a contoured foam pillow with a cutout for the dependent ear. The patient's head is protected with a folded towel. The lower extremities are protected with pillows between the legs and foam padding beneath the dependent leg and ankle. The fibular head should be checked to make certain that there is no pressure around the peroneal nerve. An electrical grounding pad is applied to a muscular area, preferably the thigh, which has been shaved, if necessary, for good skin contact. After preparing the skin of the shoulder and arm, if alcohol is used, it should all be blotted dry from the field to avoid potential fire hazard.

Arm Suspension and Traction

Traction is required to support the arm in the lateral decubitus surgical position. The suspension system chosen should allow a firm hold on the arm so that the traction rope can safely support the extremity. The surgeon should choose this suspension system carefully, since there have been reports of injury to the superficial radial nerve from compression near the radial styloid.[1,2] Blistering of the skin can occur if adhesive tape is applied directly to the thin skin of a patient with rheumatoid arthritis or other steroid-dependent conditions. Additionally, a tourniquet effect is possible in a person with a compromised peripheral vascular blood flow when the hand is suspended and a snug wrap is placed around the forearm. For these reasons, we advise the following safe techniques: After the surgical preparation is completed, and the patient has been draped, the arm is placed in a sterilized soft foam traction sleeve. An ideal suspension system developed by the Arthrex Company (Naples, Florida) includes the sterile foam arm sleeve with the appropriate connector loops and ropes to permit the application of either one- or two-point traction (STaR Sleeve). Since there is extra padding on the hand end of the device, the area of the superficial branch of the radial nerve can be double-padded. The additional straps can then be secured on the forearm, with the two most proximal straps tightened above the elbow.

This method serves to distribute the traction pull throughout the extremity rather than isolating it in one area around the wrist. In addition, there is not the significant risk of skin damage that accompanies the use of adhesive-type materials. It is not recommended to wrap the foam sleeve with an elastic wrap or other bandage that might induce a tourniquet effect, unless the arm is extremely small.

When arthroscopy is performed for shoulder instability, it is helpful to use a double traction system as described by Gross and Fitzgibbons[3] (see Chaps. 3 and 12). Traction is applied to the *proximal* humerus to distract the humeral head laterally from the socket, using a sling around the upper arm. The median and ulnar nerves are at risk during this maneuver; care must be taken to ensure that the traction cuff around the arm is as smooth and wide as possible. In addition, the weight applied should be the minimum necessary to allow visualization and performance of the surgical procedure. From 10 to 15 lb of upward traction usually is adequate. Traction applied to the hand-end of the suspension apparatus should be just enough to balance the arm. A force of 5 lb usually is adequate. A helpful device for applying vertical traction is a sterilized soft cervical collar. The traction rope can also be sterilized to ensure a sterile operating field. If the Arthrex STaR Sleeve is used, it can be connected directly to the overhead rope, obviating the need for the cervical collar (Fig. 15-1). All traction should be removed as soon as possible at the completion of the operation.

Support of the Arm

Early in the history of shoulder arthroscopy there were several reports of injury caused to the upper-extremity nerves by arm support mechanisms. It has been reported by Olson and Fu, and also by Klein, that the amount and direction of traction used during arthroscopy could cause injury to the nerves of the brachial plexus.[4,5] They determined that although the 90-degree forward flexion position caused the least brachial plexus strain, it did not permit adequate glenohumeral visualization. They recommend using

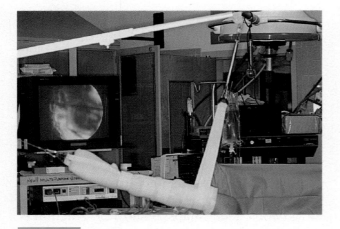

Figure 15-1
The Anthrex STaR Sleeve is used to safely apply two-point traction for shoulder positioning during instability surgery.

a position of 45 degrees of flexion with 0 to 90 degrees of abduction, depending on the desired area of visualization. By using an arm support device connected either to a strain gauge or to a free-turning pulley mechanism, appropriate weight can be applied in a controlled fashion. A weight of 10 lb provides adequate support for most patients (body weights between 130 and 200 lb). For smaller individuals this weight should be decreased appropriately. When an arm is extremely heavy, adding up to 15 lb of weight may be necessary during the arthroscopic evaluation and surgery. In the "bursoscopy position" a little more weight may be used, since the arm is abducted only 10 to 15 degrees. A weight of 15 lb has been safe in average-sized individuals; slightly lower or higher weights can be used if necessary. Once the surgical procedure has been completed, all unnecessary weight is removed immediately. It is acceptable to leave 3 to 5 lb of weight to support the arm during the final skin closure and application of bandages.

Risks During Portal Development

Outlining of the bony anatomy with a skin marker helps the surgeon determine the safest positions in which to create the arthroscopic portals (see Chap. 4). The anatomical structures at risk for the posterior portals are the axillary nerve and the descending branch of the suprascapular nerve. The axillary nerve is located approximately 6 to 7 cm distal to the posterolateral corner of the acromion and spine. Since this distance is 3 to 4 cm below the usual posterior portal, the axillary nerve should not be significantly at risk. On the other hand, the descending branch of the suprascapular nerve, which supplies the infraspinatus muscle, is located 1.5 to 2 cm medial to the edge of the glenoid just below the spinoglenoid notch.[6] This nerve can be injured quite easily when a sharp-tipped trochar is used during the initial shoulder puncture. By using a blunt-tipped obturator and palpating the humeral head first, thus avoiding pressure over the glenoid neck, injury to this nerve should be avoided.

When the spinal needle or cannula is initially inserted into the posterior aspect of the shoulder, it is possible to injure the articular cartilage of the posterior humeral head. Care must be taken to avoid repeated penetrations into the joint with the needle. By using very gentle insertional techniques and angling the tip of the needle away from the posterior head the cartilage can be spared. The cannula should be inserted using only the *blunt*-tipped obturator. If a sharp trochar is used to penetrate the capsule, there is a risk of damaging the articular surface or actually penetrating the soft bone of the posterior humeral head (Fig. 15-2). Using the blunt tip of the obturator within the cannula to carefully ballot the humeral head ensures that the correct location will be found for penetration of the capsule. The tip can be angled slightly medially and proximally to enter the joint in the appropriate space between the glenoid and the humeral head. Care must also be taken to avoid tunneling through the posterior rotator cuff; this can be avoided by angling the cannula to penetrate perpendicularly through the capsule and into the joint.

Anterior Portal Risks
The shoulder arthroscopist must be well aware of the anterior shoulder anatomy at

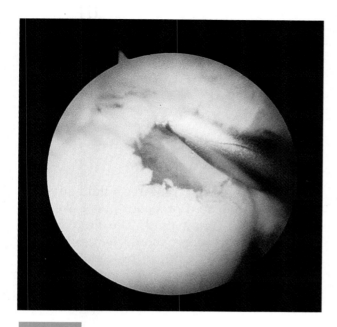

Figure 15-2
A sharp trochar, used to enter the glenohumeral joint, has inadvertently damaged the articular cartilage of the humerus.

mm incision is made through the skin (never into the muscle, where the cephalic vein might be lacerated), and the rod is passed out anteriorly. A snug-fitting cannula placed over the guide rod is worked back into the joint using a twisting motion.

We prefer to make the anterior midglenoid portal from outside in. Since the position of this portal is critical when performing instability surgery (see Chap. 12), and since the cephalic vein and the axillary and mucocutaneous nerves are more at risk with this portal, it should be reserved for the experienced arthroscopist who has performed cadaver laboratory evaluation (Fig. 15-3). One technique for safe joint entry involves making a skin incision at a point approximately 2 cm distal from the anterior superior portal, remaining

risk before developing any anterior portals.[7] There is a "safe triangle," located between the lower edge of the biceps tendon and the upper edge of the subscapularis tendon, where one or two cannulae may be safely inserted. If a cannula is placed inferior to the upper edge of the subscapularis tendon, the axillary and musculocutaneous nerves are at risk. In addition, since the brachial plexus, and especially the lateral cord, are located medial to the coracoid process, this area should be avoided.

To create the anterior portals safely, one of two methods can be used. We prefer the inside-out technique for the anterior superior portal. The "safe triangle" is located while viewing with the arthroscope from the posterior portal. The arthroscope is maneuvered to the desired position, usually just inferior to the biceps tendon, and then held in place against the anterior capsule while the scope is removed. Using a tapered-tipped transarticular rod passed down the posterior cannula, the anterior capsule in the rotator interval is punctured. The rod tip is directed to a location beneath the skin approximately 1 cm below the anterior edge of the acromion. A 4-

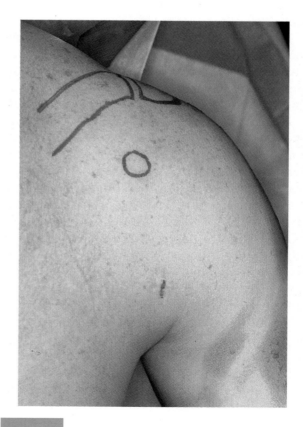

Figure 15-3
An extremely low anterior axillary puncture site for shoulder instability surgery was used in this patient to insert a metallic staple. The portal is in an extremely dangerous position, threatening injury to the axillary nerves and vessels.

lateral to the coracoid tip. Once the puncture wound is made in the skin, a cannula with a *blunt*-tipped obturator is gently worked through the deltoid muscle. The obturator tip is visualized with the scope as it indents the anterior capsule. When the desired entry point is located—usually adjacent to the subscapularis tendon—the joint is entered. This technique, using only blunt instruments with the outside-in approach, seems to be safe; no complications have been encountered.

Risks With Additional Arthroscopy Portals

An additional posterior portal can be developed 2 cm inferior to the original posterior portal. The main anatomical areas at risks are the axillary and infraspinatus nerves and the posterior aspect of the humeral head. By using the techniques described above for the superior posterior portal, these risks are minimized.

The supraclavicular notch portal was once recommended for an auxiliary inflow cannula. Currently, with the use of an arthroscopic pump or adjustable arthroscopic fluid tower, this superior portal is not necessary. The cannula usually passes through the muscular fibers of the supraspinatus and probably does not often damage the rotator cuff tendon. Souryal and Baker found in their cadaver study that the tendon fibers may be damaged if the superior portal is created with the arm abducted more than 45 degrees or flexed more than 15 degrees.[8] The suprascapular nerve is present just medial to the superior rim of the glenoid as it descends toward the spinoglenoid notch; it can be traumatized during creation of the supraclavicular notch portal. Additionally, cartilage on the superior aspect of the humeral head can easily be scarred during development of this portal. Since we do not advocate using the supraclavicular portal, no further attempt will be made to discuss it.

The lateral subacromial portal is used when performing an arthroscopic subacromial decompression, Mumford procedure, or rotator cuff repair. The correct location of this portal is 3 to 4 cm lateral from the lateral acromial border, in line with the posterior edge of the

AC joint. The axillary nerve can be damaged if this portal is placed more than 5 cm lateral, especially if the arm is in an abducted position. As with all portal development, the cannula should be inserted using a blunt-tipped obturator.

Arthroscopic Fluids

Shoulder arthroscopy requires a fluid environment. A complicated procedure may use 20 L or more of irrigation fluid. The fluid chosen for use in arthroscopy should be appropriate for the intended surgical procedure. Since electrosurgery and motorized mechanical instruments are often used together during shoulder arthroscopy, an ideal irrigation fluid is one that can be used during all surgical procedures. This fluid would be non-ionic (no electrical conductivity), isosmotic, Ph-balanced, nontoxic, clear, colorless, and non-antigenic. At the same time it should be able to support and encourage cartilage metabolism. A universal fluid, Synovisol (isosmolar glycerol, Baxter Travenol, Inc.), fits all of these criteria and has proved safe and effective in the animal models,[9] in living tissue cultures,[10] and in human clinical trials.[11] This solution has the added advantage of having a slightly slippery nature that lubricates the cannulas and portals to minimize tissue trauma during repeated insertions. Because Synovisol is non-ionic, electrosurgery can be used with various electrode tips while using a very low-power setting on the generator. Since the power setting determines the amount of tissue damage related to the electrosurgical procedure, the surgeon must keep the setting as low as possible.[12]

Laboratory, as well as clinical, studies have demonstrated the potential for damage to the delicate intra-articular cells if a hyposmotic solution, such as sterile water or, to a lesser extent, glycine (193 mosm), is used.[13] Synovisol has an osmolarity of 280 mosm, similar to that of the intracellular fluid; hence, minimal transfer of free water across cell boundaries occurs.

Glycine 1.5% is the next-best fluid for electrosurgery if Synovisol is not available. The glycine solution contains an amino acid that has been used in urological procedures where electrosurgery is needed. Several noteworthy complications should be considered when using glycine. Transient visual disturbances, including blindness, have been reported in the urological literature and, less frequently, in the orthopaedic literature.[14] The hyposmolarity of glycine may also cause an intracranial fluid imbalance, with swelling of the brain tissues. The post-TURP syndrome presents as confusion, restlessness, and agitation, with possible respiratory depression.[15] Although this has not been reported after arthroscopy, the potential should be considered. The surgeon should be aware that glycine has *not* been approved by the Food and Drug Administration for use during arthroscopy.

If no electrosurgery is planned, Ringer's lactate solution is acceptable. This solution is osmotically and pH-balanced, and has no significant toxic effects on the articular cartilage.[16] Although some surgeons use electrosurgery with a specialized plastic-coated electrode in Ringer's lactate, it has been demonstrated unequivocally that much higher power settings are necessary and that inadvertent tissue damage may result when attempting to coagulate bleeding vessels or cut tissue in and around the rotator cuff or deltoid muscle.[17]

Complications Resulting from Intra-Articular Surgery of the Shoulder

Once the arthroscopic portals have been safely established, the next area for potential iatrogenic injury is the use of various operative tools. As in knee arthroscopy, the mechanical shaving devices are often the primary instruments used for tissue resection. The surgeon should choose the shaver with the smallest possible diameter that will perform the resection. A 4.5-mm full-radius resector is usually adequate. Aggressive cutting tools and those with angled teeth should be avoided.

While debriding labral, biceps, or cuff lesions, the surgeon should be extremely cautious and conservative. Knowledge of the intra-articular anatomical variations, such as the Buford complex, the sublabral hole, the rotator cuff ridge, and the SLAP lesion, will help the surgeon avoid iatrogenic damage to these and other normal structures (see Chap. 4). Overzealous shaving can convert a frayed labrum into an instability lesion, or a partial-thickness rotator cuff tear into a full-thickness defect.

Complications Associated with Arthroscopic Repair of Shoulder Instability

No aspect of shoulder arthroscopy is more apt to result in complications than the surgical procedures for shoulder instability.[18–20] The types of potential complication include (1) neurovascular complications secondary to anterior inferior or medial portal placement; (2) complications related to implantable hardware, such as anchors, staples, and screws; (3) damage to the posterior soft tissue and neurological structures caused by transglenoid drilling; and (4) failure of the procedure, with recurrent instability. Each of these areas deserves careful discussion.

As mentioned above, under "Anterior Portal Risks," the anterior inferior portal is the one most often associated with complications. Since the classic Bankart labral avulsion often extends to the inferior aspect of the glenoid, it is necessary to reach this area during glenoid and labral debridement. It may be necessary to use fixation techniques at these lower glenoid levels as well. When the surgeon develops a portal that allows the best access to this area, it often must be medial to the coracoid or inferior to the leading edge of the subscapularis tendon. A portal in this location risks damage to the musculocutaneous nerve as it enters the conjoined tendon below, and medial to, the coracoid process.[19] In addition, the axillary nerve travels across the musculotendinous junction of the subscapularis before it passes below the anterior inferior shoulder capsule. Damage to either of these structures will cause devastating consequences. For this reason, the steps in developing this portal and the anatomy at risk should be perfectly understood by the operating surgeon. It is strongly recommended that a "blunt-only" instrumentation technique be used. The risk of damage, even by inserting a spinal needle from outside in, should be avoided. If an inside-out technique is used with the help of a guide rod, the location of the exit point for that rod should be carefully gauged prior to penetration of the capsule. In addition, the tip of the guide rod should be blunted. If the cephalic vein is speared with a sharpened rod, considerable bleeding will occur before the vein clots.

Hardware Complications

The initial arthroscopic surgical procedures developed to repair avulsed labral tissue consisted of the implantation of metal staples or screws to hold the avulsed tissues in an appropriate position on the anterior neck of the glenoid until healing occurred. The first-generation staples were constructed with a prominent head that protruded about 4 mm away from the bone when completely implanted. These staples also had very soft metal tines which frequently bent, or even broke, if they were not aligned properly with the bone surface into which they were being placed. The bent or broken staples would not anchor well in the glenoid bone, and were subject to later displacement or migration throughout the shoulder environment. Removal of these staples was sometimes extremely difficult, because they were difficult to find when encased in soft tissue and sometimes were located outside the articular environment—sometimes perilously close to the neurovascular structures (Fig. 15-4). At other times damage occurred when a loose staple migrated into the glenohumeral joint. Additionally, the head of a properly placed staple was known to cause irritation, particularly to the overlying subscapularis tendon. If the staples were placed too near the articular surface, the humeral head could contact the head of the staple, either dislodging it or damaging the articular cartilage of the head. For these reasons, the popularity of staples and metal screws in the shoulder has been declining in favor of the lower-risk suture procedures and absorbable implants.

The cannulated screw technique for anterior labral fixation had some of the same problems as the staples. The screw technique has never been popular, because it is technically very difficult to insert the screw. The potential risks were also not so high as those for the staple. The screws, once fixed in the glenoid

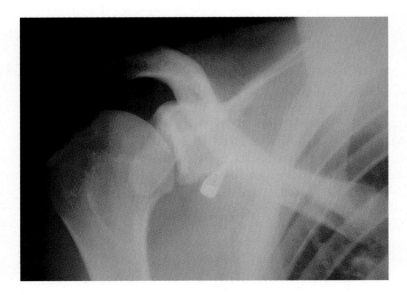

Figure 15-4
An arthroscopic staple has been improperly placed on the inferior medial aspect of the glenoid. This loose staple was extremely difficult to remove and required an open procedure.

neck, were very secure and seldom bent, loosened, or migrated. The difficulty occurred with placing the screw in the appropriate position on the neck of the glenoid. If the screw was too close to the surface of the joint it risked impingement by the humeral head; if it was placed too far medially it might not seat the capsular tissues correctly adjacent to the articular margin. Additionally, since the screws were relatively large, it was difficult to place more than one in any given instability case. Having only one point of capsular fixation often did not allow adequate tensioning; therefore, inadequate stability occurred.

An additional problem with the screw was that the prominent head sometimes irritated the subscapularis tendon. For this reason a second surgery for screw removal was often necessary, and removal was frequently very difficult. Since the screws were very securely fixed to the bone, the head of the screw could strip or the screwdriver tip could break (Fig. 15-5), making removal difficult with arthroscopic techniques. If a well-fixed screw did not strip, the weak lag shank of the screw

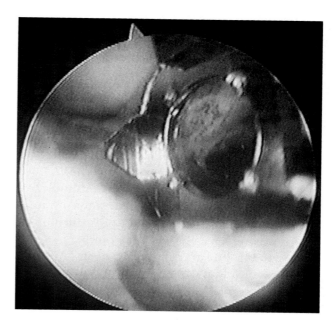

Figure 15-6
This arthroscopically placed screw head broke off during an attempted removal, allowing the spiked washer to fall into the subscapularis recess.

could fracture, resulting in a free fragment from the head and washer in the joint (Fig. 15-6).

Complications from Suturing Techniques

Several popular techniques have been developed for the use of suture material to attach the avulsed labrum and ligaments to the neck of the glenoid to allow healing. Several of the earlier techniques used various methods for passing the sutures through the capsular structures anteriorly, and then pulling the sutures out posteriorly through a transglenoid drill hole. The sutures could be either tied over a skin bolster or tied together beneath the skin, over the posterior muscle tissues.

The potential risks using this transglenoid drilling technique include possible injury to the descending branch of the suprascapular nerve, and pain and scarring at the site of the posterior suture fixation, with possible stran-

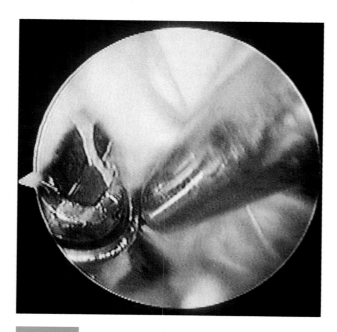

Figure 15-5
When attempting to remove a labral fixational screw, the tip of the OSI screwdriver broke off inside the hex head of the screw.

gulation of muscle tissue. The outside skin anchor technique was seldom used because of the potential risk of infection. An additional potential risk with transglenoid drilling was of damage to the glenoid articular surface if the pin was misdirected.

Additionally, a case of a drilling pin migrating and breaking off in the scapulothoracic space has been reported.[21] This was thought to have occurred because during the drilling the pin did not penetrate the posterior cortex, but instead bent into the cancellous bone of the scapula and then fractured during attempts to remove it. An open surgical procedure was needed to remove the pin. Another reported problem was that of a synovial cyst that formed posteriorly over a mass of nonabsorbable subcutaneous suture material.[22] This required open debridement. If absorbable suture material had been used, this cyst probably would not have occurred.

There are now a number of suture anchor devices being used for arthroscopic anterior instability surgery. These anchors can be placed very near the articular cartilage edge,

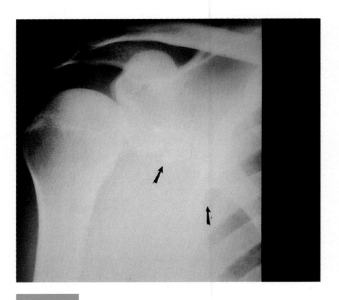

Figure 15-8
Several anchors have been passed through the neck of the glenoid and have been caught in the soft tissue posterior to the scapula.

allowing the capsule and labral tissues to be approximated in a nearly anatomical position. One risk with this technique is the potential damage to the articular surface when the anchor holes are drilled. Additionally, an anchor can dislodge in the joint during insertion or postoperatively, resulting in an intra-articular loose body (Fig. 15-7). If the drill hole penetrates the glenoid posteriorly or inferiorly, the anchor may pass through the bone and lodge in the soft tissue (Fig. 15-8). In repairing a SLAP lesion, the risk of overdrilling the superior glenoid must be avoided. In inserting the anchors, care must be taken to insert the anchor only to the seating mark on the insertion tool. If the anchor is impacted too deeply, it may lodge in the suprascapular fossa, causing irritation to the muscle (Fig. 15-9). With the absorbable anchors this loose-body phenomenon is not considered a significant problem, but with metal anchors it may lead to joint damage and, certainly, difficulty in locating and removing the small loose anchor in the joint and soft tissues. To avoid these problems when using metallic suture anchors, the manufacturers' guidelines should be carefully followed. Drill guides help in locating and con-

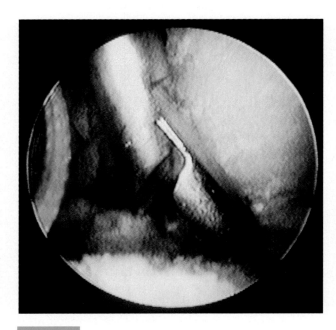

Figure 15-7
A Mitek anchor has dislodged from the insertion tool and may be difficult to retrieve. A safety suture should be used to control the anchor until it is seated.

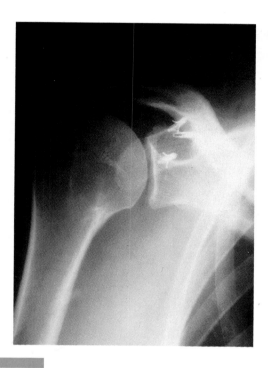

the soft tissue prior to insertion, and should be tapped only as deep as the seating mark on the insertion tool. A safety suture should always attach the anchor to the insertion tool, so that if the anchor comes loose it will not fall into the joint.[23]

Risks of Surgery in the Subacromial Space

Arthroscopy in the subacromial space is most often used for evaluation and shaving of the bursal side of the rotator cuff—sometimes with subacromial decompression, Mumford procedure, or rotator cuff repair. The potential risks of surgery specific to the subacromial space are usually related to the surgeon's disorientation, or to inadequate presurgical planning and subsequent overaggressive or inadequate bone or soft tissue debridement (Figs. 15-10 and 15-11).

Risks of Subacromial Decompression Surgery

During subacromial decompression, the surgeon first must remove the soft tissues from beneath the acromion. Electrosurgical tools are often very helpful and, in some cases, in-

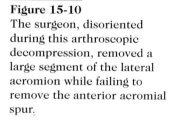

Figure 15-9
A SLAP lesion was repaired with three suture anchors, one of which appears to be lodged in the suprascapular area above the glenoid.

trolling the proper drilling position, and in avoiding overpenetration of the glenoid. The anchor should always be inserted through an appropriate cannula to prevent its snagging in

Figure 15-10
The surgeon, disoriented during this arthroscopic decompression, removed a large segment of the lateral acromion while failing to remove the anterior acromial spur.

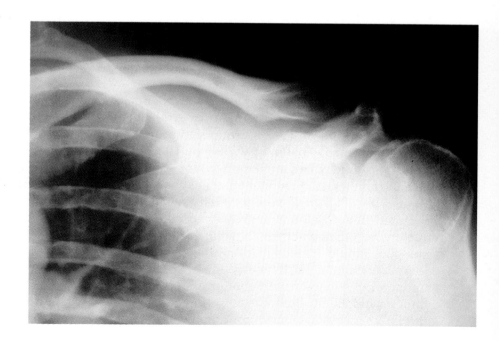

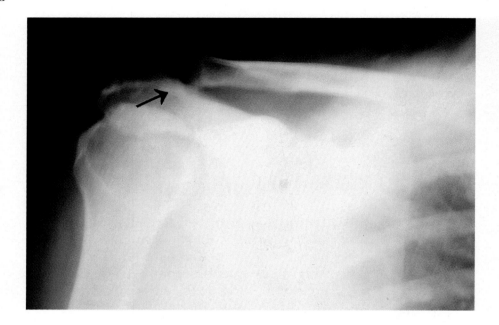

valuable, especially when bleeding occurs. Risks associated with electrosurgery per se (see "Arthroscopic Fluids," above) involve inadvertent damage to the surrounding soft tissues. When using electrosurgery, the lowest possible power setting should be employed to minimize tissue damage. A nonconductive irrigating solution, such as Synovisol or glycine, is recommended, along with an insulated electrosurgical operating tip. The surgeon should be very careful when coagulating bleeding sites around the deltoid muscle or the rotator cuff tendon. The vessel itself should be cauterized precisely, under direct vision, to minimize injury to adjacent tissues.

Risks of Bony Decompression

The thickness of the acromion varies significantly from person to person. In a study by Snyder and Wuh, it was determined that in 34 percent of female patients with type III acromial morphology (an anterior hook or spur on the acromion) the acromial thickness was less than 8 mm.[24] During acromioplasty a patient with a thin acromion is at greater risk of inadvertent acromial fracture[25,26] (Fig. 15-12). The surgeon should insist on a technically excellent subacromial outlet x-ray for all patients undergoing subacromial decompression. That film should be studied carefully for acromial thickness as well as for contour, and should be

present in the operating room for reference during the resection. The arthroscopic burr used during the resection should be sized according to the predetermined acromial thickness. For the thin acromion a small-diameter burr is adequate; for an acromion larger than 12 mm a larger-diameter burr can be used (see Chap. 11).

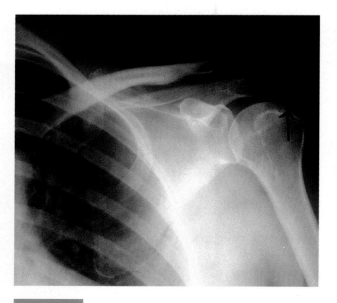

Figure 15-12
When the acromion is very thin it may be at high risk of fracture during subacromial decompression. Fracture occurred in this case.

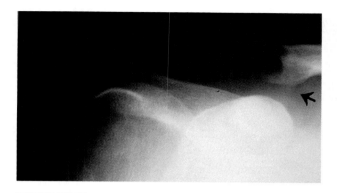

Figure 15-13
Overzealous resection of the clavicle can damage the coracoclavicular ligaments and destabilize the clavicle.

Resection of the distal clavicle can be difficult at first, particularly if the surgeon is disoriented. The potential for clavicular fracture or damage to the coracoclavicular ligaments is present with overzealous medial burring (Figs. 15-13 and 15-14). By insistence on proper orientation of the scope and maintenance of a clear visual field, this operation should seldom have complications.

Risks of Rotator Cuff Repair

Complete arthroscopic repair of the rotator cuff is a new procedure that has just become

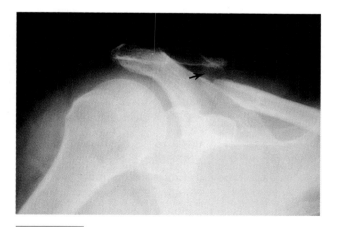

Figure 15-14
Fracture of the end of the clavicle may occur when the surgeon is disoriented during a decompression or a Mumford procedure.

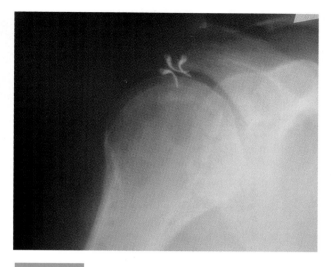

Figure 15-15
This surgeon attempted to repair a rotator cuff with miniature metal anchors, which were not adequate to hold the rotator cuff for healing.

feasible with the development of suture shuttle relays and specialized suture anchors. One obvious source of potential problems is the failure of the suture anchors to hold the rotator cuff tendon in place until healing occurs. Several anecdotal reports have been made by pioneers with these techniques, and further long-term clinical evaluations, as well as laboratory pull-out tests, are required before any definitive recommendations can be made[27] (Fig. 15-15).

Conclusion

Despite these potential risks associated with shoulder arthroscopic surgery, very few complications do occur, except in shoulder stabilization procedures. If the operating surgeon is attentive in the preoperative planning, rehearses the techniques, and uses good surgical judgment, shoulder arthroscopy can be a very safe form of surgery with limited numbers of complications. If the procedure becomes difficult, it can always be abandoned in favor of an open approach.

References

1. Curtis AS, Del Pizzo W, Snyder SJ, et al: Complications of shoulder arthroscopy. Presented at the American Academy of Orthopaedic Surgeons Annual Meeting, Washington, DC, 1992.

2. Ellman H: Arthroscopic subacromial decompression: Analysis of one to three year results. *Arthroscopy* 3:173, 1987.

3. Gross RM, Fitzgibbons TC: Shoulder arthroscopy: A modified approach. *Arthroscopy* 1:156, 1985.

4. Olson EJ, Fu FH: Complications and pitfalls in shoulder arthroscopy. *Operative Tech Orthop* 1(3):253, 1991.

5. Klein AH, France JC, Mutschaler TA, Fu FH: Measurements of brachial plexus strain in arthroscopy of the shoulder. *Arthroscopy* 3:45, 1987.

6. Bigliani LU, Dalsey RM, McCann PD, et al: An anatomical study of the suprascapular nerve. *Arthroscopy* 6:301, 1990.

7. Wolf EM: Anterior portals in shoulder arthroscopy. *Arthroscopy* 5:201, 1989.

8. Souryal TO, Baker CL: Anatomy of the supraclavicular fossa portal in shoulder arthroscopy. *Arthroscopy* 6:279, 1990.

9. Marshall GJ, Kirchen ME, Sweeney JR, Snyder SJ: Synovisol as an irrigant for electrosurgery of joints. *Arthroscopy* 4:187, 1988.

10. Regan BR, Zarins B, Mankin HJ: Low conductivity irrigating solutions for arthroscopy. *Arthroscopy* 7:105, 1991.

11. Baxter Travenol Synovisol study, FDA protocol. Valley Presbyterian Hospital, Van Nuys, California, 1989.

12. Rand JA, Gaffey TA: The effects of electrocautery on fresh human articular cartilage. *Arthroscopy* 1:242, 1985.

13. Mah ET, Lee WKC, Southwood RT, et al: Effects of irrigation fluid on human menisci: An experimental comparison of water, normal saline, and glycine. *Arthroscopy* 7:24, 1991.

14. Burkhart SS, Barnet CR, Snyder SJ: Transient postoperative blindness as a possible effect of glycine toxicity. *Arthroscopy* 6:112, 1990.

15. Ovassapian A, Joshi CW, Brunner EA: Visual disturbances: An unusual symptom of transurethral prostatic resection. *Anesthesiology* 57:332, 1982.

16. Regan BR, McInerny VK, Treadwell BV, et al: Irrigating solutions for arthroscopy. *J Bone Joint Surg* 65A:629, 1983.

17. Snyder SJ: Use of electrocautery for performing lateral retinacular release using the Concept Electrode [letter to the editor]. *Arthroscopy* 4:147, 1988.

18. Gross RM: Arthroscopic staple capsulorrhaphy: Does it work? *Arthroscopy* 5:495, 1989.

19. Hawkins RB: Arthroscopic stapling for shoulder instability: A retrospective study of 50 cases. *Arthroscopy* 5:122, 1989.

20. Small NC: Complications in arthroscopy—the knee and other joints. *Arthroscopy* 2:253, 1968.

21. Shea KP, Lovallo JL: Scapulothoracic penetration of a Beath pin: An unusual complication of arthroscopic Bankart suture repair. *Arthroscopy* 7:115, 1991.

22. Moran MC, Warren RF: Development of a synovial cyst after arthroscopy of the shoulder. *J Bone Joint Surg* 71A:837, 1989.

23. Wolf EM, Wilke RM, Richmond JC: Arthroscopic Bankart repair using suture anchors. *Operative Tech Orthop* 1:184, 1991.

24. Snyder SJ, Wuh HCK: A modified classification of the supraspinatus outlet view based on the configuration and the anatomic thickness of the acromion. Presented at American Shoulder and Elbow Surgeons Annual Closed Meeting, Seattle, Washington, September 1991.

25. Paulos LE, Franklin JL: Arthroscopic shoulder decompression: Development and appli-

cation. A five year experience. *Am J Sports Med* 18:235, 1990.

26. Matthews LS: Acromial fracture complicating arthroscopic subacromial decompression. A report of six cases. Presented at American Shoulder and Elbow Surgeons Annual Closed Meeting, Vail, Colorado, 1992.

27. Wolf EM: Personal communication.

Index